NEUROSCIENCE RESEARCH PROGRESS

ATAXIA

CAUSES, SYMPTOMS AND TREATMENT

ATAXIA

CAUSES, SYMPTOMS AND TREATMENT

SUNG HOI HONG

EDITOR

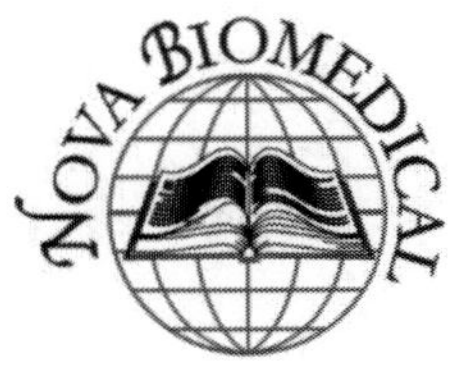

Nova Science Publishers, Inc.
New York

LIBRARY OF CONGRESS CATALOGING-IN-PUBLICATION DATA

ISBN: 978-1-61942-867-6
Library of Congress Control Number: 2011946004

Published by Nova Science Publishers, Inc. † New York

CONTENTS

PREFACE

Ataxia is a neurological sign and symptom characterized by lack of coordination of muscle movement that is due to dysfunction of the parts of the nervous system, such as motor control of the cerebellum. Although the cause of the dysfunction varies from mutations in channels for potassium and/or calcium to progressive degeneration of cerebellar tissue-specific neurons, the neurological signs and symptoms of ataxia are similar. The treatment of ataxia and its effectiveness depend on the underlying cause, and it could be managed by pharmacological treatments and through physical therapy and occupational therapy. The treatment may ameliorate the signs of ataxia, but it is not likely to eliminate them entirely. In this book, the authors present current research in the study of the causes, symptoms and treatments on ataxia.

Chapter 1 - Ataxia telangiectasia (AT) is characterized by progressive neurovascular degeneration, immunodeficiency, impaired organogenesis, premature aging, endocrine dysfunction, and cancer proneness. Dedicated efforts have greatly advanced their understanding of the complex biochemical, molecular and cellular defects associated with AT. However, there is still no cure for the disease. The gene mutated in AT, *ATM* (AT mutated), encodes a 350-kDa serine/threonine protein kinase that functions upstream in the p53 signaling pathway. Activation of the ATM-p53 pathway following exposure to biologically relevant doses of ionizing radiation results in transcriptional activation of $p21^{WAF1}$ (hereafter p21), a multifunctional protein that downregulates apoptosis and switches on the stress-induced premature senescence (SIPS) program. Recent evidence indicates that ATM interacts with p21 to counteract MDM2, the major negative regulator of p53, to positively control the specific activity of p53 as a transcription factor. ATM also plays an important role in the sustained upregulation of p21 and maintenance of the SIPS phenotype at late times after genotoxic insult. In view of these properties of ATM and p21, AT cells would be expected to primarily undergo apoptosis and not SIPS in response to genotoxic stress. To the contrary, skin fibroblasts cultured from AT patients show a low threshold for both replicative senescence and ionizing radiation-induced SIPS when compared to normal fibroblasts. In this chaper, the authors review these and related findings with AT and highlight compelling evidence that argues against the widely held notion that activation of the ATM-p53 pathway by DNA-damaging agents triggers apoptosis. In addition, they outline studies with eicosanoids and antioxidants that support therapeutic approaches for this multifaceted disorder.

Chapter 2 - Ataxia-telangiectasia (A-T) is a rare autosomal recessive disorder associated with mutations in the ATM gene. ATM plays a central role in regulating the signal-transduction pathway activated in response to DNA double-strand breaks and is involved in the control of the intracellular redox status homeostasis. The hallmarks of the disease are related to the progressive neurological dysfunction, especially affecting the cerebellum and resulting in uncoordinated and ataxic movements associated to a deterioration of gross and fine motor skills. The onset of neurological signs is usually by approximately 2-4 years of age. The overall phenotype consists of oculo-cutaneous teleangiectasia, immunodeficiency, high incidence of neoplasms and hypersensitivity to ionising radiations. The neurodegeneration is progressive and greatly impairs the quality of life, invariably leading to confinement of patients to wheelchair. The cerebellar damage is associated to dystrophic changes of dendrites and axons of Purkinje cells. Death usually occurs by the 3rd decade of life for pulmonary infections or neoplasms. Currently, there is no effective treatment for A-T, but only supportive care aimed to halt progressive neurodegenerative changes. Many attempts to relief the neurological symptoms have so far been made: antioxidants were promising, but only modest improvement has been observed. Aminoglycosides have been proposed for the correction of ATM gene function by read-through of premature termination codons, while further attempts have been made with antisense morpholino oligonucleotides to redirect and restore normal splicing. Some encouraging results on neurological symptoms have been obtained with short courses of oral betamethasone, even though the beneficial effect is drug-dependent. Aim of this chapter is to report on the molecular basis, clinical features and diagnostic process of A-T paying a special attention to the therapeutic approach so far described in the attempt to halt progressive degeneration.

Chapter 3 - Ion channels are membrane proteins that allow the selected and concerted movement of ions across cell membrane that is otherwise relatively impermeable to ions. These proteins are expressed in virtually every cell type, where they play key physiological roles. Thus, it is not surprising that ion channels dysfunction causes disease in animals and humans. The term *channelopathy* (CP) was coined less than two decades ago to identify ion channel diseases. To date, a large group of channelopathies have been identified and new ones are continuously being discovered; therefore, they represent a heavy burden on society.

Chapter 4 - Mitochondrial dysfunction has been implicated in the pathogenesis of Friedreich Ataxia and other hereditary ataxias. In some cases, mitochondrial DNA primary genetic abnormalities (i.e., myoclonic epilepsy with ragged red fibers syndrome [MERRF}; neuropathy, ataxia and pigmentary retinopathy syndrome [NARP]; Kearns-Sayre syndrome) or secondary mitochondrial dysfunction (i.e., due to mitochondrial polymerase *POLG1* gene mutation or coenzyme Q10 deficiency) can directly cause ataxia. In this chapter, the authors revise the role of mitochondrial dysfunction in hereditary ataxias, and they discuss the well-defined "mitochondrial ataxias". Mitochondrial diseases are a group of disorders caused by impairment of the mitochondrial respiratory chain. The effects of mutations which affect the respiratory chain may be multisystemic, with involvement of visual and auditory pathways, heart, central nervous system, and skeletal muscle. Genetic ataxias other from well-defined mitochondrial ataxias and Friedreich ataxia will not be extensively discussed here, but the role of mitochondrial dysfunction in some of these diseases will be briefly reviewed.

Chapter 5 - Epidemics of an acute ataxic syndrome occur annually in the rainy season in parts of West Africa, characterized by cerebellar ataxia, ocular abnormalities and impairment of consciousness, The onset of symptoms is usually shortly after a meal. The epidemics have been called the seasonal ataxic syndrome. Detailed epidemiological and dietary studies have indicated that the seasonal ataxic syndrome is a thiamine deficiency state similar to Wernicke's encephalopathy, occurring in poor, undernourished individuals who are mildly thiamine-deficient because of subsistence on a monotonous diet of cassava (*manihot esculenta*) meals. These individuals then suffer an acute exacerbation of thiamine deficiency from heat-stable thiaminases present in the *Anaphe venata* larvae, an invariable component of the last meals eaten prior to symptom onset. The annual period of availability of the *Anaphe* larvae coincides with the seasonal occurrence of the seasonal ataxic syndrome. This syndrome is the only thiamine-deficiency state known to be caused by thiaminases in insects. The epidemiology, clinical presentation, etiological mechanisms, therapy and control of the seasonal ataxic syndrome will be discussed in this chapter.

Chapter 6 - The group of hereditary ataxias is represented by different modes of inheritance, such as X-linked, mitochondrial, autosomal dominant and the autosomal recessive ataxias. This chapter will provide an overview of the autosomal recessive group, by describing those that are best defined. For each disorder, the clinical manifestations will be described, allowing a better definition and recognition of the symptoms. Then, the causative gene and the mechanisms leading to the disease will be discussed. Currently available treatments and/or potential therapeutic targets will also be outlined. The most frequent recessive ataxias will be covered: Friedreich's Ataxia, Ataxia-Telangiectasia, Autosomal Recessive Spastic Ataxia of Charlevoix-Saguenay, Autosomal Recessive Cerebellar Ataxia type 1 and type 2, Ataxia with Oculomotor Apraxia type 1 and type 2 and Ataxia with Vitamin E Deficiency.

Chapter 7 - Hereditary ataxias constitute a clinically and genetically heterogeneous group of rare neurological disorders that cannot be distinguished solely by clinical criteria, thus demanding a subtype confirmation by molecular diagnosis. Enclosed in this group are spinocerebellar ataxias (SCAs), which are autosomal dominant disorders. In several SCAs, the causative genes display age-dependent patterns of penetrance, implying that the *a posteriori* risk of being a carrier diminishes with aging of at-risk individuals that remain asymptomatic. Machado-Joseph disease (MJD), also known as SCA3, corresponds to the most frequent form of SCA. Similarly to other SCAs, named "polyglutamine" ataxias (*e.g.,* SCA1, SCA2, SCA6, SCA7, SCA17 and DRPLA), MJD is caused by an expansion of a CAG repeat motif in the coding region of its causative gene. In this particular case, more than 52 CAG repeats in exon 10 of the *ATXN3* gene (14q32.1) are necessary for disease expression. Despite the inverse correlation between the size of the CAG tract and the age at onset, the causative mutation only partially (50-75%) explains the observed variation in phenotype. Therefore, precise predictions of the age at onset are currently impossible. Results from recent research studies are pointing to the involvement of other factors, namely additional genetic variability related to the causative gene itself (*e.g.,* generated by alternative splicing) and/or modifier genes. The knowledge of such factors may not only enable improvements of phenotype predictions, but may also raise hypotheses of new targets for gene therapy. The present chapter will focus on MJD, using it as a paradigm to demonstrate multiple roles and usefulness of genetics for a vaster group of neurodegenerative disorders.

Chapter 8 - Spinocerebellar ataxia 3 (SCA3) is a clinically heterogeneous neurodegenerative disorder characterized by ataxia, ophthalmoplegia, peripheral neuropathy, pyramidal dysfunction and movement disorders. It has an autosomal dominant inheritance and it results from a CAG repeat expansion mutation in the protein coding region of the

ATXN3 gene located at chromosome 14q32. Early neuropathological and neuroimaging studies mostly concentrated on the cerebellum, brainstem, spinal cord and basal ganglia; however, recent observations have demonstrated a more widespread cerebral involvement in SCA3. Visual analysis usually displays atrophy of the pons, cerebellar peduncles, frontal and temporal lobes, globus pallidus, as well as decreased anteroposterior and transverse diameters of the midbrain and decrease anteroposterior diameter of the medulla oblongata. Brain SPECT showed perfusion abnormalities in the parietal lobes, inferior portion of the frontal lobes, mesial and lateral portions of the temporal lobes, basal ganglia, and cerebellar hemispheres and vermis, while 18F-Dopa uptake (PET) was significantly decreased in the cerebellum, brainstem and nigro-striatal dopaminergic system, cerebral cortex and the striatum. Magnetic resonance spectroscopy (MRS) of the deep white matter demonstrated changes suggestive of axonal dysfunction in normal appearing white matter. Voxel-based morphometry (VBM) studies have conflicting results probably reflecting differences in sample sizes and characteristics. Different studies using texture analysis, manual volumetry and VBM demonstrated thalamic involvement in SCA3. The objective of this review is to discuss neuroimaging findings in SCA3 and how they contribute to a better understanding of the disease pathophysiology and future research directions.

Chapter 9 - People affected by ataxia, a genetic neurological disorder, have problems with coordination. Ataxia is the principal symptom of a group of neurological disorders known as cerebellar ataxias. Most of them are progressive. In ataxia, a neurodegenerative process leads to changes in a motor cortex responsible for balance and coordination. Recently several genes that cause autosomal dominant ataxia development were identified. These abnormal genes share a common ability to produce abnormal ataxin protein sequences that affect nerve cells in the cerebellum and spinal cord. Here, using signal processing methods they analysed ataxin proteins and identified the characteristic features corresponding to their biological activities. The Resonant Recognition Model (RRM) is a physico-mathematical approach developed for analysis of protein interactions. By incorporating Smoothed Pseudo Wigner - Ville distribution (SPWV) in the RRM, the authors can predict locations of active/binding sites along the protein molecule. The findings of this study showed that their computational predictions correspond closely with the experimentally identified locations of the active regions for the selected ataxin-1 and ataxin-3 protein groups. They also present and discuss the results of possible interactions between the ataxin-1 and growth factor independent transcriptional regulator-1 (Gfi-1) proteins known to be responsible for the selective Purkinje cell degeneration in ataxia disorder. In addition, the authors demonstrate that by using their recently developed protein classification methodology, they can distinguish between different ataxin protein functional groups that correspond to different neurological disorders. By employing Hierarchical classification methodology and using the Euclidian distance as a measure of the distance between vectors representing the distribution of amino acid residues along the ataxin proteins, it is possible to extract ataxin proteins' specific features into an adjoin 10-dimensional vector that represents the distribution of electron ion potentials along a proteins' backbone, and thus classify ataxin proteins by their different functionalities. The developed classification system is tested here on known ataxin proteins. The results obtained provide a valuable insight into the functional performance of ataxin proteins. The presented novel computational approach can be used to predict unknown protein-protein interactions of ataxin with other proteins that can potentially influence its function and thus, contribute to ataxia disorder development.

Chapter 10 - The hamster Purkinje Cell Degeneration (*hm*PCD) is a line of spontaneous ataxic mutation in the Syrian hamster. *Nna1* gene expression in the *hm*PCD brain is suppressed similar to that in the authentic *pcd* mutant mice. The influence of the causal allele in the *hm*PCD is considerably milder than the previously described alleles of the *pcd* mouse strains. The homozygous mutants of *hm*PCD develop a progressive but moderate ataxia that becomes apparent within the first two months of life. The major pathology in the mutant hamster is substantial corticocerebellar atrophy, which is attributable to primary loss of Purkinje neurons. The characteristic discordant movement can be quantitatively assessed by several behavioral tests; thus, the *hm*PCD would be applicable to study the effectiveness of pharmacological agents for ataxia. Recently, the authors demonstrated that daily administrations of NK-4, a neurotrophic cyanine dye compound, considerably delayed the onset of ataxia in the *hm*PCD. The behavioral outcomes were well supported by the histological findings of the cerebellum. NK-4 significantly suppressed degenerative loss of Purkinje neurons, which resulted in reduced cerebellar atrophy. Their results suggest that the *hm*PCD is a unique animal model for validating the efficacy of drugs targeting spinocerebellar ataxia and identify NK-4 as a promising candidate.

Chapter 11 - Spinocerebellar ataxia type 1 (SCA1) is an autosomal dominant neurodegenerative disorder caused by expansion of CAG trinucleotide repeats in the ataxin-1 gene and is characterized by cerebellar ataxia and progressive motor deterioration. The ataxin-1 protein is involved in transcription and RNA processing. SCA1 pathogenesis appears to be related to a gain-of-function effect that is caused by toxic mutant ataxin-1-derived aggregates or cellular dysfunction through an abnormal interaction between mutated and normal proteins. Recent studies have clarified the molecular mechanisms of SCA1 pathogenesis, which provide direction for future treatments. Therapeutic hope has come from observations including the reduction of aggregates and alleviation of the pathogenic phenotype by the application of potent inhibitors and RNA interference. However, no treatment is currently available for SCA1 disease. In this chapter, the authors discuss the potential of stem cells as a therapeutic approach to SCA1.

In: Ataxia: Causes, Symptoms and Treatment
Editor: Sung Hoi Hong

ISBN: 978-1-61942-867-6
© 2012 Nova Science Publishers, Inc.

Chapter 1

ROLE OF THE ATAXIA TELANGIECTASIA MUTATED PROTEIN IN STRESS-INDUCED PREMATURE SENESCENCE

Razmik Mirzayans and David Murray*

Department of Oncology, Cross Cancer Institute, University of Alberta, Edmonton, Alberta, Canada

ABSTRACT

Ataxia telangiectasia (AT) is characterized by progressive neurovascular degeneration, immunodeficiency, impaired organogenesis, premature aging, endocrine dysfunction, and cancer proneness. Dedicated efforts have greatly advanced our understanding of the complex biochemical, molecular and cellular defects associated with AT. However, there is still no cure for the disease. The gene mutated in AT, *ATM* (AT mutated), encodes a 350-kDa serine/threonine protein kinase that functions upstream in the p53 signaling pathway. Activation of the ATM-p53 pathway following exposure to biologically relevant doses of ionizing radiation results in transcriptional activation of p21^{WAF1} (hereafter p21), a multifunctional protein that downregulates apoptosis and switches on the stress-induced premature senescence (SIPS) program. Recent evidence indicates that ATM interacts with p21 to counteract MDM2, the major negative regulator of p53, to positively control the specific activity of p53 as a transcription factor. ATM also plays an important role in the sustained upregulation of p21 and maintenance of the SIPS phenotype at late times after genotoxic insult. In view of these properties of ATM and p21, AT cells would be expected to primarily undergo apoptosis and not SIPS in response to genotoxic stress. To the contrary, skin fibroblasts cultured from AT patients show a low threshold for both replicative senescence and ionizing radiation-induced SIPS when compared to normal fibroblasts. In this article we review these and related findings with AT and highlight compelling evidence that argues against the widely held notion that activation of the ATM-p53 pathway by DNA-damaging agents triggers apoptosis. In addition, we outline studies with eicosanoids and antioxidants that support therapeutic approaches for this multifaceted disorder.

*Correspondence concerning this article should be addressed to Razmik Mirzayans, Tel: 780-432-8897, Fax: 780-432-8428, e-mail: razmik.mirzayans@albertahealthservices.ca.

Keywords: Ataxia Telangiectasia; Ionizing radiation; DNA damage response; Senescence

INTRODUCTION

Ataxia telangiectasia (AT) is a rare autosomal recessively inherited disorder characterized by progressive neurovascular degeneration, immunologic deficiency, impaired organogenesis, premature aging, and endocrine dysfunction [Gatti *et al.*, 1991; Brown *et al.*, 1999]. Afflicted patients are also prone to lymphoproliferative neoplasia and respond untowardly to radiotherapy for cancer treatment [Paterson and Smith, 1979; Gatti *et al.*, 1991; Khanna, 2000]. Pronounced radiosensitivity extends to the cellular level *in vitro*. On exposure to ionizing radiation, for example, cultured AT cells display hypersensitivity in the clonogenic survival assay, excessive genetic instability, impaired activation of cell cycle checkpoints, and defective DNA repair [Paterson and Smith, 1979; Brown *et al.*, 1999; Kühne *et al.*, 2004]. The disease is caused by a single gene, called *ATM* (AT mutated), which encodes a 350-kDa serine/threonine protein kinase. The ATM protein functions upstream in the DNA-damage surveillance network that is activated after exposure to ionizing radiation and other agents that induce DNA double-strand breaks (DSBs) (Figure 1). Exposure to such agents results in ATM-dependent activation of the p53 tumor suppressor, which in turn transcriptionally activates p21^{WAF1} (hereafter p21) and a host of other genes. Both p53 and p21 are multifunctional proteins and play central roles in determining the fate of a cell following genotoxic stress in terms of survival, apoptotic cell death, and a growth-arrested state called stress-induced premature senescence (SIPS). The p21 protein also participates in feedback loops that control the function of both ATM and p53.

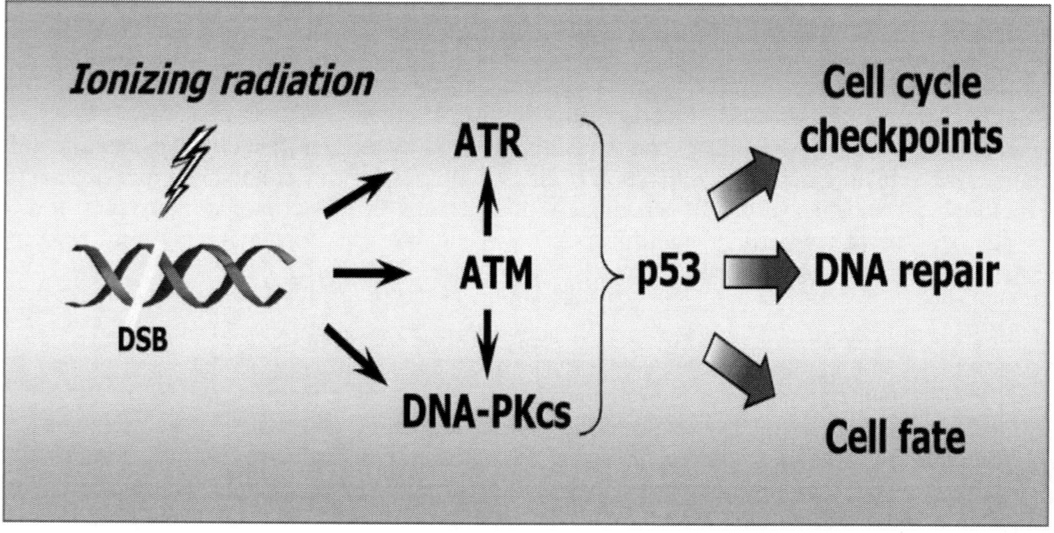

Figure 1. Responses triggered by ionizing radiation in normal human fibroblasts. DNA DSBs induced by ionizing radiation trigger the rapid activation of ATM which elicits a series of post-translational modifications on p53 that contribute to its stabilization, nuclear accumulation and biochemical activation. ATM also contributes to the activation of ATR and DNA-PKcs. Collectively, these four tumor suppressors and their downstream effectors regulate cell cycle checkpoints, DNA repair, and cell fate in terms of survival, apoptosis, and growth arrest (e.g., SIPS).

This chapter provides an overview of the current knowledge on the function of the ATM-p53-p21 signaling axis in replicative senescence and ionizing radiation-induced SIPS. We focus on findings with human normal, ATM-deficient (AT) and p53-deficient [Li-Fraumeni syndrome (LFS)] fibroblast strains. One of our objectives is to highlight studies that challenge the widely held notion that activation of the ATM network by ionizing radiation triggers apoptotic cell death. In addition, we outline discoveries that support therapeutic approaches for some of the symptoms associated with AT. Specifically, we discuss the following topics:

> ATM activation
> ATM substrates
> p53 structure, activation and function
> Roles of ATM and p53 in DNA repair
> Multiple functions of p21 in the ATM network
> Sequential waves of p53 activation by DNA damage
> ATM-dependent senescence
> ATM-independent senescence
> Role of ATM in preventing escape from SIPS: a novel tumor suppressor function beyond p53?
> Potential therapeutic approaches for the treatment of AT

ATM ACTIVATION

The C-terminal domain of ATM shares the kinase signature of the phosphatidylinositol 3-kinase (PI3K) superfamily of proteins involved in the regulation of cell cycle progression, DNA damage processing, and maintenance of genomic stability and cellular homeostasis [reviewed in Lavin and Khanna, 1999; Rotman and Shiloh, 1999; Shiloh, 2003]. The ATM- and Rad3-related (ATR) and DNA-dependent protein kinase catalytic subunit (DNA-PKcs) proteins also belong to this family of kinases and play important roles in DNA damage response pathways [Shiloh, 2003]. In unstressed cells ATM exists as a dimer, is not phosphorylated and is present throughout the nucleus. ATM is constitutively associated with protein phosphatase-2A (PP2A), presumably to ensure that ATM is not inappropriately activated [Lavin, 2008]. Activation of ATM is a complex process that involves the relaxation of chromatin as a consequence of a DNA DSB. After exposure to ionizing radiation, which leads to the formation of DSBs, PP2A dissociates from ATM and loses its activity. ATM is then rapidly monomerized post-irradiation and is autophosphorylated on at least three sites: Ser367, Ser1893 and Ser1981 [Lavin, 2008]. Some pool of ATM monomer molecules are recruited to the sites of DSBs [Bakkenist and Kastan, 2003]. The MRE11–RAD50–NBS1 (MRN) complex is of structural and functional importance during the early DSB response, by tethering DNA ends and recruiting ATM [Horejsi *et al.*, 2004; Costanzo *et al.*, 2004]. Activation of ATM can also be mediated by 53BP1 through an MRN-independent mechanism [Zgheib *et al.*, 2005].

ATM SUBSTRATES

ATM is activated in every phase of the cell cycle and phosphorylates a host of substrates on their serine or threonine residues that are followed by a glutamine. These include p53 (Ser6, Ser15, Ser20, and Ser46), CHK2 (Ser33, Ser35, Thr68), MDM2 (Ser395), WRN (Ser1058, Ser1141, Ser1292) [Ammazzalorso *et al.*, 2010], BRCA1 (Ser1387, Ser1423), the histone H2A variant H2AX (Ser139) [Kurz and Lees-Miller, 2004], and DNA-PKcs (Thr2609) [Chen *et al.*, 2007]. In addition, ATM activates ATR-CHK1 signaling, enabling the cells to respond to DNA strand breaks with coordinated, highly modulated outputs [Adams *et al.*, 2006; Cuadrado *et al.*, 2006; Jazayeri *et al.*, 2006; Myers and Cortez, 2006]. An assessment of the functions of ATM substrates and ATM interacting proteins is beyond the scope of the current article and the reader is referred to previous reviews [e.g., Shiloh, 2003; Meulmeester *et al.*, 2005; Lavin, 2008; Pichierri *et al.*, 2011]. In what follows, we outline the multiple functions of p53 and its downstream effector p21 in the ATM signaling network.

P53 STRUCTURE, ACTIVATION AND FUNCTION

Human p53 is a 393 amino acid (53 kDa) polypeptide consisting of five structural and functional domains: an N-terminal acidic transcriptional transactivation domain, a proline-rich regulatory domain, a central DNA-binding domain, a tetramerization domain, and a C-terminal domain involved in the regulation of DNA binding (Figure 2). The N-terminal domain is required for activating p53-inducible genes. The proline-rich domain is responsible for interaction with pro-apoptotic proteins, resulting in activation of apoptotic signaling. The central domain facilitates sequence-specific binding of the protein to p53 response elements in DNA. The tetramerization domain is comprised of a β-strand, a tight turn, and an α-helix, through which p53 monomers interact to form dimers, and dimers interact to form tetramers. Tetramerization is indispensable for the ability of p53 to function as a transcription factor.

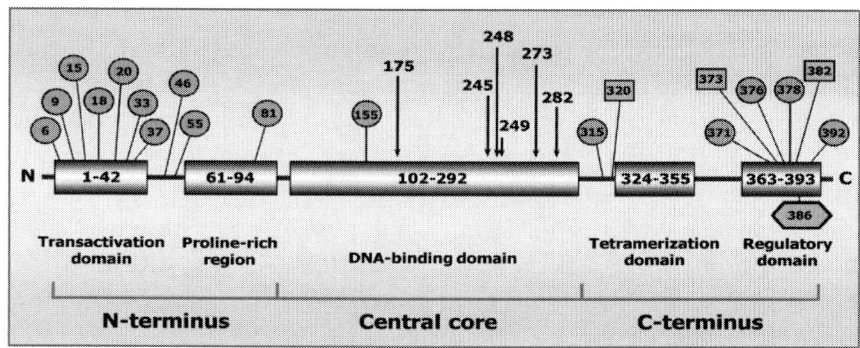

Figure 2. Structure and posttranscriptional modification of the p53 protein. Circles, Ser/Thr phosphorylation sites; squares, acetylation sites; hexagon, SUMOylation site. Arrows show the six most frequently mutated codons ("hotspots") found in the TP53 gene in human tumors [Cho et al., 1994; Bouchet et al., 2006]. The length of the arrows corresponds to the prevalence of mutations.

In normal unstressed human cells, p53 is present in a latent state and is maintained at low levels through targeted degradation by the proteasome-mediated and calpain-mediated pathways [Michael and Oren, 2003]. Turnover of p53 is mediated by ubiquitin ligases such as MDM2, MDM4, Pirh2 and Cop1 [Meek, 2004]. Each of these proteins acts as a ubiquitin E3 ligase that results in ubiquitination of p53 and its degradation.

Altered chromatin structure, DNA damage, and other forms of stress trigger a series of post-translational modifications on p53 that contribute to its stabilization, nuclear accumulation and biochemical activation [Ljungman, 2000; Meek, 2004]. Different sites in p53 undergo phosphorylation or acetylation, contributing to induction of the p53 response [Meek, 2004]. The phosphorylation sites Ser15, Thr18 and Ser20 are critical for protein stabilization. Ser15 phosphorylation primes the subsequent phosphorylation of Thr18 and Ser20, both of which lie within close proximity of the MDM2 binding site. Concomitant phosphorylation of p53 at these two sites, and of MDM2 at Ser395, mediated by ATM, interrupts MDM2-p53 interaction, thereby attenuating the inhibitory action of MDM2 on p53. Moreover, phosphorylation of p53 (Ser15, Thr18 and Ser20) stimulates recruitment of factors (e.g., p300, CBP, P/CAF) that contribute to p53 stabilization through acetylation of a cluster of C-terminal lysine residues in p53 that are normally targets for ubiquitination [Li *et al.*, 2002].

Most of the responses controlled by p53 are attributed to transcriptional activation of p53-target genes in general, and *p21* in particular [Roninson *et al.*, 2001; Lane, 2004; Mirzayans *et al.*, 2005]. As discussed below, in human fibroblast strains and solid tumor-derived cell lines, the protein encoded by this gene (p21) down-regulates apoptosis, activates cell cycle checkpoints, and switches on the SIPS program in response to DNA damage. Several other proteins that are transcriptionally regulated by p53 also influence apoptosis. These include the pro-apoptotic proteins BAX, PUMA and NOXA, and the anti-apoptotic protein BCL-2 [Akhtar *et al.*, 2006; Fuster *et al.*, 2007].

In addition to regulating gene expression, p53 directly modulates the transmission of specific signals by interacting with other cellular proteins. For example, p53 accelerates DNA repair through interacting with key players of different DNA repair pathways [Jongmans *et al.*, 1998; Sturzbecher *et al.*, 2002; Sengupta and Harris, 2005; Al Rashid *et al.*, 2005; Mirzayans *et al.*, 2006; Murray and Mirzayans, 2007], and promotes apoptosis through interaction with pro-apoptotic proteins [Asada *et al.*, 1999]. The proline-rich domain of p53 contains a motif that serves as a docking site in the transmission of signals that inhibit DNA replication, resulting in transactivation-independent growth arrest [Ruaro *et al.*, 1997].

ROLES OF ATM AND P53 IN DNA REPAIR

In the mid 1990's, we reported that p53-deficient LFS fibroblasts [Mirzayans *et al.*, 1996] and AT fibroblasts [Paterson and Mirzayans, 1993] exhibited a reduced ability to repair alkali-stable DNA lesions induced by ionizing radiation when compared to normal human fibroblasts. Since then, considerable efforts have been made to elucidate the roles of p53 and ATM in the rejoining of DSBs, which are considered to be the most deleterious lesions induced by ionizing radiation. Employing the neutral comet assay, p53-deficient murine embryo fibroblasts were shown to rejoin DSBs in response to ionizing radiation at a much slower rate than their p53-proficient counterparts [Al Rashid *et al.*, 2005]. Employing this assay, the LFS and AT fibroblast strains used in our earlier study [Mirzayans *et al.*, 1996] also exhibited an abnormally slow rate of DSB rejoining following exposure to ionizing radiation [Mirzayans *et al.*, 2006].

The reduced rate of DSB rejoining in p53-deficient cells was manifested at various times between 1 and 24 h (Figure 3) and 2 to 24 h [Al Rashid *et al.*, 2005] post-irradiation, and was attributed to absence of Ser15 phosphorylation [Al Rashid *et al.*, 2005]. Consistent with the outcome of the neutral comet assays, several groups have reported that p53 interacts with various key players in homologous recombination (HR) and nonhomologous end joining (NHEJ), the two distinct and complimentary pathways for DSB repair [e.g., Jongmans *et al.*, 1998; Sturzbecher *et al.*, 2002; Sengupta and Harris, 2005; Al Rashid *et al.*, 2005].

The reduced rate of DSB rejoining in AT fibroblasts was also manifested at early (e.g., 1 h) and late (>24 h) times after irradiation [Mirzayans *et al.*, 2006; Figure 3]. This observation was highly anticipated for three reasons. First, the AT fibroblast strains used in our studies do not exhibit p53 activation under these conditions [Enns *et al.*, 1998]. Second, ATM is required for activation of DNA-PKcs [Chen *et al.*, 2007] that is a key component of the NHEJ repair pathway [Burma and Chen, 2004]; this ATM-mediated activation is accomplished through phosphorylation of DNA-PKcs at the Thr2609 cluster [Chen *et al.*, 2007]. Third, the WRN helicase, which is activated by ATM, plays a crucial role in DSB rejoining [Chen *et al.*, 2003; Liu *et al.*, 2011]. WRN enhances both the HR and NHEJ pathways by protecting the broken DNA ends from degradation as well as recruiting other proteins involved in DSB repair.

Not all studies support a role for p53 or ATM in DSB rejoining, particularly at relatively short times (<24 h) after irradiation. Human tumor cell lines with differing p53 status, for example, have been reported to rejoin DSBs at similar rates, arguing against the involvement of p53 and p53 targets in the physical rejoining of DSBs [DiBiase *et al.*, 1999; Orre *et al.*, 2006]. In addition, AT fibroblast strains have been reported to rejoin DSBs at a rate comparable to that seen in normal fibroblasts [Kühne *et al.*, 2004]. DSB rejoining in these studies was measured by the pulsed-field gel electrophoresis assay.

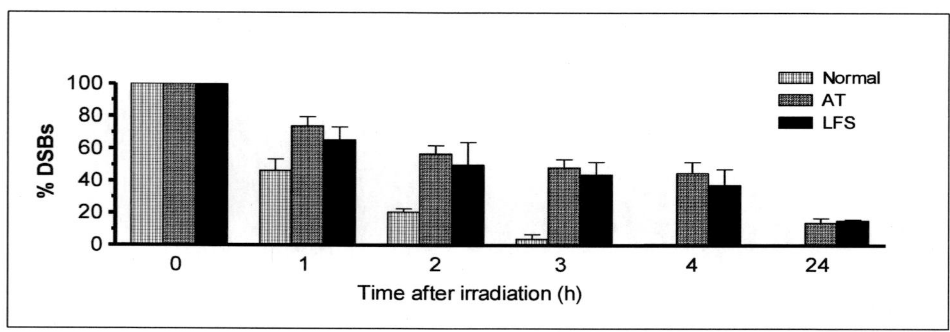

Figure 3. Comparison of the rates of DSB rejoining in human normal (GM38, GM10), AT (AT2BE, AT5BI), and LFS (2674T, 2800T) fibroblast strains after exposure to 8 Gy of γ radiation. DSBs were evaluated using the neutral comet assay as described [Mirzayans et al., 2006]. The results were re-plotted from our previous work [Mirzayans et al., 2006]. Each datum point represents the mean (±SD) of the values obtained for two strains within each group. The data are expressed as the percentage of DSBs measured immediately after exposure (set at 100%).

The reasons for the inconsistent results obtained with the neutral comet and pulsed-field gel electrophoresis assays remain unknown. However, it is important to note that the former and the latter assays were performed with relatively low doses (e.g., 8 Gy in our work) and extremely high doses (e.g., 80 Gy) of ionizing radiation, respectively. These results suggest the involvement of the ATM-p53 pathway in DSB rejoining after exposure to physiologically relevant doses of ionizing radiation but not necessarily in response to supralethal doses. Further studies are needed to test this hypothesis.

Quantification of nuclear foci associated with γ-H2AX (Ser139 phosphorylated H2A) has emerged as a widely-used marker of DSBs that are detected by the cell [Fernandez-Capetillo *et al.*, 2004]. Using this technique, we observed the rate of γ-H2AX clearance after exposure to ionizing radiation to be slower in AT and LFS fibroblast strains than in normal controls [Mirzayans *et al.*, 2006], which is in agreement with the DSB rejoining data obtained by the neutral comet assay. Similarly, Kato *et al.* [2006] observed the rate of γ-H2AX clearance post-irradiation to be slower in cells derived from Atm-deficient mice than in those from Atm-proficient mice; the slow rate of γ-H2AX clearance in both of these studies was observed at all sampling times, between 1 and 24 h after irradiation. Other groups have observed an abnormally slow rate of γ-H2AX clearance in ATM-deficient cells only at late times (>2 h) after exposure to ionizing radiation (e.g., Goodarzi *et al.*, 2008).

Irrespective of the basis for the inconsistent results reported from different laboratories, there is general agreement that a small, but significant proportion of DSBs remain unrejoined in AT cells at late times (e.g., 24 h) after exposure to different doses of ionizing radiation (between 1 and 80 Gy). Goodarzi *et al.* [2008] demonstrated that DSBs in heterochromatin are generally repaired more slowly than DSBs in euchromatin, and that ATM is preferentially required for DSB repair within heterochromatin.

MULTIPLE FUNCTIONS OF P21 IN THE ATM NETWORK

Between 1993 and 1995, different groups independently reported the identification of the human gene that encodes the p21 protein. Harper and associates isolated a gene that was found to specify a 21-kDa protein that immunoprecipitated with the G1 checkpoint proteins cyclin-dependent kinase (CDK) 2, cyclin A, cyclin D1, and cyclin E [Harper *et al.*, 1993]. They called the novel gene *CIP1* for CDK-interacting protein 1. El-Diery *et al.* [1993] identified a gene whose induction was associated with the wild-type p53 function in a human brain tumor cell line, and called it *WAF1* for wild-type p53-activated fragment 1. Noda *et al.* [1994] isolated a gene that is highly expressed in senescent human fibroblasts and called it *SDI1* for senescent cell-derived inhibitor 1. These three genes turned out to be one and the same. Three other groups also reported the identification of the p21 protein [Gu *et al.*, 1993; Xiong *et al.*, 1993a; 1993b; Jiang *et al.*, 1995]. The multiple functions of p21 became apparent from the fact that the various independent laboratories that identified this protein used unique approaches to explore distinct cell pathways.

The human p21 protein is classified as a member of the kinase inhibitor protein (KIP) family of CDK inhibitors [Sherr and Roberts, 1999]. It is transcriptionally activated by the ATM-CHK2-p53 pathway after exposure to ionizing radiation and other DNA DSB-inducing agents, and by the ATR-CHK1-p53 pathway in response to agents such as ultraviolet light that induce bulky DNA lesions [Cook, 2009]. Certain non-DNA-damaging agents (e.g., cytokines [Datto *et al.*, 1995; Li *et al.*, 1995; Hu *et al.*, 1999], glucocorticoids [Corroyer *et al.*, 1997], and retinoids [Liu *et al.*, 1996; Yang *et al.*, 1999]) are known to trigger p21 induction through p53-independent mechanisms.

Although not universally appreciated, there is compelling evidence that p21 plays different crucial roles in the ATM (and ATR) signaling network, most of which are independent of its inhibitory action on CDKs (Figure 4). Thus, in addition to activating transient cell cycle checkpoints, p21 regulates gene expression, senescence, apoptosis, p53 protein stability, p53 function, and ATM function.

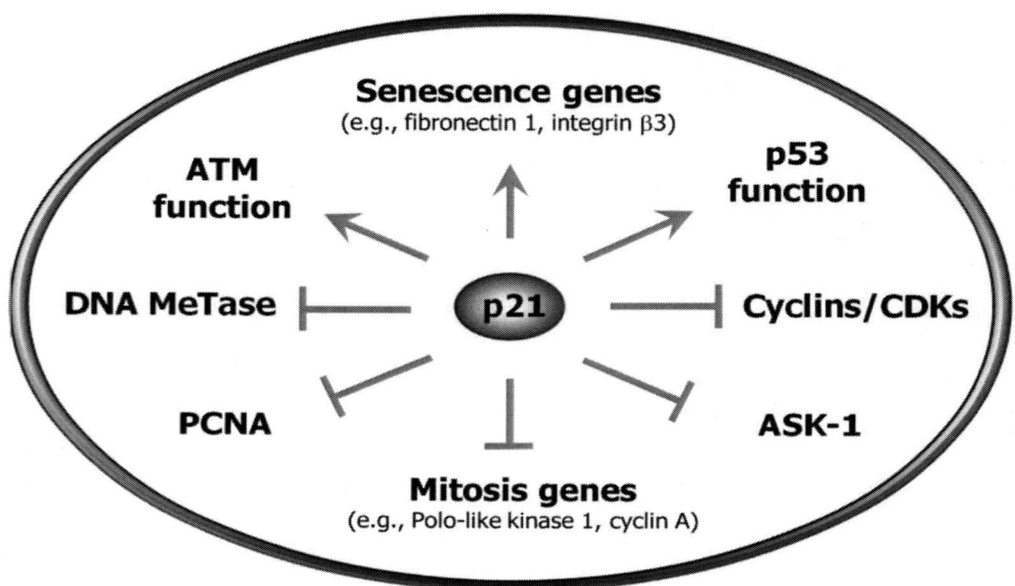

Figure 4. Multiple functions of p21. This tumor suppressor is at the hub of ATM signaling, owing to its ability to: (i) inhibit cell cycle progression by interacting with PCNA and cyclin/CDK complexes; (ii) influence gene expression indirectly, through interfering with DNA methyltransferase (MeTase) activity, and directly, by stimulating transcription of a series of genes involved in senescence and suppressing the transcription of numerous genes involved in mitosis; (iii) down-regulating apoptosis through, e.g., interacting with ASK-1; and (iv) forming positive feedback loops with both ATM and p53.

The p21 protein exerts its effect on the cell cycle by several mechanisms. The C-terminus of p21 suppresses DNA synthesis by interacting with proliferating cell nuclear antigen (PCNA), an auxiliary factor for DNA polymerase δ [Rousseau *et al.*, 1999]. The N-terminus of p21 binds to CDKs and inhibits their ability to phosphorylate the retinoblastoma protein (pRB), an event that is required for progression of cells from G1 to S phase [Rousseau *et al.*, 1999]. Induction of p21 also activates the G2/M checkpoint following genotoxic stress [Bunz *et al.*, 1998; Gillis *et al.* 2009]. According to Gillis *et al.* [2009], the latter effect is caused by p21-mediated degradation of the G2-associated cyclin, cyclin B1. It is noteworthy that not all checkpoints are dependent on the p53-p21 axis. The ionizing radiation-induced S-phase checkpoint, which is defective in AT cells, is not dependent on p53 [Mirzayans *et al.*, 1995; Enns *et al.*, 1999] or p21 [Guo *et al.*, 1999].

In 1997 it was reported that p21 negatively regulates the enzyme DNA-methyltransferase [Chuang *et al.*, 1997]. This finding raised the intriguing possibility that p21 might influence the expression of the many human genes that contain CpG islands within their transcription start sites [Baylin, 1997]. Subsequent studies reported from various laboratories established an active role for p21 in the regulation of genes involved in growth arrest, senescence, and aging. Specifically, p21 down-regulates a series of genes involved in mitosis, and up-regulates numerous genes associated with senescence [Chang *et al.*, 2000; Roninson *et al.*, 2003]. p21 also represses the activity of the transcription factors E2F [Delavaine and La Thangue, 1999] and c-myc [Kitaura *et al.*, 2000] that directly participate in the expression of genes that control cell cycle progression.

Another major function of p21 in many cell types is to suppress apoptosis by acting at different levels of the death cascade. Thus, p21 suppresses apoptosis by interacting with apoptosis signal-regulating kinase 1 (ASK-1) [Asada *et al.*, 1999; Zhou and Hung, 2002], forming a complex with procaspase-3 and suppressing its activation by masking the protease cleavage site [Suzuki *et al.*, 1999], inhibiting activation of caspase-9 [Sohn *et al.*, 2006], inhibiting cytochrome *c* release from mitochondria [Le *et al.* 2005], and lowering the level of the wild-type p53 protein [Javelaud and Besaçon, 2002].

Suppression of p21 function in p53 wild-type human solid tumor-derived cells is known to be associated with increased p53 protein levels without exposure to genotoxic agents [Javelaud and Besaçon, 2002]. In addition, p21 deficiency leads to elevated expression of p14^{ARF} (hereafter ARF) which is known to stabilize p53 by antagonizing MDM2 [Zhang *et al.*, 1998; Pomerantz *et al.*, 1998]. These findings led Javelaud and Besaçon to propose that increased ARF levels in p21-deficient cells may increase the steady-state levels of p53 by interrupting the MDM2-mediated degradation of p53. Suppression of p21 in p53 wild-type human cells renders them highly sensitive to undergoing apoptosis after exposure to ionizing radiation [Wouters *et al.*, 1997; Tian *et al.*, 2000], which is consistent with the pro-apoptotic and anti-apoptotic properties of p53 and p21, respectively. All of these studies measured global p53 protein levels by Western blotting.

Recently, Pang *et al.* [2011] demonstrated that regulation of p53 by p21 is more complex than originally believed, and it also involves ATM. In that study, p21-null solid tumor-derived cells exhibited compromised p53-mediated transcription (despite containing high constitutive levels of global p53 protein) that was linked to a p53 protein shift from chromatin into the cytoplasm; complementation of p21-null cells with the *p21* gene restored nuclear localization of p53. Inhibition of ATM function in p53 and p21 wild-type cells resulted in nuclear exclusion of p53, suggesting a positive interaction between ATM and p21.

These observations highlighted the interaction between two p53-regulated proteins, one of which (MDM2) is a negative regulator of p53 and promotes p53 degradation, and the other (p21) is a positive effector and maintains both nuclear localization of p53 and the ATM-dependent DNA damage response.

SEQUENTIAL WAVES OF P53 ACTIVATION BY DNA DAMAGE

The discovery of the involvement of p53 in the DNA damage response in the early 1990's led to a model in which the p53-p21 pathway either promotes survival by activating cell cycle checkpoints to facilitate repair, or eliminates injured cells through apoptotic cell death [e.g., Enoch and Norbury, 1995]. In 1998, we reported studies with human fibroblasts which led us to propose a "two wave" model for activation of the p53/p21 response by ionizing radiation and UV (254 nm) [Barley *et al.*, 1998]. According to our model for fibroblasts, while the rapid activation of the p53-p21 pathway (first wave) causes transient activation of cell cycle checkpoints and facilitates DNA repair, the persistence of genomic lesions (e.g., DNA damage, chromosome breaks) provides the critical signal for the late activation of the p53-p21 pathway (second wave), leading to p21-mediated SIPS or p53-mediated apoptosis, depending on the extent of genomic injury. For both agents, the primary mode of clonogenic "death" (i.e., inability of a cell to form a colony of at least 50 cells) was shown to be SIPS and not apoptosis. In fact, apoptosis was observed only after exposure to supralethal doses of UV (>30 J/m^2) which produce sufficient numbers of bulky DNA lesions to block transcription of genes such as *p21* [Barley *et al.*, 1998]. Accordingly, we have focused our studies on "survival-curve-range" doses of DNA-damaging agents (i.e., doses that cause no more that 90% cell kill in the clonogenic assay). Under these conditions, we have shown that the principal mode of clonogenic death is SIPS and not apoptosis in human normal and DSB-repair deficient (AT and LFS) fibroblast strains exposed to ionizing radiation [Mirzayans *et al.*, 2010], and in human normal and nucleotide excision repair-deficient (xeroderma pigmentosum and Cockayne syndrome) fibroblast strains exposed to UV [Mirzayans *et al.*, 2008].

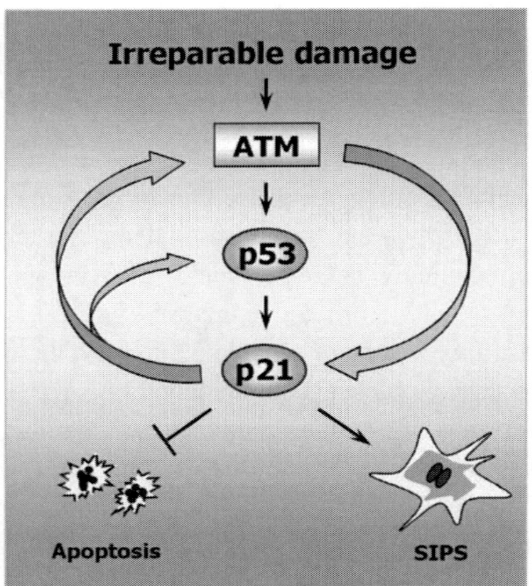

Figure 5. Sequential waves of p53 signaling in normal human fibroblasts exposed to ionizing radiation. [A] Exposure to ionizing radiation results in ATM-dependent activation of numerous proteins (e.g., p53, WRN, DNA-PKcs) that play key roles in DSB repair, as well as p53-mediated activation of p21 which suppresses apoptosis and activates the G1/S and G2/M checkpoints. Proper activation of these early events provides time for removal of potentially cytotoxic and mutagenic DNA lesions. [B] Persistence of DNA damage (i.e., irreparable damage) at late times (>24 h) post-irradiation results in sustained nuclear accumulation of p21 which suppresses apoptosis and induces "permanent" growth arrest through SIPS. Positive feedback loops between ATM and p21 and between p53 and p21 ensure the maintenance of the SIPS response.

The sequential waves of p53 signaling have now been documented for human solid tumor-derived cell lines [Lahav *et al.*, 2008; Batchelor *et al.*, 2008; Zhang *et al.*, 2011]. Batchelor *et al.* [2008] proposed the same outcome at each wave of the DNA damage response, i.e., p21-mediated G1/S checkpoint activation and p53-mediated apoptosis. More recently, Zhang *et al.* [2011] suggested that p53 may first be partially activated by primary modifications such as phosphorylation at Ser15 and Ser20 to induce cell cycle checkpoints, and if the damage is beyond repair, p53 may be fully activated by further modifications at Ser46 to trigger apoptosis. Neither model considers the pivotal role of p21 in suppressing apoptosis and inducing SIPS.

The well-established multifunctional nature of p21 described above is consistent with our original model, with different p21-mediated outcomes from early and late waves, the former activating checkpoints to facilitate repair, and the latter suppressing apoptosis and triggering SIPS, primarily through regulating gene expression independent of its influence on early cell cycle checkpoints [Barley *et al.*, 1998]. In view of the recent discovery of the ATM-p21 and p53-p21 regulatory loops [Pang *et al.*, 2011] alluded to earlier, our original model needs to be revised to incorporate the role of p21 in maintaining the DNA damage response (Figure 5).

ATM-DEPENDENT SENESCENCE

When normal human cells are explanted in culture they proliferate for several generations and ultimately enter a state of growth arrest called replicative or cellular senescence. This phenomenon was first observed with human diploid fibroblasts half a century ago [Haff and Swim, 1956], and was subsequently reported for keratinocytes, endothelial cells, and other cell types [reviewed in Cristofalo and Pignolo, 1993]. Major characteristics of senescent cells include an enlarged and flattened morphology, positive staining for senescence-associated β-galactosidase (SA-β-Gal), and loss of proliferating capacity. Senescence is not merely a passive growth arrest. Cells undergoing senescence remain metabolically active and influence their environment and neighboring cells through an active secretory program. Senescence can also be induced in some types of proliferating (young) human cells by different means, including exposure to DNA damaging agents (i.e., SIPS) and overexpression of p21, p16^{INK4a} (hereafter p16) and other tumor suppressors [Xu *et al.*, 1997; Kato *et al.*, 1998; McConnell *et al.*, 1998; Chen *et al.*, 2005].

Replicative senescence results primarily from the shortening of telomeres as a function of culture age. Telomere shortening is believed to destabilize or even prevent the capping of chromosome ends by telomerases, triggering replicative senescence [Shay, 1999]. On the other hand, SIPS in young human fibroblasts is triggered by nonspecific genome-wide DNA damage, independent of telomere status and telomerase function [Chen *et al.*, 2001; Roninson, 2003; Shay and Roninson, 2004]. In normal human fibroblasts, both replicative senescence [Sedelnikova *et al.*, 2004; Mirzayans *et al.*, 2010] and SIPS [di Fagagna *et al.*, 2003; Fernandez-Capetillo *et al.*, 2004; Mirzayans *et al.*, 2008; 2010] are accompanied by nuclear foci containing γ-H2AX molecules, signifying the presence of irreparable DNA DSBs.

Although overexpression of p16 triggers senescence in some cell types, the role of endogenous p16 in different types of senescence has been contentious [Mirzayans *et al.*,

2010, and references therein]. Some reports suggested a sequential involvement of p21 and p16 in senescence [Alcorta *et al.*, 1996; Stein *et al.*, 1999], and other reports did not support a role for p16 in senescence [Herbig *et al.*, 2004; Freedman and Folkman, 2005]. Our recent studies with LFS fibroblasts led us to propose the model presented in Figure 6 for the fibroblast background, in which p16 serves as a backup regulator of replicative senescence and SIPS, triggering these responses only in the absence of wild-type p53 function [Mirzayans *et al.*, 2010]. Our model is consistent with the properties of both p53 and p16, with the former functioning as a negative regulator of p16 [Jacobs and De Lange, 2005; Hernández-Vargas *et al.*, 2006; De Lange *et al.*, 2009], and the latter capable of suppressing apoptosis [Al-Mohanna *et al.*, 2004; Lau *et al.*, 2007] and triggering senescence [Zhang, 2007]. The role of ATM in the induction of p16 in different p53-deficient cell types undergoing replicative senescence and ionizing radiation-induced SIPS remains to be determined.

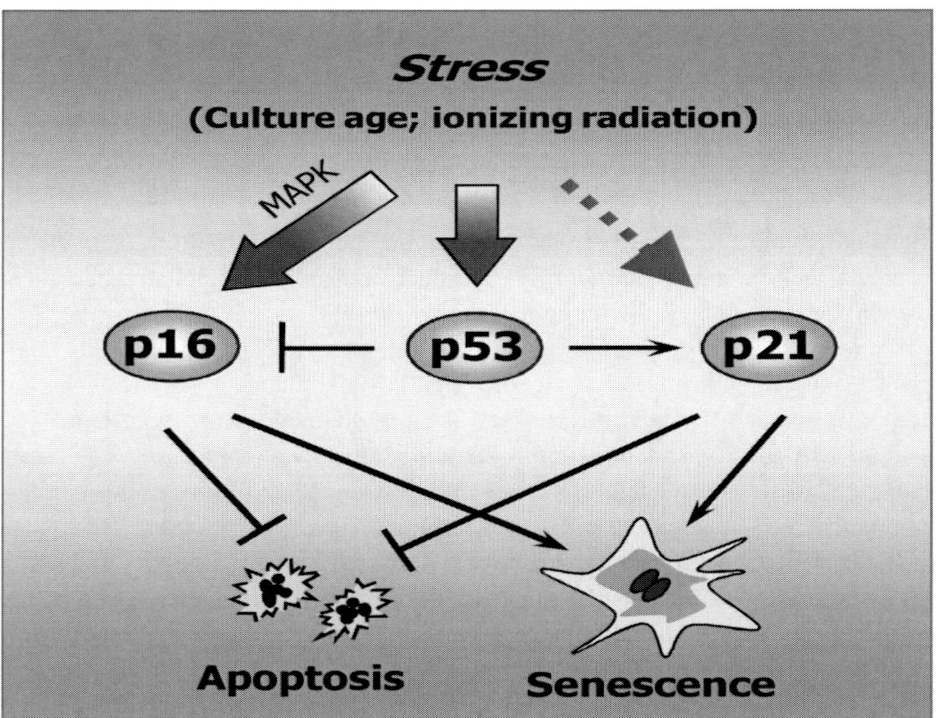

Figure 6. Model for the roles of p16, p53 and p21 in replicative senescence and DNA damage-induced SIPS in human fibroblast cultures. In p53 wild-type (normal and AT) fibroblasts, exposure to DNA-damaging agents or telomere shortening as a result of culture age results in activation of p53, which suppresses p16 and induces p21. The latter protein represses apoptosis and triggers senescence. On the other hand, p53-deficient (LFS) fibroblasts respond to stress by upregulation of p16 which serves to repress apoptosis and to activate senescence.

ATM-INDEPENDENT SENESCENCE

Skin fibroblasts cultured from AT patients exhibit elevated levels of spontaneous chromosomal instability coupled with premature replicative senescence when compared to normal fibroblasts [Wood *et al.*, 2001]. Consistent with these observations, ATM is known to contribute to telomere maintenance [Wong *et al.*, 2003; Chan and Blackburn, 2003]. We have confirmed the early onset of replicative senescence in AT fibroblasts, and further demonstrated that this response is associated with nuclear accumulation of p21 independent of p16 expression [Mirzayans *et al.*, 2010].

As mentioned above, the AT fibroblast strains used by us do not activate p53 at early times (between 3 and 24 h) after exposure to ionizing radiation [Enns *et al.*, 1998]. It was of interest to determine whether ionizing radiation exposure would elicit SIPS in these strains, and if so, whether this response would involve p16 (and not p21) as we have documented for p53-deficient LFS fibroblasts [Mirzayans *et al.*, 2010]. Exposure to a given dose of γ-rays induced SIPS in a much higher proportion of cells within young cultures of AT fibroblasts than those of normal fibroblasts [Mirzayans *et al.*, 2010]. Unexpectedly, the ionizing radiation-induced SIPS in AT fibroblasts correlated with a robust induction of p21 but not of p16. Furthermore, immunofluorescence microscopy revealed that ionizing radiation exposure caused nuclear accumulation of p53 in AT fibroblasts when measured several days post-irradiation, but not at earlier times (within 2 days) post-irradiation.

Further studies are warranted to elucidate the mechanisms by which ionizing radiation exposure triggers a delayed (>2 days) wave of p53-p21 activation in AT fibroblasts, and to determine whether this ATM-independent wave constitutes an integral part of the normal DNA damage surveillance machinery, or whether it reflects the involvement of a redundant pathway (e.g., mediated by ATR and/or DNA PKcs) operating only in the absence of ATM function.

ROLE OF ATM IN PREVENTING ESCAPE FROM SIPS: A NOVEL TUMOR SUPPRESSOR FUNCTION BEYOND P53?

In the original model of the p53-mediated surveillance network [Meyn, 1995; Enoch and Norbury, 1995], the mechanism by which p53 eliminates injured cells was hypothesized to be through apoptosis. This model still continues to be widely cited. However, numerous studies with non-transformed skin fibroblast strains [Barley *et al.*, 1998; Mirzayans *et al.*, 2008; 2010] and p53 wild-type solid tumor-derived cell lines [Han *et al.*, 2002; Mirzayans *et al.*, 2005; Sohn *et al.*, 2006; Crescenzi *et al.*, 2008; Gewirtz *et al.*, 2008; Sliwinska *et al.*, 2009] have now established that SIPS, and not apoptosis, is the predominant (if not exclusive) response triggered by "survival-curve-range" doses of DNA-damaging agents in such cell types. Although cells undergoing SIPS do not form macroscopic colonies and hence are scored as "dead" in clonogenic assays, it is becoming increasingly evident that under some conditions SIPS might not be a permanent growth-arrested state. Thus, a proportion of cells exhibiting features of SIPS can escape the proliferation block and give rise to giant cells with extensive genetic abnormalities (e.g., multinucleation) [Rajaraman *et al.*, 2006; Sliwinska *et al.*, 2009]. In addition, loss of p53 function is now universally accepted to be permissive for the development of such giant cells after exposure to ionizing radiation and other cancer therapeutic agents [Illedge *et al.*, 2000; Erenpreisa and Cragg, 2001; Rajaraman *et al.*, 2006; Vakifahmetoglu *et al.*, 2008; Ianzini *et al.*, 2009].

What is the fate of such giant cells? It is well documented that multinucleation /polyploidy may provide a radiation-survival mechanism in some mammalian cell types. Giant cells with such genetic abnormalities may give rise to rapidly proliferating offspring by depolyploidization through meiotic or pseudo-meiotic pathways [Ianzini *et al.*, 2009; Erenpreisa *et al.*, 2009], as well as neosis, an ill-defined parasexual somatic reduction division which resembles division of the budding yeast [Rajaraman *et al.*, 2006; Sliwinska *et al.*, 2009; Mansilla *et al.*, 2009] (also see Figure 7). Through these complex processes, giant cells can give rise to rapidly proliferating descendants that can exhibit stem cell-like properties and resistance to cancer therapeutic agents [reviewed in Rajaraman *et al.*, 2006]. The Aurora B kinase, a key regulator of chromosome segregation and cytokinesis [Warner *et al.*, 2003], has been identified as the gatekeeper between life and death of multinucleated/polyploid giant cells. Endogenous expression of catalytically active Aurora B kinase promoted the survival of giant cells, whereas its absence was associated with giant-cell apoptosis [Erenpreisa *et al.*, 2008].

Does ATM play a role in determining the fate of giant cells? The mitotic kinases Aurora A and Aurora B are inhibited by DNA damage to ensure blocking of mitosis [reviewed in Bensimon *et al.*, 2011]. This inhibition is accomplished through dephosphorylation and is dependent on protein phosphatase 1 (PP1) [Satinover *et al.*, 2004; Tang *et al.*, 2008; Bhatia *et al.*, 2010]. Intriguingly, PP1 is known to act as an ATM effector to control Aurora kinases as well as other kinases. Specifically, Tang *et al.* [2008] determined that ionizing radiation induces the dissociation of PP1 from its regulatory subunit (inhibitor-2), which results in activation of PP1, inhibition of Aurora B kinase, and down-regulation of histone H3 Ser10 phosphorylation, leading to mitotic arrest.

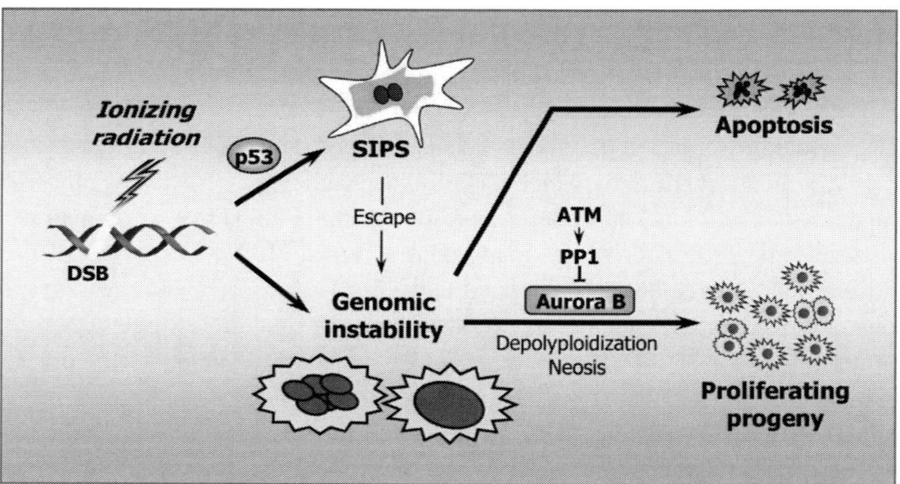

Figure 7. Fate of multinucleated and polyploid giant cells. DNA-damaging agents trigger the development of such giant cells within p53-deficient cultures. In addition, a small proportion of cells within p53-proficient cultures "escape" from the SIPS response after DNA damage and give rise to giant cells. While some giant cells may die through apoptosis, others may retain viability and undergo complex genome reduction processes (e.g., depolyploidization; neosis), ultimately resulting in the generation of rapidly proliferating progeny. The mitotic kinase Aurora B plays a key role in the survival of giant cells. We propose that ATM prevents the propagation of giant cells and their descendants through activating PP1 and inhibiting Aurora B kinase activity.

In short, as illustrated in Figure 7, one of the tumor suppressor functions of ATM might be associated with its ability to prevent the growth of multinucleated/polyploid giant cells through activating the PP1-mediated G2/M checkpoint pathway at late times (several days) post-irradiation.

POTENTIAL THERAPEUTIC APPROACHES FOR THE TREATMENT OF AT

The growing complexity of the molecular and cellular events regulated by ATM discussed above, in concert with the presence of different mutations within the gene among AT patients [Lavin, 2008], indicate that complete cure for AT patients will require gene replacement which must be tailored to specific mutations [Lavin, 2008]. This strategy, however, has met with a number of obstacles which need to be addressed before it could be used in the clinic [reviewed in Lavin, 2008]. Alternative strategies have been proposed that might be effective for managing or alleviating some of the symptoms associated with the disease. One such strategy exploits the bystander effect of ionizing radiation, and another makes use of antioxidants. These strategies are outlined below.

The term "bystander effect" in the field of radiobiology refers to the detection of radiation-like effects in cells that have not received a direct radiation "hit". In addition to ionizing radiation-associated bystander effects, we reported another form of cell-to-cell communication between non-irradiated normal and AT fibroblast cultures, resulting in correction of the AT phenotype [Paterson and Mirzayans, 1993; Mirzayans and Paterson, 2001]. Employing the alkaline sucrose velocity sedimentation technique, AT fibroblasts were shown to be defective in repairing alkali-stable DNA lesions after exposure to ionizing radiation or the radiomimetic carcinogen 4-nitroquinoline 1-oxide [Paterson *et al.*, 1976; Mirzayans *et al.*, 1989; Paterson and Mirzayans, 1993]. Interestingly, this repair deficiency could be corrected by co-cultivation of AT fibroblasts with normal fibroblasts in the absence of somatic cell fusion [Paterson and Mirzayans, 1993]. These and related studies (published before cloning of the *ATM* gene) led us to propose that the product of the gene mutated in AT must function upstream in various signaling pathways [Mirzayans *et al.*, 1988; 1989; Mirzayans and Paterson, 1991].

We next focused our attention on correcting the "radioresistant DNA synthesis" (RDS) phenotype of AT cells, which has often been taken as a molecular hallmark of AT. RDS reflects the failure of AT cells to exhibit inhibition of *de novo* DNA synthesis immediately after ionizing radiation exposure. We demonstrated that: (i) the radiation-responsive S-phase checkpoint operating in normal human fibroblasts is mediated by a p53-independent signaling pathway involving Ca^{2+}/calmodulin-dependent protein kinase II (CaMKII) [Mirzayans *et al.*, 1995; Enns *et al.*, 1999]; (ii) this p53-independent pathway is activated by a heat-labile diffusible factor [Mirzayans *et al.*, 1997]; and (iii) the RDS phenotype of AT cells is associated with failure to activate the CaMKII-dependent S-phase arrest [Mirzayans *et al.*, 1995]. We further reported that the RDS phenotype of AT fibroblasts can be rectified in the absence of ectopic expression of functional ATM [Paterson and Mirzayans, 1999; Mirzayans and Paterson, 2001]. Correction of RDS was observed when: (i) AT fibroblasts were co-incubated with normal fibroblasts under conditions in which the two different cell cultures shared the same medium but were completely separated physically; (ii) AT fibroblasts were incubated with conditioned medium collected from exponentially-growing (non-irradiated) normal fibroblasts; and (iii) AT fibroblasts were briefly incubated with an eicosanoid (e.g., prostaglandin E_2) in the absence of normal feeder cells/conditioned medium.

Collectively, these results indicated that exogenous factors, including some eicosanoids, are capable of compensating for aspects of the ATM function in AT cells. Accordingly, such factors have been proposed to potentially provide a practical strategy for the management of AT patients and probably AT carriers (heterozygotes) without the need for *ATM* gene therapy [Paterson and Mirzayans, 1999]. The clinical ramifications of eicosanoids in this context remain to be explored.

Other groups have taken the advantage of antioxidants in an attempt to formulate treatments for AT [reviewed in Lavin *et al.*, 2007; Reliene and Schiestl, 2008]. Several observations led to this approach. For example, antioxidant capacity is reduced in the serum of AT patients, cultured AT cells show evidence of increased oxidative stress, and ATM-mediated inhibition of oxidative stress is required for self-renewal of haematopoietic stem cells. Thus, it was hypothesized that unusually increased oxidative stress in AT might lead to increased macromolecular damage and in turn to genome instability, cancer and neurodegeneration [Lavin *et al.*, 2007]. Studies with *Atm* deficient mice revealed that several antioxidants were effective in suppressing genome rearrangement, increasing life span, and reducing both the incidence and multiplicity of lymphoma [Reviewed in Reliene and Schiestl, 2008]. The antioxidants tested in these studies included N-acetyl-L-cysteine (NAC), desferrioxamine, and 5-carboxy-1,1,3,3-tetramethylisoindolin-2-yloxyl. Among these compounds, only NAC has wide clinical applications due to safety and efficacy. It is also available as an over-the-counter dietary supplement. Therefore, NAC was proposed to have a strong potential to emerge as a dietary supplement for the management of some symptoms associated with AT [Reliene and Schiestl, 2008].

CONCLUSION

In the mid 1990's, it was proposed that activation of the p53 pathway by DNA-damaging agents might lead to either cell cycle arrest or apoptosis, the former promoting cell survival by facilitating DNA repair, and the latter resulting in the removal of irreparably damaged cells from the proliferating population [e.g., Meyn, 1995; Enoch and Norbury, 1995]. This model still provides the impetus for numerous studies. However, compelling recent evidence has revealed that the primary response of human fibroblasts to DNA damaging agents is SIPS and not apoptosis. Similarly, many p53 wild-type human solid tumor cell lines respond to ionizing radiation and chemotherapeutic agents by undergoing SIPS [Chang *et al.*, 1999a; 1999b; Mirzayans *et al.*, 2005; Afshar *et al.* 2006; Sohn *et al.* 2006], and targeting either p53 or p21 switches the treatment-induced response from SIPS to apoptosis [Han *et al.*, 2002; Tian *et al.*, 2002; Crescenzi *et al.*, 2008; Gewirtz *et al.*, 2008; Li *et al.*, 2011]. The p21 protein is at the hub of ATM signaling because of the ability of this multifunctional protein to activate transient cell cycle checkpoints, suppress apoptosis, control gene expression, positively regulate ATM and p53, and induce SIPS. An improved understanding of the function of the ATM-p53-p21 signaling axis is crucial for designing effective approaches not only for the outcome of cancer therapy, but also for the treatment of AT patients.

ACKNOWLEDGMENTS

The authors wish to thank Bonnie Andrais and April Scott for technical assistance. This work was supported in part by the Canadian Institute of Health Research and the Canadian Breast Cancer Foundation-Prairies/NWT region.

REFERENCES

Adams, K. E., Medhurst, A. L., Dart, D. A. & Lakin, N. D. (2006). Recruitment of ATR to sites of ionising radiation-induced DNA damage requires ATM and components of the MRN protein complex. *Oncogene, 25,* 3894–3904.

Afshar, G., Jelluma, N., Yang, X., Basila, D., Arvold, N. D., Karlsson, A., Yount, G. L., Dansen, T. B., Koller, E. & Haas-Kogan, D. A. (2006). Radiation-induced caspase-8 mediates p53-independent apoptosis in glioma cells. *Cancer Res., 66,* 4223–4232.

Akhtar, R. S., Geng, Y., Klocke, B. J., Latham, C. B., Villunger, A. W., Michalak, E. M., Strasser, A., Carroll, S. L. & Roth, K. A. (2006). BH3-Only proapoptotic Bcl-2 family members Noxa and Puma mediate neural precursor cell death. *J. Neurosci., 26,* 7257–7264.

Alcorta, D. A., Xiong, Y., Phelps, D., Hannon, G., Beach, D. & Barrett, J. C. (1996). Involvement of the cyclin-dependent kinase inhibitor p16 (INK4a) in replicative senescence of normal human fibroblasts. *Proc. Natl. Acad. Sci. USA, 93,* 13742–13747.

Al-Mohanna, M. A., Manogaran, P. S., Al-Mukhalafi, Z. A., Al-Hussein, K. & Aboussekhra, A. (2004). The tumor suppressor p16^{INK4a} gene is a regulator of apoptosis induced by ultraviolet light and cisplatin. *Oncogene, 23,* 201–212.

Al Rashid, S. T., Dellaire, G., Cuddihy, A., Jalali, F., Vaid, M., Coackley, C., Folkard, M., Xu, Y., Chen, B. P., Chen, D. J., Lilge, L., Prise, K. M., Bazett-Jones, D. P. & Bristow, R. G. (2005). Evidence for the direct binding of phosphorylated p53 to sites of DNA breaks *in vivo. Cancer Res., 65,* 10810–10821.

Ammazzalorso, F., Pirzio, L. M., Bignami, M., Franchitto, A. & Pichierri, P. (2010). ATR and ATM differently regulate WRN to prevent DSBs at stalled replication forks and promote replication fork recovery. *EMBO J., 29,* 3156–3169.

Asada, M., Yamada, T., Ichijo, H., Delia, D., Miyazono, K., Fukumuro, K. & Mizutani, S. (1999). Apoptosis inhibitory activity of cytoplasmic p21$^{Cip1/WAF1}$ in monocytic differentiation. *EMBO J., 18,* 1223–1234.

Batchelor, E., Mock, C. S., Bhan, I., Loewer, A. & Lahav, G. (2008). Recurrent initiation: a mechanism for triggering p53 pulses in response to DNA damage. *Mol. Cell, 9,* 277–289.

Bakkenist, C. J. & Kastan, M. B. (2003). DNA damage activates ATM through intermolecular autophosphorylation and dimer dissociation. *Nature, 421,* 499-506.

Barley, R. D. C., Enns, L., Paterson, M. C. & Mirzayans, R. (1998). Aberrant *p21^{WAF1}*-dependent growth arrest as the possible mechanism of abnormal resistance to ultraviolet light cytotoxicity in Li-Fraumeni syndrome fibroblast strains heterozygous for *TP53* mutations. *Oncogene, 17*, 533–543.

Baylin, S. B. (1997). Tying it all together: epigenetics, genetics, cell cycle, and cancer. *Science, 277*, 1948–1949.

Bensimon, A., Aebersold, R. & Shiloh, Y. (2011). Beyond ATM: the protein kinase landscape of the DNA damage response. *FEBBS Lett., 585*, 1625–1639.

Bhatia, P., Menigatti, M., Brocard, M., Morley, S. J. & Ferrari, S. (2010). Mitotic DNA damage targets the Aurora A/TPX2 complex. *Cell Cycle, 9*, 4592–4599.

Bond, J., Jones, C., Haughton, M., DeMicco, C., Kipling, D. & Wynford-Thomas, D. (2004). Direct evidence from siRNA-directed "knock down" that p16^{INK4a} is required for human fibroblast senescence and for limiting ras-induced epithelial cell proliferation. *Exp. Cell Res., 292*, 151–156.

Brookes, S., Rowe, J., Gutierrez Del Arroyo, A., Bond, J. & Peters, G. (2004). Contribution of p16^{INK4a} to replicative senescence of human fibroblasts. *Exp. Cell Res., 298*, 549–559.

Brown, K. D., Barlow, C. & Wynshaw-Boris, A. (1999). Multiple ATM-dependent pathways: an explanation for pleiotropy. *Am. J. Hum. Genet., 64*, 46–50.

Bunz, F., Dutriaux, A., Lengauer, C., Waldman, T., Zhou, S., Brown, J. P., Sedivy, J. M., Kinzler, K. W. & Vogelstein, B. (1998). Requirement for p53 and p21 to sustain G2 arrest after DNA damage. *Science, 282*, 1497–501.

Burma, S. & Chen, D. J. (2004). Role of DNA-PK in the cellular response to DNA double-strand breaks. *DNA Repair (Amst.), 3*, 909–918.

Chan, S. W. & Blackburn, E. H. (2003). Telomerase and ATM/Tel1p protect telomeres from nonhomologous end joining. *Mol. Cell, 11*, 1379–1387.

Chang, B. D., Broude, E. V., Dokmanovic, M., Zhu, H., Ruth, A., Xuan, Y., Kandel, E. S., Lausch, E., Christov, K. & Roninson, I. B. (1999a). A senescence-like phenotype distinguishes tumor cells that undergo terminal proliferation arrest after exposure to anticancer agents. *Cancer Res., 59*, 3761–3767.

Chang, B. D., Xuan, Y., Broude, E. V., Zhu, H., Schott, B., Fang, J. & Roninson, I. B. (1999b). Role of p53 and p21$^{waf1/cip1}$ in senescence-like terminal proliferation arrest induced in human tumor cells by chemotherapeutic drugs. *Oncogene, 15*, 4808–4818.

Chang, B. D., Watanabe, K., Broude, E. V., Fang. J., Poole, L. C., Kalinchenko, T. & Roninson, I. B. (2000). Effects of p21$^{Waf1/Cip1/Sdi1}$ on cellular gene expression: Implications for carcinogenesis, senescence, and age-related diseases. *Proc. Natl. Acad. Sci. USA, 97*, 4291–4296.

Chen, Q. M., Prowse, K. R., Tu, V. C., Purdom, S. & Linskens, M. H. (2001). Uncoupling the senescent phenotype from telomere shortening in hydrogen peroxide-treated fibroblasts. *Exp. Cell Res., 265*, 294–303.

Chen, L., Huang, S., Lee, L., Davalos, A., Schiestl, R. H., Campisi, J. & Oshima, J. (2003). WRN, the protein deficient in Werner syndrome, plays a critical structural role in optimizing DNA repair. *Aging Cell, 2*, 191–199.

Chen, C. R., Wang, W., Rogoff, H. A., Xiaotong, L., Mang, W. & Li, C. J. (2005). Dual induction of apoptosis and senescence in cancer cells by Chk2 activation: checkpoint activation as a strategy against cancer. *Cancer Res., 65*, 6017–6021.

Chen, B. P., Uematsu, N., Kobayashi, J., Lerenthal, Y., Krempler, A., Yajima, H., Löbrich, M., Shiloh, Y. & Chen, D. J. (2007). Ataxia telangiectasia mutated (ATM) is essential for

DNA-PKcs phosphorylations at the Thr-2609 cluster upon DNA double strand break. *J. Biol. Chem., 282,* 6582–6587.

Cho, Y., Gorina, S., Jeffrey, P. D. & Pavletich, N. P. (1994). Crystal structure of a p53 tumor suppressor-DNA complex: understanding tumorigenic mutations. *Science, 265,* 346–355.

Chuang, L., Ian, H. I., Koh, T. W., Ng, H. H., Xu, G. & Li, B. F. (1997). Human DNA-(cytosine-5) methyltransferase-PCNA complex as a target for p21^{WAFl}. *Science, 277,* 1996–2000.

Cook , J. G. (2009). Replication licensing and the DNA damage checkpoint. *Front. Biosci., 14,* 5013–5030.

Corroyer, S., Nabeyrat, E. & Clement, A. (1997). Involvement of the cell cycle inhibitor CIP1/WAF1 in lung alveolar epithelial cell growth arrest induced by glucocorticoids. *Endocrinology, 138,* 3677–3685.

Costanzo, V., Paull, T., Gottesman, M. & Gautier, J. (2004). Mre11 assembles linear DNA fragments into DNA damage signaling complexes. *PLoS Biol., 2,* E110.

Crescenzi, E., Palumbo, G., de Boer, J. & Brady, H. J. (2008). Ataxia telangiectasia mutated and p21^{CIP1} modulate cell survival of drug-induced senescent tumor cells: implications for chemotherapy. *Clin. Cancer Res., 14,* 1877–1887.

Cristofalo, V. J. & Pignolo, R. J. (1993). Replicative senescence of human fibroblast-like cells in culture. *Physiol. Rev., 73,* 617–638.

Cuadrado, M., Martinez-Pastor, B., Murga, M., Toledo, L. I,, Gutierrez-Martinez, P., Lopez, E. & Fernandez-Capetillo, O. (2006). ATM regulates ATR chromatin loading in response to DNA double-strand breaks. *J. Exp. Med., 203,* 297–303.

Datto, M. B., Li, Y., Panus, J. F., Howe, D. J., Xiong, Y. & Wang, X. F. (1995). Transforming growth factor beta induces the cyclin-dependent kinase inhibitor p21 through a p53-independent mechanism. *Proc. Natl. Acad. Sci., USA, 92,* 5545–5549.

De Leong, W. F., Chau, J. F. L. & Li, B. (2009). p53 deficiency leads to compensatory up-regulation of p16^{INK4a}. *Mol. Cancer Res., 7,* 354–360.

Delavaine, L. & La Thangue, N. B. (1999). Control of E2F activity by p21$^{Wafl/Cip1}$. *Oncogene, 18,* 5381–5392.

di Fagagna, F. d'A., Reaper, P. M., Clay-Farrace, L., Fiegler H., Carr P., von Zglinicki, T., Saretzki G., Carter N. P. & Jackson S. P. (2003). A DNA damage checkpoint response in telomere-initiated senescence. *Nature, 426,* 194–198.

DiBiase, S. J., Guan, J., Curran, W. J. & Iliakis, G. (1999). Repair of DNA double-strand breaks and radiosensitivity to killing in an isogenic group of p53 mutant cell lines. *Int. J. Radiat. Oncol. Biol. Phys., 45,* 743–751.

Dickson, M. A., Hahn, W. C., Ino, Y., Ronfard, V., Wu, J. Y., Weinberg, R. A., Louis, D. N., Li, F. P. & Rheinwald, J. G. (2000). Human keratinocytes that express hTERT and also bypass a p16^{INK4a}-enforced mechanism that limits life span become immortal yet retain normal growth and differentiation characteristics. *Mol. Cell. Biol., 20,* 1436–1447.

El Deiry, W. S., Tokino, T., Velculescu, V. E., Levy, D. B., Parsons, R., Trent, J. M., Lin, D., Mercer, W. E., Kinzler, K. W. & Vogelstein, B. (1993). WAF1, a potential mediator of p53 tumor suppression. *Cell, 75,* 817–825.

Enoch, T. & Norbury, C. (1995). Cellular responses to DNA damage: cell-cycle checkpoints, apoptosis and the roles of p53 and ATM. *Trends Biochem. Sci., 20,* 426–430.

Enns, L., Barley, R. D., Paterson, M. C. & Mirzayans, R. (1998) Radiosensitivity in ataxia telangiectasia fibroblasts is not associated with deregulated apoptosis. *Radiat. Res., 150,* 11–16.

Enns, L., Murray, D. & Mirzayans, R. (1999). Effects of the protein kinase inhibitors wortmannin and KN62 on cellular radiosensitivity and radiation-activated S phase and G1/S checkpoints in normal human fibroblasts. *Br. J. Cancer, 81,* 959–965.

Erenpreisa, J. & Cragg, M. S. (2001). Mitotic death: a mechanism of survival? A review. *Cancer Cell Int., 1,* 1–7.

Erenpreisa, J., Ivanov, A., Wheatley, S. P., Kosmacek, E. A., Ianzini, F., Anisimov, A. P., Mackey, M., Davis, P. J., Plakhins. G. & Illidge, T. M. (2008). Endopolyploidy in irradiated p53-deficient tumour cell lines: persistence of cell division activity in giant cells expressing Aurora-B kinase. *Cell. Biol. Int., 32,* 1044–1056.

Erenpreisa, J., Cragg, M. S., Salmina, K., Hausmann, M. & Scherthan, H. (2009). The role of meiotic cohesin REC8 in chromosome segregation in γ irradiation-induced endopolyploidtumour cells. *Exp. Cell Res., 315,* 2593–2603.

Fernandez-Capetillo, O., Lee, A., Nussenzweig, M. & Nussenzweig, A. (2004). H2AX: the histone guardian of the genome. *DNA Repair (Amst.), 3,* 959–967

Ford, J. M. (2005). Regulation of DNA damage recognition and nucleotide excision repair: another role for p53. *Mutat. Res., 577,* 195–202.

Freedman, D. A. & Folkman, J. (2004). CDK2 translational down-regulation during endothelial senescence. *Exp. Cell Res., 307,* 118–130.

Fuster, J. J., Sanz-González, S. M., Moll, U. M. & Andres, V. (2007). Classic and novel roles of p53: prospects for anticancer therapy. *Trends Mol. Med., 13,* 192-199.

Gatti, R. A., Boder, E., Vinters, H. V., Sparkes, R. S., Norman, A. & Lange, K. (1991). Ataxia-telangiectasia: an interdisciplinary approach to pathogenesis. *Medicine, 70,* 99–117.

Gewirtz, D. A., Holt, S. E. & Elmore, L. W. (2008). Accelerated senescence: an emerging role in tumor cell response to chemotherapy and radiation. *Biochem. Pharmacol., 76,* 947–957.

Gillis, L. D., Leidal, A. M., Hill, R. & Lee, P. W. (2009). p21$^{Cip1/WAF1}$ mediates cyclin B1 degradation in response to DNA damage. *Cell Cycle, 8,* 253-256.

Goodarzi, A. A., Noon, A. T., Deckbar, D., Ziv, Y., Shiloh, Y., Löbrich, M. & Jeggo, P. A. (2008). ATM signaling facilitates repair of DNA double-strand breaks associated with heterochromatin. *Mol. Cell, 31,* 167–177.

Gu, Y., Turck, C. W. & Morgan, D. O. (1993). Inhibition of CDK2 activity in vivo by an associated 20K regulatory subunit. *Nature, 366,* 707–710.

Guo, C. Y., D'Anna, J. A., Li, R. & Larner, J. M. (1999). The radiation-induced S-phase checkpoint is independent of CDKN1A. *Radiat. Res., 151,* 125–965.

Haff, R. F. & Swim, H. E. (1956). Serial propagation of 3 strains of rabbit fibroblasts: their susceptibility to infection with vaccinia virus. *Proc. Soc. Exp. Biol. Med., 93,* 200–204.

Han, Z., Wei, W., Dunaway, S., Darnowski, J. W., Calabresi, P., Sedivy, J., Hendrickson, E. A., Balan, K. V., Pantazis, P. & Wyche, J. H. (2002). Role of p21 in apoptosis and senescence of human colon cancer cells treated with camptothecin. *J. Biol. Chem., 277,* 17154–17160.

Harper, J. W., Adami, G. R., Wei, N., Keyomarsi, K. & Elledge, S. J. (1993). The p21 Cdk-interacting protein Cip1 is a potent inhibitor of G1 cyclin-dependent kinases. *Cell, 75,* 805–816.

Herbig, U., Jobling, W. A., Chen, B. P., Chen, D. J. & Sedivy, J. M. (2004). Telomere shortening triggers senescence of human cells through a pathway involving ATM, p53, and p21^{CIP1}, but not p16^{INK4a}. *Mol. Cell, 14,* 501–513.

Hernández-Vargas, H., Ballestar, E., Carmona-Saez, P., von Kobbe, C., Bañón-Rodríguez, I., Esteller, M., Moreno-Bueno, G. & Palacios, J. (2006). Transcriptional profiling of MCF7 breast cancer cells in response to 5-Fluorouracil: relationship with cell cycle changes and apoptosis, and identification of novel targets of p53. *Int. J. Cancer, 119,* 1164–1175.

Horejsi, Z., Falck, J., Bakkenist, C. J., Kastan, M. B., Lukas, J. & Bartek, J. (2004). Distinct functional domains of Nbs1 modulate the timing and magnitude of ATM activation after low doses of ionizing radiation. *Oncogene, 23,* 3122–3127.

Hu, P. P., Shen, X., Huang, D., Liu, Y., Counter, C. & Wang, X. F. (1999). The MEK pathway is required for stimulation of p21$^{WAF1/CIP1}$ by transforming growth factor-beta. *J. Biol. Chem., 274,* 35381–35387.

Ianzini, F., Kosmacek, E. A., Nelson, E. S., Napoli, E., Erenpreisa, J., Kalejs, M. & Mackey, M. A. (2009). Activation of Meiosis-Specific Genes Is Associated with Depolyploidization of Human Tumor Cells following Radiation-Induced Mitotic Catastrophe. *Cancer Res., 69,* 2296–2304.

Illidge, T. M., Cragg, M. S., Fringes, B., Olive, P. & Erenpresia, J. A. (2000). Polyploid giant cells provide a survival mechanism of p53 mutant cells after DNA damage. *Cell Biol. Int., 24,* 621–633.

Itahana, K., Zou, Y., Itahana, Y., Martinez, J. L., Beausejour, C., Jacobs, J. J., Van Lohuizen, M., Band, V., Campisi, J. & Dimri, G. P. (2003). Control of the replicative life span of human fibroblasts by p16 and the polycomb protein Bmi-1. *Mol. Cell. Biol., 23,* 389-401.

Jacobs, J. J. & de Lange, T. (2005). p16^{INK4a} as a second effector of the telomere damage pathway. *Cell Cycle, 4,* 1364–1368.

Javelaud, D. & Besançon, F. (2002). Inactivation of p21^{WAF1} sensitizes cells to apoptosis *via* an increase of both p14^{ARF} and p53 levels and an alteration of the Bax/Bcl-2 ratio. *J. Biol. Chem., 277,* 37849–37954.

Jazayeri, A., Falck, J., Lukas, C., Bartek, J., Smith, G. C., Lukas, J. & Jackson, S. P. (2006). ATM- and cell cycle-dependent regulation of ATR in response to DNA double-strand breaks. *Nat. Cell Biol., 8,* 37–45.

Jiang, H., Lin, J., Su, Z. Z., Herlyn, M., Kerbel, R. S., Weissman, B. E, Welch, D. R. & Fisher, P. B. (1995). The melanoma differentiation-associated gene mda-6, which encodes the cyclin-dependent kinase inhibitor p21, is differentially expressed during growth, differentiation and progression in human melanoma cells. *Oncogene, 10,* 1855–1864.

Jongmans, W., Vuillaume, M., Kleijer, W. J., Lakin, N. D. & Hall J. (1998). The p53-mediated DNA damage response to ionizing radiation in fibroblasts from ataxia-without-telangiectasia patients. *Int. J. Radiat. Biol., 74,* 287–295.

Kato, D., Miyazawa, K., Ruas, M., Starborg, M., Wada, I., Oka, T., Sakai, T., Peters, G. & Hara, E. (1998). Features of replicative senescence induced by direct addition of antennapedia-p16^{Ink4A} fusion protein to human diploid fibroblasts. *FEBS Lett., 427,* 203–208.

Kato, T. A., Nagasawa, H., Weil, M. M., Genik, P. C., Little, J. B. & Bedford, J. S. (2006). γ-H2AX foci after low-dose-rate irradiation reveal *atm* haploinsufficiency in mice. *Radiat. Res., 166*, 47–54.

Khanna, K. K. (2000). Cancer risk and the ATM gene: a continuing debate. *JNCI, 92*, 795–802.

Kitaura, H., Shinshi, M., Uchikoshi, Y., Ono, T., Iguchi-Ariga, S. M. & Ariga, H. (2000). Reciprocal regulation via protein-protein interaction between c-Myc and p21[cip1/waf1/sdi1] in DNA replication and transcription. *J. Biol. Chem., 275*, 10477–10483.

Kiyono, T., Foster, S. A., Koop, J. I., McDougall, J. K., Galloway, D. A. &. Klingelhutz, A. J. (1998). Both Rb/p16[INK4a] inactivation and telomerase activity are required to immortalize human epithelial cells. *Nature, 396*, 84–88.

Kühne, M., Riballo, E., Rief, N., Rothkamm, K., Jeggo, P. A. & Löbrich, M. (2004). A double-strand break repair defect in ATM-deficient cells contributes to radiosensitivity. *Cancer Res., 64*, 500–508.

Kurz, E. U. & Lees-Miller, S. P. (2004). DNA damage-induced activation of ATM and ATM-dependent signaling pathways. *DNA Repair, 3*, 889–900.

Lahav, G., Rosenfeld, N., Sigal, A., Geva-Zatorsky, N., Levine, A. J., Elowitz, M. B. & Alon, U. (2008). Dynamics of the p53-Mdm2 feedback loop in individual cells. *Nat. Genet., 36*, 147–150.

Lane, D. P. (2004). p53 from pathway to therapy. *Carcinogenesis, 25*, 1077–1081.

Lau, W. M., Ho, T. H. & Hui, K. M. (2007). p16[INK4A]-silencing augments DNA damage-induced apoptosis in cervical cancer cells. *Oncogene, 26*, 6050–6060.

Lavin, M. F. (2008). Ataxia-telangiectasia: from a rare disorder to a paradigm for cell signalling and cancer. *Nat. Rev. Mol. Cell Biol. 9*, 759–769.

Lavin, M. F. & Khanna, K. K. (1999). ATM: the protein encoded by the gene mutated in the radiosensitive syndrome ataxia-telangiectasia. *Int. J. Radiat. Biol., 75*, 1201–1214.

Lavin, M. F., Gueven, N., Bottle, S. & Gatti, R. A. (2007). Current and potential therapeutic strategies for the treatment of ataxia-telangiectasia. *Br. Med. Bull., 81–82*, 129–147.

Le, H. V., Minn, A. J. & Massague, J. (2005). Cyclin-dependent kinase inhibitors uncouple cell cycle progression from mitochondrial apoptotic functions in DNA-damaged cancer cells. *J. Biol. Chem., 280*, 32018-32025.

Li, C. Y., Suardet, L. & Little, J. B. (1995). Potential role of WAF1/Cip1/p21 as a mediator of TGF-beta cytoinhibitory effect. *J. Biol. Chem., 270*, 4971–4974.

Li, M., Luo, J., Brooks, C. L. & Gu, W. (2002). Acetylation of p53 inhibits its ubiquitination by Mdm2. *J. Biol. Chem., 277*, 50607–50611.

Li, Q., Zhao, L. Y., Zheng, Z., Yang, H., Santiago, A. & Liao, D. (2011). Inhibition of p53 by adenovirus type 12 E1B-55K deregulates cell cycle control and sensitizes tumor cells to genotoxic agents. *J. Virol., 85*, 7976–7988.

Liu, M., Iavarone, A. & Freedman, L. P. (1996). Transcriptional activation of the human p21(WAF1/CIP1) gene by retinoic acid receptor. Correlation with retinoid induction of U937 cell differentiation. *J. Biol, Chem., 271*, 31723–31728.

Liu, J., Song, Y., Qian, J., Liu, B., Dong, Y., Tian, B. & Sun, Z. (2011). Promyelocytic leukemia protein interacts with werner syndrome helicase and regulates double-strand break repair in γ-irradiation-induced DNA damage responses. *Biochemistrey (Mosc.), 76*, 550–554.

Ljungman, M. (2000). Dial 9-1-1 for p53: Mechanisms of p53 activation by cellular stress. *Neoplasia, 2,* 208–225.

Mansilla, S., Bataller, M. & Portugal, J. (2009). A nuclear budding mechanism in transiently arrested cells generates drug-sensitive and drug-resistant cells. *Biochem. Pharmacol., 78,* 123–132.

McConnell, B. B., Starborg, M., Brookes, S. & Peters, G. (1998). Inhibitors of cyclin-dependent kinases induce features of replicative senescence in early passage human diploid fibroblasts. *Curr. Biol., 8,* 351–354.

Meek, D. W. (2004). The p53 response to DNA damage. *DNA Repair, 3,* 1049–1056.

Meulmeester, E., Pereg, Y., Shiloh, Y. & Jochemsen, A. G. (2005). ATM-Mediated Phosphorylations Inhibit Mdmx/Mdm2 Stabilization by HAUSP in Favor of p53 Activation. *Cell Cycle, 4,* 1166–1170.

Meyn, M. S. (1995). Ataxia-telangiectasia and cellular response to DNA damage. *Cancer Res., 55,* 5991–6001.

Michael, D. & Oren, M. (2003). The p53-Mdm2 module and the ubiquitin system. *Semin. Cancer Biol., 13,* 49–58.

Mirzayans, R. & Murray, D. (1997). Cellular senescence: Implications for cancer therapy. In: Garvey RB Ed. *New Research on Cell Aging.* Hauppauge, NY, Nova Science Publishers, Inc.; pp. 1–64.

Mirzayans, R. & Paterson, M. C. (1991). Lack of correlation between hypersensitivity to cell killing and impaired inhibition of DNA synthesis in ataxia telangiectasia fibroblasts treated with 4-nitroquinoline 1-oxide. *Carcinogenesis, 12,* 19–24.

Mirzayans, R. & Paterson, M. C. (2001). Correction of radioresistant DNA synthesis in ataxia telangiectasia fibroblasts by prostaglandin E_2 treatment. *Environ. Mol. Mutagen., 38,* 191–199.

Mirzayans, R., Sabour, M. & Paterson, M. C. (1988). Enhanced bioreduction of 4-mtroquinoline 1-oxide by cultured ataxia telangiectasia cells. *Carcinogenesis, 9,* 1711–1715.

Mirzayans, R., Smith, B. P. & Paterson, M. C. (1989). Hypersensitivity to cell killing and faulty repair of 1-β-D-arabinofuranosylcytosine-detectable sites in human (ataxia-telangiectasia) fibroblasts treated with 4-nitroquinoline 1-oxide. *Cancer Res., 49,* 5523–5529.

Mirzayans, R., Famulski, K., Enns, L., Fraser, M. & Paterson, M. C. (1995). Characterization of the signal transduction pathway mediating γ ray-induced inhibition of DNA synthesis in human cells: indirect evidence for involvement of calmodulin but not protein kinase C nor p53. *Oncogene, 11,* 1597–1605.

Mirzayans, R., Enns, L., Dietrich, K., Barley, R. D. & Paterson, M. C. (1996). Faulty DNA polymerase δ/ε-mediated excision repair in response to γ radiation or ultraviolet light in p53-deficient fibroblast strains from affected members of a cancer-prone family with Li-Fraumeni syndrome. *Carcinogenesis, 17,* 691–698.

Mirzayans, R., Enns, L. & Paterson, M. C. (1997). Inhibition of DNA synthesis and G_1/S transition in normal human fibroblast cultures elicited by a heat-labile trans-acting factor in γ-irradiated HeLa cell extracts. *Radiat. Res., 147,* 13–21.

Mirzayans, R., Scott, A., Cameron, M. & Murray, D. (2005). Induction of accelerated senescence following exposure to ionizing radiation in human solid tumor-derived cell lines expressing wild-type *TP53*. *Radiat. Res., 163*, 53–62.

Mirzayans, R., Severin, D. & Murray, D. (2006). Relationship between DNA double strand break rejoining and cell survival following exposure to ionizing radiation in human fibroblast strains with differing ATM/p53 function: implications for the evaluation of clinical radiosensitivity. *Int. J. Radiat. Oncol. Biol. Phys., 66*, 1498–1505.

Mirzayans, R., Scott, A., Andrais, B., Pollock, S. & Murray, D. (2008). Ultraviolet light exposure triggers nuclear accumulation of $p21^{WAF1}$ and accelerated senescence in human normal and nucleotide excision repair-deficient fibroblast strains. *J. Cell. Physiol., 215*, 55–67.

Mirzayans, R., Andrais, B., Scott, A., Paterson, M. C. & Murray, D. (2010). Single-cell analysis of $p16^{INK4a}$ and $p21^{WAF1}$ expression suggests distinct mechanisms of senescence in normal human and Li-Fraumeni Syndrome fibroblasts. *J. Cell. Physiol., 223*, 57–67.

Morris, M., Hepburn, P. & Wynford-Thomas, D. (2002). Sequential extension of proliferative lifespan in human fibroblasts induced by over-expression of CDK4 or 6 and loss of p53 function. *Oncogene, 21*, 4277–4288.

Munro, J., Steeghs, K., Morrison, V., Ireland, H. & Parkinson, E. K. (2001). Human fibroblast replicative senescence can occur in the absence of extensive cell division and short telomeres. *Oncogene, 20*, 3541–3552.

Murray, D. & Mirzayans, R. (2007). Role of p53 in the repair of ionizing radiation-induced DNA damage. In: Landseer BR Ed. *New Research on DNA Repair*. Hauppauge, NY, Nova Science Publishers, Inc.; pp. 325–373.

Myers, J. S. & Cortez, D. (2006). Rapid activation of ATR by ionizing radiation requires ATM and Mre11. *J. Biol. Chem., 281*, 9346–9350.

Noda, A., Ning, Y., Venable, S. F., Pereira-Smith, O. M. & Smith, J. R. (1994). Cloning of senescent cell-derived inhibitors of DNA synthesis using an expression screen. *Exp. Cell Res., 211*, 90–98.

Pang, L. Y., Scott, M., Hayward, R. L., Mohammed, H., Whitelaw, C. B., Smith, G. C. & Hupp, T. R. (2011). $p21^{WAF1}$ is component of a positive feedback loop that maintains the p53 transcriptional program. *Cell cycle, 10*, 932–950.

Paterson, M. C. & Mirzayans, R. (1993). Correction of post-γ ray DNA repair deficiency in ataxia-telangiectasia complementation group A fibroblasts by cocultivation with normal fibroblasts. In: R. A. Gatti, & R. B. Painter (Eds.), *Ataxia-Telangiectasia: NATO ASI series*. Berlin, Springer-Verlag. Vol 77, pp. 117–126.

Paterson, M. C. & Mirzayans, R. (1999). *Methods and compositions for the treatment of ataxia telangiectasia.* US Patent Serial No. 5,990,168.

Paterson, M. C. & Smith, P. J. (1979). Ataxia telangiectasia: an inherited human disorder involving hypersensitivity to ionizing radiation and related DNA-damaging chemicals. *Annu. Rev. Genet., 13*, 291–318.

Paterson, M. C., Smith, B. P., Lohman, P. H. M., Anderson, A. K. & Fishman, L. (1976). Defective excision repair of γ-ray-damaged DNA in human (ataxia telangiectasia) fibroblasts. *Nature, 260*, 444–447.

Pichierri, P., Ammazzalorso, F., Bignami, M. & Franchitto, A. (2011). The Werner syndrome protein: linking the replication checkpoint response to genome stability. *Aging (Albany NY), 3,* 311–318.

Pomerantz, J., Schreiber-Agus, N., Liegeois, N. J., Silverman, A., Alland, L., Chin, L., Potes, J., Chen, K., Orlow, I., Lee, H. W., Cordon-Cardo. C. & DePinho, R. A. (1998). The *Ink4a* tumor suppressor gene product, p19[Arf], interacts with MDM2 and neutralizes MDM2's inhibition of p53. *Cell, 92,* 713–723.

Orre, L. M., Stenerlow, B., Dhar, S., Larsson, R., Lewensohn, R. & Lehtio, J. (2006). p53 is involved in clearance of ionizing radiation-induced RAD51 foci in a human colon cancer cell line. *Biochem. Biophys. Res. Commun., 342,* 1211–1217.

Rajaraman, R., Guernsey, D. L., Rajaraman, M. M. & Rajaraman, S. R. (2006). Stem cells, senescence, neosis and self-renewal in cancer. *Cancer Cell Int., 6,* 25.

Ramirez, R. D., Morales, C. P., Herbert, B. S., Rohde, J. M., Passons, C., Shay, J. W. & Wright, W. E. (2001). Putative telomere-independent mechanisms of replicative aging reflect inadequate growth conditions. *Genes Dev., 15,* 398–403.

Reliene, R. & Schiestl, R. H. (2008). Experimental antioxidant therapy is ataxia telangiectasia. *Clin. Med. Oncol., 2,* 431–436.

Roninson, I. B. (2003). Tumor cell senescence in cancer treatment. *Cancer Res., 63,* 2705–2715.

Roninson, I. B., Broude, E. V. & Chang, B. D. (2001). If not apoptosis, then what? Treatment-induced senescence and mitotic catastrophe in tumor cells. *Drug Resist. Updates, 4,* 303–313.

Rotman, G. & Shiloh, Y. (1999). ATM: a mediator of multiple responses to genotoxic stress. *Oncogene, 18,* 6135–6144.

Rousseau, D., Cannella, D., Boulaire, J., Fitzgerald, P., Fotedar, A. & Fotedar, R. (1999) Growth inhibition by CDK-cyclin and PCNA binding domains of p21 occurs by distinct mechanisms and is regulated by ubiquitin-proteasome pathway. *Oncogene, 18,* 4313–4325.

Ruaro, E. M., Collavin, L., Sal, G. D., Haffner, R., Oren, M., Levine, A. J. & Schneider, C. (1997). A proline-rich motif in p53 is required for transactivation-independent growth arrest as induced by Gas1. *Proc. Natl. Acad. Sci. USA, 94,* 4675–4680.

Satinover, D. L., Leach, C. A., Stukenberg, P. T. & Brautigan, D. L. (2004). Activation of Aurora-A kinase by protein phosphatase inhibitor-2, a bifunctional signaling protein. *Proc. Natl. Acad. Sci. USA, 101,* 8625–8630.

Sedelnikova, O. A., Horikawa, I., Zimonjic, D. B., Popescu, N. C., Bonner, W. M. & Barrett J. C. (2004). Senescing human cells and ageing mice accumulate DNA lesions with unrepairable double-strand breaks. *Nat. Cell Biol., 6,* 168–170.

Sengupta, S. & Harris, C. C. (2005). p53: traffic cop at the crossroads of DNA repair and recombination. *Nat. Rev. Mol. Cell Biol., 6,* 44–55.

Shay, J. W. (1999). At the end of the millennium, a view of the end. *Nat. Genet., 23,* 382-383.

Shay, J. W. & Roninson, I. B. (2004). Hallmarks of senescence in carcinogenesis and cancer therapy. *Oncogene, 23,* 2929–2933.

Sherr, C. J. & Roberts, J. M. (1999). CDK inhibitors: positive and negative regulators of G1-phase progression. *Genes Dev., 13,* 1501–1512.

Shiloh, Y. (2003). ATM and related protein kinases: safeguarding genome integrity. *Nat. Rev. Cancer, 3,* 155–168.

Sliwinska, M. A., Mosieniak, G., Wolanin, K., Babik, A., Piwocka, K., Magalska, A., Szczepanowska, J., Fronk, J. & Sikora, E. (2009). Induction of senescence with doxorubicin leads to increased genomic instability of HCT116 cells. Mech. *Ageing Dev., 130*, 24–32.

Sohn, D., Essmann, F., Schulze-Osthoff, K. & Jänicke, R. U. (2006). p21 blocks irradiation-induced apoptosis downstream of mitochondria by inhibition of cyclin-dependent kinase-mediated caspase-9 activation. *Cancer Res., 66*, 11254–11262.

Stein, G. H., Drullinger, L. F., Soulard, A. & Dulic, V. (1999). Differential roles for cyclin-dependent kinase inhibitors p21 and p16 in the mechanisms of senescence and differentiation in human fibroblasts. *Mol. Cell Biol., 19*, 2109–2117.

Sturzbecher, H. W., Donzelmann, B., Henning, W., Knippschild, U. & Buchhop, S. (1996). p53 is linked directly to homologous recombination processes via RAD51/RecA protein interaction. *EMBO J., 15*, 1992–2002.

Suzuki, A., Tsutomi, Y., Yamamoto, N., Shibutani, T. & Akahane, K. (1999). Mitochondrial regulation of cell death: mitochondria are essential for procaspase 3-p21 complex formation to resist Fas-mediated cell death. *Mol. Cell. Biol., 19*, 3842–3847.

Tang, X., Hui, Z. G., Cui, X. L., Garg, R., Kastan, M. B. & Xu. B. (2008). A novel ATM-dependent pathway regulates protein phosphatase 1 in response to DNA damage. *Mol. Cell. Biol., 28*, 2559–2566.

Tasdemir, E., Maiuri, M. C., Galluzzi, L., Vitale, I., Djavaheri-Mergny, M., D'Amelio, M., Criollo, A., Morselli, E., Zhu, C., Harper, F., Nannmark, U., Samara, C., Pinton, P., Vicencio, J. M., Carnuccio, R., Moll, U. M., Madeo, F., Paterlini-Brechot, P., Rizzuto, R., Szabadkai, G., Pierron, G., Blomgren, K., Tavernarakis, N., Codogno, P., Cecconi, F. & Kroemer, G. (2008). Regulation of autophagy by cytoplasmic p53. *Nat. cell Biol., 10*, 676–687.

Tian, H., Wittmack, E. K. & Jorgensen, T. J. (2000). p21[WAF1/CIP1] antisense therapy radiosensitizes human colon cancer by converting growth arrest to apoptosis. *Cancer Res., 60*, 679–684.

Vakifahmetoglu, H., Olsson, M. & Zhivotovsky, B. (2008). Death through a tragedy: mitotic catastrophe. *Cell Death Differ., 15*, 1153–1162.

Warner, S. L., Bearss, D. J., Han, H. & Von Hoff, D. D. (2003). Targeting Aurora-2 kinase in cancer. *Mol. Cancer Ther., 2*, 589–595.

Wei, W., Herbig, U., Wei, S., Dutriaux, A. & Sedivy, J. M. (2003). Loss of retinoblastoma but not p16 function allows bypass of replicative senescence in human fibroblasts. *EMBO Rep., 4*, 1061–1066.

Wong, K. K., Maser, R. S., Bachoo, R. M., Menon, J., Carrasco, D. R., Gu, Y., Alt, F. W. & DePinho, R. A. (2003). Telomere dysfunction and Atm deficiency compromises organ homeostasis and accelerates ageing. *Nature, 421*, 643–648.

Wood, L. D., Halvorsen, T. L., Dhar, S., Baur, J. A., Pandita, R. K., Wright, W. E., Hande, M. P., Calaf, G., Hei, T. K., Levine, F., Shay, J. W., Wang, J. J. & Pandita, T. K. (2001). Characterization of ataxia telangiectasia fibroblasts with extended life-span through telomerase expression. *Oncogene, 20*, 278–288.

Wouters, B. G., Giaccia, A. J., Denko, N. C. & Brown, J. M. (1997). Loss of p21[Waf1/Cip1] sensitizes tumors to radiation by an apoptosis-independent mechanism. *Cancer Res., 57*, 4703–4706.

Xiong, Y., Hannon, G. J., Zhang, H., Casso, D., Kobayashi, R. & Beach, D. (1993a). p21 is a universal inhibitor of cyclin kinases. *Nature, 366*, 701–704.

Xiong, Y., Zhang, H. & Beach, D. (1993b). Subunit rearrangement of the cyclin-dependent kinases is associated with cellular transformation. *Genes Dev., 7*, 1572–1583.

Xu, H. J., Zhou, Y., Ji, W., Perng, G. S., Kruzelock, R., Kong, C. T., Bast, R. C., Mills, G. B., Li, J. & Hu, S. X. (1997). Reexpression of the retinoblastoma protein in tumor cells induces senescence and telomerase inhibition. *Oncogene, 15*, 2589–2596.

Yang, W. L., Zeng, Y. X., El Deiry, W. S., Nason-Burchenal, K., Dmitrovsky, E. & Chin, K. V. (1999). Transcriptional activation of the cyclin-dependent kinase inhibitor p21 by PML/RARalpha. *Mol. Cell Biol. Res. Commun., 1*, 125–131.

Zgheib, O., Huyen, Y., DiTullio, R. A. Jr., Snyder, A., Venere, M., Stavridi, E. S. & Halazonetis, T. D. (2005). ATM signaling and 53BP1. *Radiother. Oncol., 76*, 119–122.

Zhang, H. (2007). Molecular signaling and genetic pathways of senescence: its role in tumorigenesis and aging. *J. Cell Physiol., 210*, 567–574.

Zhang, Y., Xiong, Y. & Yarbrough, W. G. (1998). ARF promotes MDM2 degradation and stabilizes p53: *ARF-INK4a* locus deletion impairs both the Rb and p53 tumor suppression pathways. *Cell, 92*, 725–734.

Zhang, X. P., Liu, F. & Wang, W. (2011). Two-phase dynamics of p53 in the DNA damage response. *Proc. Natl. Acad. Sci. USA, 108*, 8990–8995.

Zhou, B. P. & Hung, M. C. (2002). Novel targets of Akt, p21Cip1/WAF1, and MDM2. *Semin. Oncol. 29*, 2–70.

Chapter 2

ATAXIA TELANGIECTASIA: MOLECULAR BASIS, DIAGNOSIS AND TREATMENT

T. Broccoletti, G. Aloj, G. Giardino and C. Pignata[*]
Department of Pediatrics, "Federico II" University, Naples, Italy

ABSTRACT

Ataxia-telangiectasia (A-T) is a rare autosomal recessive disorder associated with mutations in the ATM gene. ATM plays a central role in regulating the signal-transduction pathway activated in response to DNA double-strand breaks and is involved in the control of the intracellular redox status homeostasis. The hallmarks of the disease are related to the progressive neurological dysfunction, especially affecting the cerebellum and resulting in uncoordinated and ataxic movements associated to a deterioration of gross and fine motor skills. The onset of neurological signs is usually by approximately 2-4 years of age. The overall phenotype consists of oculo-cutaneous teleangiectasia, immunodeficiency, high incidence of neoplasms and hypersensitivity to ionising radiations. The neurodegeneration is progressive and greatly impairs the quality of life, invariably leading to confinement of patients to wheelchair. The cerebellar damage is associated to dystrophic changes of dendrites and axons of Purkinje cells. Death usually occurs by the 3rd decade of life for pulmonary infections or neoplasms. Currently, there is no effective treatment for A-T, but only supportive care aimed to halt progressive neurodegenerative changes. Many attempts to relief the neurological symptoms have so far been made: antioxidants were promising, but only modest improvement has been observed. Aminoglycosides have been proposed for the correction of ATM gene function by read-through of premature termination codons, while further attempts have been made with antisense morpholino oligonucleotides to redirect and restore normal splicing. Some encouraging results on neurological symptoms have been obtained with short courses of oral betamethasone, even though the beneficial effect is drug-dependent. Aim of this chapter is to report on the molecular basis, clinical features

---

[*]Correspondence: Claudio Pignata, M.D., Ph.D., Professor of Pediatrics, Department of Pediatrics, Unit of Immunology, "Federico II" University, via S. Pansini 5-80131, Naples, Italy, Tel.: +39-081-7464340; Fax: +39-081-5451278, E-mail address: pignata@unina.it

and diagnostic process of A-T paying a special attention to the therapeutic approach so far described in the attempt to halt progressive degeneration.

INTRODUCTION

Ataxia-telangiectasia (A-T) is a rare autosomal recessive multisystem disorder characterized by progressive neurological dysfunction, especially in the cerebellum, with motor impairments secondary to a neurodegenerative process, oculo-cutaneous telangiectasia, immunodeficiency, high incidence of neoplasms and hypersensitivity to ionising radiations [1, 2]. The disease is caused by mutations of the ataxia telangiectasia mutate (ATM) gene, localized on chromosome 11q22-23, a member of a family of phosphatidylinositol-3-kinase (PI3K)-related genes involved in cellular response to DNA damage and cell cycle control through checkpoints. Thus, the disease is considered the prototype of the DNA-repair defect syndromes [3]. The prevalence of A-T in the US is 1: 40.0000-1:100.000 live births. Over the past 20 years, the expected life span of A-T patients has increased considerably. Median survival of patients with A-T remains actually 19-25 years with a wide range but most affected individuals now live beyond age 25-30 years [4, 5]. Of note, as for some other neurodegenerative diseases, life expectancy does not well correlate with the severity of neurological impairment [5]. On the contrary the quality of life is dramatically dependent on the neurological deterioration [6]. The progressive neurodegeneration and subsequent pulmonary failure with or without identifiable pneumonia are a frequent cause of death in patients with A-T. Immunodeficiency is variable and usually affects both humoral and cellular responses. However, severe infections are uncommon in A-T [7]. A-T shows progressive neuronal degeneration due to loss of Purkinje cells in the cerebellum. Purkinje cells are thought to be selectively depleted, then resulting in the progressive cerebellar atrophy of the cortex associated with significant thinning of the molecular layer, as revealed by autopsy and biopsy studies [8, 9]. Figure 1 illustrates an exemplificative Magnetic resonance imaging (MRI) examination showing diffuse atrophy of vermis and cerebellar hemispheres.

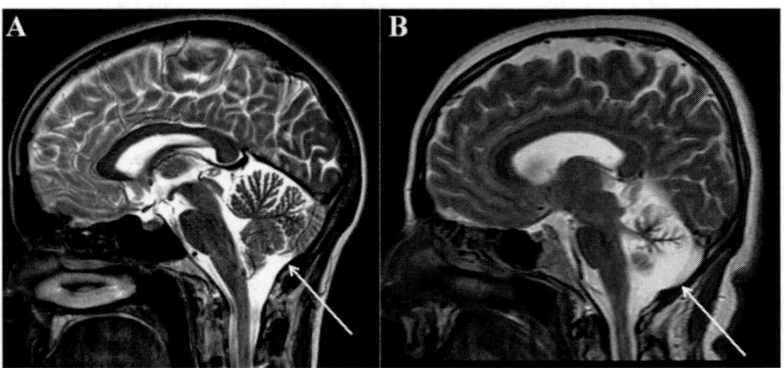

Figure 1. Brain structural MRI in an A-T patient and a control (T2-weighed sagittal section). (A) The arrow indicates a normal cerebellum in an unaffected subject; (B) The arrow indicates severe cerebellar and vermian atrophy in an A-T patient.

CLINICAL FEATURES OF A-T

Neurological Phenotype and Cutaneous Manifestations

The main neurological features of A-T are: i) cerebellar symptoms as ataxia, seating, head (head tilting) and postural instability, essential tremor, dysmetria, dysarthria, adiadochokinesia, slurred speech; ii) extrapyramidal symptoms as choreiform movements of hands and feet, multifocal and chaotic myoclonus, tics; iii) other symptoms as oculomotor apraxia, crewing and swallowing difficulty, drooling, hypomimea, axonal polyneuropathy with decreased or absent deep tendon reflex (Table 1) [8, 10]. A-T is a multisystem disease but is stereotyped by its neurological symptoms. A-T individuals have normal mental skills and IQ tests are normal [11-13].

Table 1. A-T clinical features

Involved district	Clinical Features
Neurologic system	**Cerebellar symptoms** Ataxia Seating, head (head tilting) and postural instability Essential tremor Dysmetria Dysarthria **Adiadochokinesia** Slurred speech Extrapyramidal symptoms Choreiform movements of hands and feet Multifocal and chaotic myoclonus Tics Other symptoms Oculomotor apraxia Crewing and swallowing difficulty Drooling Hypomimea Axonal polyneuropathy with decreased or absent deep tendon reflex Ocular signs Oculomotor apraxia Deficient accommodation Impaired smooth pursuit Hypometric saccades Nystagmus Absence of optokinetic nystagmus Frequent blinking Photophobia
Immune system	Humoral defects Cellular defects
Other features	Predisposition to cancer especially leukemia and lymphoma Radiosensitivity **Telangiectasias** Pulmonary manifestations Elevated aFP

The neurological phenotype of A-T is dramatically conditioned by the cerebellar gait and truncal ataxia with onset between age one and four years, associated with deterioration of gross and fine motor skills occurring by approximately four years of age. The cerebellar ataxia is the clinical hallmark of the syndrome, invariably present in all cases, progressive and spreading to affect the extremities and then the speech as well as peripheral coordination. Eventually, most of the affected children are confined to a wheelchair by age of ten [14].

Ocular abnormalities are an early and progressive feature of A-T and include oculomotor apraxia, deficient accommodation, impaired smooth pursuit, hypometric saccades, nystagmus, absence of optokinetic nystagmus, frequent blinking and photophobia (Table 1) [15]. Oculomotor apraxia associated to slurred speech often leads to impassive facies. This feature may be misdiagnosed as cerebral palsy or mental retardation. Oculomotor apraxia is the main sign helpful in the early recognition of the patients [16]. When children try to fix an object, the head is turned rapidly toward the object. Thereafter, while maintaining fixation, the head is moved back to the target. The head-turning technique, by using the vestibulo-ocular reflex, allows the patient to compensate for the difficulty in initiating voluntary refixation eye movements (saccades) [15]. No alterations of visual acuity, pupillary response and funduscopic examination are usually seen. Reading difficulties are often observed in patients with A-T due to abnormalities of accommodation and eye movements [12]. However, these alterations are quite variable.

In addition, a peripheral axonal neuropathy may be found and leads to decreased deep tendon reflexes [8].

The second major clinical manifestation of A-T is represented by telangiectasias (dilated blood vessels), occurring later between two and eight years of age. They appear predominantly in the eye's sclerae (ocular telangiectasia), the skin of face, neck, antecubital, or popliteal fossae and ears (cutaneous telangiectasia). Occasionally, they appear on the dorsum of the hands and feet. On the conjunctiva, a "bloodshot" appearance is usual, leading to fine, bright, red streaks. In a few cases, the dermatological features, including hypo/hyperpigmentation may be evident later in life up to the second decade. Further cutaneous manifestations include cutaneous atrophy, partial albinism and premature graying of hair. Follicular keratosis, dry skin and scleroderma-like lesions may also be observed in these patients [17]. Cutaneous granulomatosis has also been recently described in children with A-T [18].

Immunodeficiency and Pulmonary Complications

A variable immunodeficiency, affecting the humoral and cellular systems (Table 1), has been long documented in patients with A-T. Immune defects are present in 60 to 80% of patients with A-T. The immunodeficiency is not progressive, variable and does not correlate well with the frequency, severity or spectrum of infections [7, 19, 20].

The most common humoral defects are low or even absent IgA, IgE, and IgG2 serum levels, inconstantly associated with impaired antibody responses to vaccines. The most common defects of the cell-mediated branch are low CD4 counts resulting in reversed CD4/CD8 ratio and impaired lymphoproliferative responses to common mitogens and antigens [7]. Lymphopenia is frequently present. Moreover, at autopsy, all individuals have a small not fully developed thymus [10, 21]. A defect in recombination or DNA rearrangement may explain the defects in both T and B cell differentiation. However, unlike most immunodeficiency disorders, severe infections are uncommon in A-T and the spectrum of infections in individuals with A-T does not comprise opportunistic infections but predisposition to sinopulmonary infections [22]. Some individuals develop chronic bronchiectasis and the frequency and severity of infections correlates more with general nutritional status than with the immune status [10].

Morbidity and mortality in these patients are related to pulmonary manifestations, as recurrent sinopulmonary disease and bronchiectasis, interstitial lung disease and pulmonary fibrosis [23]. Unfortunately, so far the evaluation of the severity of the lung involvement does not rely on specific guidelines that would help manage such patients. Treatment with bronchodilators and steroids may be required [24]. Individuals with frequent and severe infections appear to benefit from intravenous immunoglobulin (IVIG) replacement therapy; however, longevity has increased substantially even in individuals not receiving IVIG [7, 10].

The impaired coordination of swallowing, the increased risk of aspiration, the reduced respiratory capacity and the propensity to infections make the anesthesia risky for these patients [25].

Given the severity of laboratory impairment of cell-mediated and humoral immunity, the fact that only a minority of patients have an increased susceptibility to severe clinical manifestations of infectious diseases is quite surprising. This discordance still remains unexplained [7]. A defect in a DNA processing with persistence of some double-strand breaks (DSBs) would best explain the immunodeficiency and the lymphoid malignancies seen in A-T.

Predisposition to Cancer and Chromosomal Instability

A-T patients have a risk of cancer more than 100 times that of controls [26, 27]. The prevalence of cancer in A-T is 10-30%, representing the second cause of death [28, 29]. Leukemia and lymphoma account for about 85% of malignancies [28]. Most leukemias are of T-cell origin, while lymphomas are usually of B-cell type. Other solid tumors including ovarian cancer, breast cancer, gastric cancer, melanoma and gonadic cancer have been described. The predisposition to develop tumors is best explained by genome instability due to altered repair of double-strand breaks [30]. An increased risk of cancer, particularly of breast cancer, has also been described among A-T heterozygotes [31-34].

Patients with A-T also show an increased sensitivity to ionizing radiations. In vitro, radiosensitivity is expressed as reduced colony forming ability (CFA) following exposure to ionizing radiations or radiomimetic chemicals [20, 35]. Because of this increased sensitivity conventional doses are dangerous in individuals with A-T and the use of radiotherapy and some radiomimetic chemotherapeutic agents should be monitored carefully. Sometimes, the doses of these chemotherapeutic agents must be reduced by 25%-50% to prevent side effects, which may also be lethal. It now seems clear that there is also an increased susceptibility for early death in heterozygote carriers of the ATM gene mutations (about 1% of the population). In a careful analysis, heterozygote carriers had an increased mortality rate from the second to the eighth decade, with a progression with the age, mainly due to cancer, particularly breast cancer, or ischemic heart disease. On average, carriers died seven to eight years earlier than non carriers [36-38].

Endocrine Dysfunction

The most common endocrine manifestations are: growth failure, hypogonadism and insulin-resistant diabetes mellitus [39].

PATHOGENESIS AND MOLECULAR DEFECT

The disease is associated with mutations in the ATM gene encoding for a serine/threonine kinase, which shares sequence similarities with the catalytic subunit of phosphatidyl-inositol-3-kinase. The ATM gene is large, spanning 150 kb of genomic DNA and encoding a ubiquitously expressed transcript of approximately 13 kb, consisting of 66 exons, giving a 350 kDa protein of 3056 amino acids. The classic form of the disease is associated to two truncating ATM mutations, leading to total loss of function of the protein. Milder forms of the disease are associated with leaky splice site mutation or to the presence of missense mutations, which allow some expression of the protein exerting residual kinase activity [40].

A-T is considered the prototype of the DNA-repair defect syndromes. In fact, ATM represents the central component of the signal-transduction pathway responding to DNA double-strand breaks (DSBs) caused by ionizing radiations (IR), endogenous and exogenous DNA damage agents [41, 42]. In response to DSB formation, ATM, several DNA-repair and cell cycle checkpoint proteins are activated, leading to cell cycle arrest and DNA repair [43-45]. The activation of ATM kinase involves autophosphorylation of serine 1981 of the protein and subsequent dissociation of inactive ATM dimers into active monomers [46]. Chromosomal DSBs are potentially one of the most dangerous forms of DNA damage that, if left unrepaired, can result in chromosomal aberrations, deletions, or translocations. Such abnormal process could also account for the high incidence of chromosomal rearrangements involving primarily the chromosomes 7 and 14 [47, 48], corresponding to the sites of the immune system genes [49]. Defects in DSBs repair are linked to cell death and tumorigenesis [50].

ATM is also involved in immune cell maturation, which requires gene rearrangements and therefore leads to DSBs [51, 52]. However, ATM deficiency does not result in a profound block in lymphocyte development. Differently, VDJ recombination may be affected. In B cells, this altered process leads to a defect in class switch recombination (CSR) from IgM to other classes, demonstrating the central role of ATM in class switching [53].

The pleiotropic clinical manifestations of the syndrome are all related to the critical roles of ATM for the cellular response to DNA double-strand breaks (DSBs) in different tissues [54].

ATM and Neurodegeneration

A-T provides a well-characterized example of the relationships between repair defects and neurodegenerative disease. In the nervous system defective DNA repair leads to neurodegeneration. Several mechanisms by which deficient DNA repair in neurons triggers their apoptosis have been proposed. Neurons among our myriad of cells types exert unique properties. They are terminally differentiated, are post-mitotic cells and they are also extremely active. Since they are irreplaceable and should survive as long as the organism does, they need to elaborate stringent defense mechanisms to ensure their longevity [55]. The post-mitotic status of differentiated neurons may make them more vulnerable to DNA damage than cells in the active proliferation status. Genetic deficiencies in enzymes involved in the DNA repair process can induce neuronal apoptosis or make neurons more sensitive to further genotoxic stresses. Even though the progressive neurodegeneration is a common hallmark of many progressive neurologic syndromes, all sharing a defective DSBs responses in their pathogenesis, the disease-specific differences in the onset and course of neurodegeneration likely reflect selective DNA repair requirements in the different areas of the nervous system [55, 56]. There are two major DNA repair pathways for the DSBs damages. Homologous recombination repair (HR) is an important process mainly during early embryogenesis; where proliferation is at its maximal expression leading to the development of stem cells and progenitors. This complex machinery requires genomic integrity. Non-homologous end-joining (NHEJ) recombination repair is active mainly in the brain. In the mature nervous system, a different pathway repairs DNA single-strand breaks (SSBs) [57, 58]. In the nervous system, ATM signaling appears to function predominantly in immature and post-mitotic neural cells, suggesting that ATM responds to DNA DSB utilizing NHEJ. In the absence of ATM, neurons survive and populate the Purkinje neuron layer and only later they degenerate as a result of DNA damage experienced during development. This would explain the reason by which ATM is an important signaling molecule only in a selective region of the nervous system [59]. Knocking out ATM does not interfere with neuronal differentiation, but it abolishes the ATM-mediated response to DNA damage [59].

Neither the normal function of ATM in the nervous system nor the biological basis of the degeneration in A-T is known. The pathological features of A-T are predominated by the selective Purkinje cell depletion and granule neurons with partial thinning of the granule cell layer. Progressive atrophy of the cerebellar cortex is a hallmark of A-T, characterized by the appearance of abnormal Purkinje cells in the molecular layer of the cerebellum with abnormal smooth dendrites, reduced arborizations and finally, ectopic cells [60, 61].

Although ATM is known to be neuroprotective in the tissue undergoing oxidative stress and apoptosis, the molecular mechanisms of its function in the nervous system are uncertain. ATM dependent apoptosis may be important for the elimination of neural cells that have accumulated genomic damage [62]. Experimental evidence in ATM-/- mice indicates that these mice lose the ability to induce apoptosis in differentiating neuronal cells, but not in proliferating neuroblasts, in response to DNA damage [63, 64].

ATM and Oxidative Stress

In neurons oxidative stress is associated to the intensive metabolic activity. In various neurodegenerative disorders a deregulated oxidative stress has been frequently described [65-68].

Oxidative stress has been long considered a causative factor in genomic instability in the brain.

Moreover, oxidative stress contributes to accumulation of DNA damage favoring the neurodegeneration in A-T. During neurogenesis, increased endogenous production of reactive oxygen species, not counteracted by protective repair systems, leads to DNA damage, resulting in cell apoptosis. Neurodegeneration probably results from altered cell homeostasis subsequent to the loss of these cells from the differentiating brain tissue. ATM is certainly involved in sensing and modulating intracellular redox status, even though it is not clear whether ATM itself is directly involved in reactive oxygen species (ROS) production [69, 70]. There is also evidence supporting that ATM deficiency leads to increased oxidative stress production within the cerebellum [70-72]. These data would suggest that ATM kinase activity is required to counteract the progressive accumulation of oxidative DNA lesions.

DIAGNOSIS AND TREATMENT

Diagnosis of A-T relies on clinical phenotype, family history and is usually supported by laboratory findings that include: i) elevated serum α-phetoprotein (AFP); ii) immunological deficiencies; iii) cerebellar atrophy at MRI (Figure 1); iv) chromosome analysis (7;14 translocation) on lymphocytes of peripheral blood; v) in vitro radiosensitivity assay; vi) absent or markedly decreased intracellular ATM protein levels by Western Blotting; vii) deficient phosphorylation of ATM substrates through ATM serine/threonine kinase activity. Finally, the diagnosis of A-T is confirmed by molecular genetic analysis of ATM gene [1, 73].

Unfortunately, there is currently no treatment for A-T except for supportive therapy of secondary symptoms. The treatment of A-T remains based both in medical management of immunodeficiency, sinopulmonary infections, neurologic dysfunction and malignancy, both neurorehabilitation (physical, occupational, and speech/swallowing therapy; adaptive equipment; and nutritional counseling). In particular, A-T is a multisystem disease requiring intervention to: (i) halt progressive neurodegenerative changes; (ii) reduce the risk of tumours; (iii) prevent severe infections due to the immunodeficiency; (iv) ameliorate respiratory functionality.

Unfortunately, no effective disease-modifying therapy is presently available for any of the major problems of the syndrome. Since the greatest mortality is caused by sinopulmonary infections, antibiotics based prophylactic regimens are often used although no formal demonstration of their usefulness is available [74]. In addition, intravenous gamma globulin is sometimes used, but again there are not clinical trials to document the benefit of these therapies [74]. Supportive therapy is available in preventing muscular contractures and in minimising lung infections and the subsequent chronic bronchopneumopathy [74]. Physical therapy certainly helps reduce long-term respiratory impairment. In particular, speech therapy has been proven useful in improving enunciation, thus ameliorating school performances and social relationships [73]. There is no cure for the progressive neurodegeneration, but medications directed to partially control drooling and tremors. Attempts to relief the neurological symptoms of A-T have so far been made with L-DOPA derivatives or dopamine agonists to correct basal ganglia dysfunction. Amantadine, fluoxetine or buspiron may be useful in improving loss of balance, speech and coordination [75-77]. Tremors are often controlled by gabapentin, clonazepan or propanalol.

Since incorporation of myo-inositol into phosphoinositides, as well as free myo-inositol content, is low in some A-T fibroblasts and phospholipid metabolism is less active in A-T as compared to normal cells, as well, a potential effect of myo-inositol has been postulated on neurological and immune functions in A-T [78]. However, although some promising results were observed in certain immune cells in a few A-T children (www.treatAT.org) in a first A-T clinical study, the sample size was not large enough to allow a conclusive interpretation of the data.

Since theoretically, the most effective treatment for A-T would either slow the progressive neurodegeneration or reduce the risk of lymphoid malignancies, thus far, the more promising fields of innovative therapeutic approaches are the usage of antioxidants and the development of innovative drugs designed to target specific mutations in the ATM gene in situ. Antioxidant therapies were expected to simultaneously slow the progression of the neurological deterioration and to reduce the risk of cancer, as well. At a preclinical level, administration of the antioxidant 5-carboxy-1,1,3,3-tetramethylisoindolin-2-yloxyl (CTMIO) to *Atm*-deficient mice reduced the rate of cell death of Purkinje cells and enhanced dendritogenesis to wild-type levels, suggesting a protective role against neurodegeneration. Recent evidence also indicates that CTMIO dramatically delays the onset of thymic lymphomas in ATM-/- mice [79].

Despite these encouraging preliminary results, in humans only a modest improvement has been achieved with antioxidant agents. A second group of antioxidant molecules, alpha-lipoic acid and a poly ADP-ribose polymerase (PARP) inhibitor, nicotinamide, has been tested at Johns Hopkins Hospital (Baltimore, MD, USA) by a randomized, double blind, double dummy trial. Two oxidative stress markers, levels of urine total alkanes and serum fast oxygen reduced adsorbance capacity (ORAC), improved in comparison with the baseline, in particular when a combined therapy with both the antioxidants was used. It is noteworthy that a trend toward increased lymphocyte counts was observed when subjects took both drugs, even though the difference did not reach a statistical significance. This finding deserves careful consideration in that lymphocytes exhibit cell biology defects intimately related to ATM deficiency and differently from Purkinje cells may be easily monitored during a study to explore the site of action of drugs. Concerning the multiple neurologic parameters evaluated in this trial (quantitative evaluation of tremor, tone, saccadic latency and A-T index score) and pulmonary function through spirometry, no positive significant change was found [45].

Overall, all attempts with anti-oxidant agents failed to halt the progressive nature of the disease [80]. As for the correction of ATM gene function by read-through of premature termination codons, Lai et al. employed aminoglycosides to achieve read-through expression of functional ATM protein [81]. In principle, these drugs bind to the RNA decoding site, inducing a conformational change that compromises the integrity of the codon–anticodon proofreading and allowing translation through an otherwise terminating codon. Gatti's group showed that geneticin and gentamycin produced detectable 'readthrough' ATM protein, as well [82]. As a proof of principle, this methodology is very promising; however, it requires the use of aminoglycosides that are toxic to cells and humans at concentrations that would be effective for read-through. Further attempts have been made with antisense morpholino oligonucleotides (AMOs) to redirect and restore normal splicing in the ATM gene [83], by targeting aberrant splice sites and enabling expression of normally spliced full-length ATM mRNA. Again, while this method provides proof of concept, a number of issues need to be addressed before it could be employed as a human therapeutic.

Symptomatic treatment can greatly improve the poor quality of life of these patients and prevent complications that could lead to death. Treatment of the symptoms of cerebellar ataxia should be symptom-focused (imbalance/incoordination/dysarthria, cerebellar tremor) and monitored with a few simple reproducible and semiquantitative measures of performance [84].

Recently, the potential benefits of glucocorticoids for A-T have been considered. A single case report pointed out that steroids produced in a child a short-term improvement in ataxia [85]. Recent clinical reports extended this observation and documented a clear cut beneficial effect of such therapy that was inversely correlated with the extent of cerebellar atrophy [86, 87]. The parents of A-T patients receiving glucocorticoids noted a reduction, sometimes dramatic, of neurological symptoms during treatment. This beneficial effect was also inversely correlated with the age of the patients [88]. In addition, a beneficial effect was also documented at very low dosages of drug as 0.01 mg/kg/day of oral betamethasone [87]. Of note, this effect was strictly drug dependent, in that the drug withdrawal paralleled the worsening of the neurological signs [86]. Intriguingly, during the short steroid trial, a paradoxical effect on the proliferative response to mitogen stimulation was documented, differently to what expected on the basis of the drug-induced immune suppression. This finding would potentially imply a direct effect of betamethasone on the intimate altered pathogenetic mechanism in A-T [87].

As for the mechanism underlying this effect of corticosteroids on neurological symptoms in A-T, any definitive explanation is currently available. The interaction with specific receptor proteins in target tissues have been shown to regulate the expression of corticosteroid-responsive genes. Several lines of evidence indicate that steroids have remarkable effects through both non-genomic and genomic mechanisms, the latter well documented also in neural system [89, 90]. The classical genomic mechanism of glucocorticoid (GC) action is cytoplasmic glucorticoid receptor (GR) mediated. GC bind and induce GR activation, followed by the GR translocation to nucleus and subsequent binding to glucocorticoid responsive element (GRE), thus modulating the transcription of a variety of genes including glucocorticoid-induced leucine zipper (GILZ). GILZ is known as a marker of GC transcriptional activity, rapidly induced by GC, able to regulate T lymphocytes activity, including T cell survival [91, 92]. A possible mechanism implicated in the beneficial effect of steroids is the suppression of inflammation [93]. If this is the case, GC would not interfere in the underlying cause of the disease, even though suppression of inflammation may be of some clinical utility [93].

An alternative explanation of the beneficial effect of betamethasone in A-T could be a potential activity of this molecule as an antioxidant. This mechanism was addressed by in a pilot study of our group, where intracellular glutathione levels, reactive oxygen species (ROS) production, and lipid peroxidation were measured in A-T patients receiving betamethasone [88]. A marked reduction, but drug-dependent, of ROS levels in the more drug responsive patient was noted. It is noteworthy that the neurological improvement was observed by 1 week of treatment. The previous observation that older patients failed to respond suggests that a threshold level of Purkinje cells number or other cerebellar hard-wiring may be a prerequisite for successful steroid therapy in A-T [88]. Thus, on the basis of very limited studies, it is mandatory that further evidence have to be gathered as to their potential role as disease-modifying agents.

The other question raised by our findings is whether long-term corticosteroid use would be a good option for patients who are already immunocompromised. It should be mentioned that differently from other congenital immunodeficiencies, severe infections are not common in A-T. Moreover, infections are almost exclusively localized in the respiratory tract, thus suggesting a non-immunological explanation for this problem [94]. As for the risk of malignancies, data are available that 10% to 30% of patients with A-T will develop cancer and, in particular, lymphoproliferative disorders, for which treatment regimens usually include steroids [28]. In conclusion, a randomized clinical trial is mandatory to definitively prove the efficacy of this new therapeutic opportunity.

CONCLUSION

Differently from other forms of primary immunodeficiencies whose clinical phenotype is predominated by the increased susceptibility to infections, A-T is the prototype of more complex syndromes in which the immunodeficiency is only one of the multiple components of the disease. The clinical phenotype is mainly characterized by a progressive neurodegenerative process, especially affecting the cerebellum. A-T is associated with mutations in the ATM gene, which is also expressed in Purkinje cells. It is to note that, unlike lymphocytes, whose turn-over is continuous, Purkinje cells are mature and differentiated cells which are not subject to turnover [49, 95]. Other clinical features are oculo-cutaneous telangiectasia, predisposition to cancer and chromosomal instability. The quality of life in A-T patients is dramatically affected by the neurological impairment, which almost invariably confines these patients to wheelchair by the age of ten years. Death occurs in the second or third decade of life.

All the phenotypic features of A-T are attributed to abnormal events after DNA-DSBs. Neurodegeneration results from accumulated DNA damage during development of nervous system. The immune dysfunction reflects the need of ATM for the physiological genomic rearrangement that occurs during V(D)J recombination [1, 96]. Furthermore, the cancer occurring in A-T, primarily leukemia and lymphoma, generally is a consequence of chromosomal instability. Thus, DNA damage responses, that engage the ATM signaling pathway, are important in ensuring that certain types of genotoxic stress are relieved during development. Recently, increasing attention has being paid to the role of oxidative stress in the pathogenesis of A-T. The cerebellum has been proven to be a target for oxygen damage resulting in the pathological macroscopic changes of A-T patients [71]. In ATM-/- mice, enhanced oxidative stress reduces life span and makes cells more sensitive to radiations, thus suggesting that free radicals are important cofactors in the expression of A-T clinical features [97]. In keeping with this observation administration of an antioxidant clearly prevented Purkinje cell death in *Atm*-deficient mice [98]. Although ATM seems to be neuroprotective in the tissue undergoing oxidative stress and apoptosis, the intimate molecular mechanism of its property is still uncertain. Overall, all attempts to treat A-T with anti-oxidant agents failed to halt the progressive nature of the disease [80].

Unfortunately, currently there is no effective treatment to cure or prevent the progress of neurological deterioration in A-T, but only supportive care of neurological symptoms and the exit usually occurs during about the second or third decade of life. Recently a drug dependent improvement of neurological signs in A-T patients, during a short-term treatment with oral betamethasone has been documented [86, 87]. As for the intimate molecular mechanism by which betamethasone led to this effect it is not possible to give a definitive interpretation, given that the pathogenesis of neurodegeneration itself is still far from being clear. Of note, the understanding of the implicated mechanisms may open an important window on novel, less dangerous therapeutic agents which may mime the effect of betamethasone on A-T.

REFERENCES

[1]   Chun, HH and Gatti, RA. Ataxia-telangiectasia, an evolving phenotype. *DNA Repair,* 2004, 3, 1187-1196.

[2]   Sedgwick, RP and Boder, E. Ataxia-Telangiectasia. In: Vinken, P, Bruyn, G and Klawans, H. *Handbook of Clinical Neurology.* New York: Elsevier; 1991; 347-423.

[3]   Savitsky, K; Bar-Shira, A; Gilad, S; Rotman, G; Ziv, Y; Vanagaite, L, et al. A single ataxia telangiectasia gene with a product similar to PI-3 Kinase. *Science,* 1995, 268, 1749-1753.

[4]   Dork, T; Bendix-Waltes, R; Wegner, RD and Stumm, M. Slow progression of ataxia telangiectasia with double missense and in frame splice mutations. *Am J Med Genet,* 2004, 126, 272-277.

[5]   Crawford, TO; Skolasky, RL; Fernandez, R; Rosquist, KJ and Lederman, HM. Survival probability in ataxia telangiectasia. *Arch Dis Child,* 2006, 91, 610-611.

[6]   Woods, CG and Taylor, AMR. Ataxia telangiectasia in the British Isles: the clinical and laboratory features of 70 affected individuals. *Q J Med,* 1992, 82, 169-179.

[7]   Nowak-Wegrzyn, A; Crawford, TO; Winkelstein, JA; Carson, KA and Lederman, HM. Immunodeficiency and infections in ataxia-telangiectasia. *J Pediatr,* 2004, 144, 505-511.

[8]   Crawford, TO. Ataxia telangiectasia. *Semin Pediatr Neurol,* 1998, 5, 287-294.

[9]   Yang, Y and Herrup, K. Loss of neuronal cell cycle control in ataxia-telangiectasia: a unified disease mechanism. *J Neurosci,* 2005, 25, 2522-2529.

[10]   Gatti, RA. Ataxia-Telangiectasia. In: Pagon, RA, Bird, TD, Dolan, CR and Stephens, K. *GeneReviews [Internet].* Seattle (WA): U.S. National Library of Medicine; 2010; 1993-1999.

[11]   Lewis, RF; Lederman, HM and Crawford, TO. Ocular motor abnormalities in ataxia telangiectasia. *Ann Neurol,* 1999, 46, 287-295.

[12]   Farr, AK; Shalev, B; Crawford, TO; Lederman, HM; Winkelstein, JA and Repka, MX. Ocular manifestations of ataxia-telangiectasia. *Am J Ophthalmol,* 2002, 134, 891-896.

[13]   Onodera, O. Spinocerebellar ataxia with ocular motor apraxia and DNA repair. *Neuropathology,* 2006, 26, 361-367.

[14]   Gatti, RA. Speculations on the Ataxia-telangiectasia defect. *Clin Immunol Immopathol,* 1991, 61, 10-15.

[15] Riise, R; Ygge, J; Lindman, C; Stray-Pedersen, A; Bek, T; R¿dningen, OK, et al. Ocular findings in Norwegian patients with ataxia-telangiectasia: a 5 year prospective cohort study. *Acta Ophthalmol Scand,* 2007, 85, 557-562.

[16] Baloh, RW; Yee, RD and Boder, E. Eye movements in ataxia-telangiectasia. *Neurology,* 1978, 28, 1099-1104.

[17] Reed, WB; Epstein, WL; Boder, E and Sedgwick, R. Cutaneous manifestations of ataxia-telangiectasia. *JAMA,* 1966, 195, 746-753.

[18] Folgori, L; Scarselli, A; Angelino, G; Ferrari, F; Antoccia, A; Chessa, L, et al. Cutaneous granulomatosis and combined immunodeficiency revealing Ataxia-Telangiectasia: a case report. *Ital J Pediatr,* 2010, 36, 29.

[19] Pashankar, F; Singhal, V; Akabogu, I; Gatti, RA and Goldman, FD. Intact T cell responses in ataxia telangiectasia. *Clin Immunol,* 2006, 120, 156-162.

[20] Gatti, RA; Becker-Catania, S; Chun, HH; Sun, X; Mitui, M; Lai, CH, et al. The pathogenesis of ataxia-telangiectasia. Learning from a Rosetta Stone. *Clin Rev Allergy Immunol,* 2001, 20, 87-108.

[21] Waldmann, TA; Broder, S; Goldman, CK; Frost, K; Korsmeyer, SJ and Medici, MA. Disorders of B cells and helper T cells in the pathogenesis of the immunoglobulin deficiency of patients with ataxia telangiectasia. *J Clin Invest,* 1983, 71, 282-295.

[22] Boder, E and Sedgwick, JB. Ataxia-telangiectasia: a review of 101 cases. In: Walsh G, e. *Little Club Clinics in Developmental Medicine.* Heineman Medical Books; 1963; 110-118.

[23] McGrath-Morrow, SA; Gower, WA; Rothblum-Oviatt, C; Brody, AS; Langston, C; Fan, LL, et al. Evaluation and management of pulmonary disease in ataxia-telangiectasia. *Pediatr Pulmonol,* 2010, 45, 847-859.

[24] Berkun, Y; Vilozni, D; Levi, Y; Borik, S; Waldman, D; Somech, R, et al. Reversible airway obstruction in children with ataxia telangiectasia. *Pediatr Pulmonol,* 2010, 45, 230-235.

[25] McGrath-Morrow, S; Lefton-Greif, M; Rosquist, K; Crawford, T; Kelly, A; Zeitlin, P, et al. Pulmonary function in adolescents with ataxia telangiectasia. *Pediatr Pulmonol,* 2008, 43, 59-66.

[26] Ball, LG and Xiao, W. Molecular basis of ataxia telangiectasia and related diseases. *Acta Pharmacol Sin,* 2005, 26, 897-907.

[27] Lavin, MF. Radiosensitivity and oxidative signalling in ataxia telangiectasia: an update. *Radiother Oncol,* 1998, 47, 113-123.

[28] Taylor, AM; Metcalfe, JA; Thick, J and Mak, YF. Leukemia and lymphoma in ataxia telangiectasia. *Blood,* 1996, 87, 423-438.

[29] Liyanage, M; Weaver, Z; Barlow, C; Coleman, A; Pankratz, DG; Anderson, S, et al. Abnormal rearrangement within the alpha/delta T-cell receptor locus in lymphomas from Atm-deficient mice. *Blood,* 2000, 96, 1940-1946.

[30] Swift, M; Morrell, D; Massey, RB and Chase, CL. Incidence of cancer in 161 families affected by ataxia-telangiectasia. *N Engl J Med,* 1991, 325, 1831-1836.

[31] Einarsdottir, K; Rosenberg, LU; Humphreys, K; Bonnard, C; Palmgren, J; Li, Y, et al. Comprehensive analysis of the ATM, CHEK2 and ERBB2 genes in relation to breast tumour characteristics and survival: a population-based case-control and follow-up study. *Breast Cancer Res,* 2006, 8, R67.

[32] Renwick, A; Thompson, D; Seal, S; Kelly, P; Chagtai, T; Ahmed, M, et al. ATM mutations that cause ataxia-telangiectasia are breast cancer susceptibility alleles. *Nat Genet,* 2006, 38, 873-875.

[33] PylkŠs, K; Tommiska, J; SyrjŠkoski, K; Kere, J; Gatei, M; Waddell, N, et al. Evaluation of the role of Finnish ataxia-telangiectasia mutations in hereditary predisposition to breast cancer. *Carcinogenesis,* 2007, 28, 1040-1045.

[34] Concannon, P; Haile, RW; B¿rresen-Dale, AL; Rosenstein, BS; Gatti, RA; Teraoka, SN, et al. Variants in the ATM gene associated with a reduced risk of contralateral breast cancer. *Cancer Res,* 2008, 68, 6486-6491.

[35] McKinnon, PJ. Ataxia-telangiectasia: an inherited disorder of ionizing-radiation sensitivity in man. Progress in the elucidation of the underlying biochemical defect. *Hum Genet,* 1987, 75, 197-208.

[36] Su, Y and Swift, M. Mortality rates among carriers of ataxia-telangiectasia mutant alleles. *Ann Intern Med,* 2000, 133, 770-778.

[37] Janin, N; Andrieu, N; Ossian, K; LaugŽ, A; Croquette, MF; Griscelli, C, et al. Breast cancer risk in ataxia telangiectasia (AT) heterozygotes: haplotype study in French AT families. *Br J Cancer,* 1999, 80, 1042-1045.

[38] Meyn, MS. Ataxia-telangiectasia, cancer and the pathobiology of the ATM gene. *Clin Genet,* 1999, 55, 289-304.

[39] Blevins, LSJ and Gebhart, SS. Insulin-resistant diabetes mellitus in a black woman with ataxia-telangiectasia. *South Med J,* 1996, 89, 619-621.

[40] Rotman, G and Shiloh, Y. ATM: from gene to function. *Hum Mol Genet,* 1998, 7, 1555-1563.

[41] Su, TT. Cellular responses to DNA damage: one signal, multiple choices. *Annu Rev Genet,* 2006, 40, 187-208.

[42] Zhou, BB and Elledge, SJ. The DNA damage response: putting checkpoints in perspective. *Nature,* 2000, 408, 433-439.

[43] Iliakis, G; Wang, Y; Guan, J and Wang, H. DNA damage checkpoint control in cells exposed to ionizing radiation. *Oncogene,* 2003, 22, 5834-5847.

[44] Shiloh, Y. ATM and related protein kinases: safeguarding genome integrity. *Nat Rev Cancer,* 2003, 3, 155-168.

[45] Lavin, MF; Gueven, N; Bottle, S and Gatti, RA. Current and potential therapeutic strategies for the treatment of ataxia-telangiectasia. *Br Med Bull,* 2007, 81-82, 129-147.

[46] Bakkenist, CJ and Kastan, MB. DNA damage activates ATM through intermolecular autophosphorylation and dimer dissociation. *Nature,* 2003, 421, 499-506.

[47] Aurias, A; Dutrillaux, B; Buriot, D and Lejeune, J. High frequencies of inversions and translocations of chromosomes 7 and 14 in ataxia telangiectasia. *Mutat Res,* 1980, 69, 369-374.

[48] Regueiro, JR; Porras, O and Lavin, M. Ataxia-telangiectasia: a primary immunodeficiency revisited. *Immunol Allergy Clin North Am,* 2000, 20, 177-206.

[49] Biton, S; Barzilai, A and Shiloh, Y. The neurological phenotype of ataxia-telangiectasia: solving a persistent puzzle. *DNA Repair,* 2008, 7, 1028-1038.

[50] Burma, S; Chen, BP and Chen, DJ. Role of non-homologous end joining (NHEJ) in maintaining genomic integrity. *DNA Repair,* 2006, 5, 1042-1048.

[51] Reina-San-Martin, B; Chen, HT; Nussenzweig, A and Nussenzweig, MC. ATM is required for efficient recombination between immunoglobulin switch regions. *J Exp Med,* 2005, 200, 1103-1110.

[52] Xu, Y; Ashley, T; Brainerd, EE; Bronson, RT; Meyn, MS and Baltimore, D. Targeted disruption of ATM leads to growth retardation, chromosomal fragmentation during meiosis, immune defects, and thymic lymphoma. *Genes Dev,* 1996, 10, 2401-2410.

[53] McCarthy, JV. Apoptosis and development. *Essays Biochem,* 2003, 39, 11-24.

[54] Shiloh, Y. Ataxia-telangiectasia and the Nijmegen breakage syndrome: related disorders but genes apart. *Annu Rev Genet,* 1997, 31, 635-662.

[55] Barzilai, A; Biton, S and Shilol, Y. The role of the DNA damage response in neuronal development, organization and maintenance. *DNA Repair,* 2008, 7, 1010-1027.

[56] Katyal, S and McKinnon, PJ. DNA repair deficiency and neurodegeneration. *Cell Cycle,* 2007, 6, 2360-2365.

[57] McKinnon, PJ. DNA repair deficiency and neurological disease. *Nat Rev Neurosci,* 2009, 10, 100-112.

[58] Lees-Miller, SP and Meek, K. Repair of DNA double strand breaks by non-homologous end joining. *Biochimie,* 2003, 85, 1161-1173.

[59] Biton, S; Gropp, M; Itsykson, P; Pereg, Y; Mittelman, L; Johe, K, et al. ATM-mediated response to DNA double strand breaks in human neurons derived from stem cells. *DNA Repair,* 2007, 6, 128-134.

[60] Vinters, HV; Gatti, RA and Rakic, P. Sequence of cellular events in cerebellar ontogeny relevant to expression of neuronal abnormalities in ataxia-telangiectasia. *Kroc Found Ser,* 1985, 19, 233-255.

[61] McKinnon, PJ and Caldecott, KW. DNA strand break repair and human genetic disease. *Annu Rev Genom Human Genet,* 2007, 8, 37-55.

[62] Lee, Y; Chong, MJ and McKinnon, PJ. Ataxia Telangiectasia mutated-dependent apoptosis after genotoxic stress in the devoloping nervous system is determined by cellular differentiation status. *J Neurosci,* 2001, 21, 6687-6693.

[63] Herzog, KH; Chong, MJ; Kapsetaki, M; Morgan, JI and McKinnon, PJ. Requirement for Atm in ionizing radiation-induced cell death in the developing central nervous system. *Science,* 1998, 280, 1089-1091.

[64] McConnell, MJ; Kaushal, D; Yang, AH; Kingsbury, MA; Rehen, SK; Treuner, K, et al. Failed clearance of aneuploid embryonic neural progenitor cells leads to excess aneuploidy in the Atm-deficient but not the Trp53-deficient adult cerebral cortex. *J Neurosci,* 2004, 24, 8090-8096.

[65] Trushina, E and McMurray, CT. Oxidative stress and mitochondrial dysfunction in neurodegenerative diseases. *Neurosci,* 2007, 145, 1233-1248.

[66] Halliwell, B. Oxidative stress and neurodegeneration: where are we now? *J Neurochem,* 2006, 97, 1634-1658.

[67] Ryter, SW; Kim, HP; Hoetzel, A; Park, JW; Nakahira, K; Wang, X, et al. Mechanisms of cell death in oxidative stress. *Antioxid Redox Signal,* 2007, 9, 49-89.

[68] Perry, JJ; Fan, L and Tainer, JA. Developing master keys to brain pathology, cancer and aging from the structural biology of proteins controlling reactive oxygen species and DNA repair. *Neurosci,* 2007, 145, 1280-1299.

[69] Liu, N; Stoica, G; Yan, M; Scofield, VL; Qiang, W; Lynn, WS, et al. ATM deficiency induces oxidative stress and endoplasmic reticulum stress in astrocytes. *Lab Invest,* 2005, 85, 1471-1480.

[70] Barzilai, A; Rotman, G and Shiloh, Y. ATM deficiency and oxidative stress: a new dimension of defecive response to DNA damage. *DNA Repair,* 2002, 1, 3-25.

[71] Barlow, C; Dennery, PA; Shigenaga, MK; Smith, MA; Morrow, JD; Roberts, LJ, et al. Loss of the ataxia-telangiectasia gene product causes oxidative damage in target organs. *Proc Natal Acad Sci USA,* 1999, 96, 9915-9919.

[72] Kamsler, A; Daily, D; Hochman, A; Stern, N; Shiloh, Y; Rotman, G, et al. Increased oxidative stress in Ataxia Telangiectasia evidenced by alternations in redox state of brains from Atm-deficient mice. *Cancer Res,* 2001, 61, 1849-1854.

[73] Perlman, S; Becker-Catania, S and Gatti, RA. Ataxia-telangiectasia: diagnosis and treatment. *Semin Pediatr Neurol,* 2003, 10, 173-182.

[74] Spacey, SD; Gatti, RA and Bebb, G. The molecular basis and clinical management of ataxia telangiectasia. *Can J Neurol Sci,* 2000, 27, 184-191.

[75] Botez, MI; Botez-Marquard, T; Elie, R; Pedraza, OL; Goyette, K and Lalonde, R. Amantadine hydrochloride treatment in heredodegenerative ataxias: a double blind study. *J Neurol Neurosurg Psychiatry,* 1996, 61, 259-264.

[76] Trouillas, P; Xie, J; Adeleine, P; Michel, D; Vighetto, A; Honnorat, J, et al. Buspirone, a 5-hydroxytryptamine1A agonist, is active in cerebellar ataxia. Results of a double-blind drug placebo study in patients with cerebellar cortical atrophy. *Arch Neurol,* 1997, 54, 749-752.

[77] Seliger, GM and Hornstein, A. Serotonin, fluoxetine, and pseudobulbar affect. *Neurology,* 1989, 39, 1400.

[78] Yorek, MA; Dunlap, JA; Manzo-Fontes, A; Bianchi, R; Berry, GT and Eichberg, J. Abnormal myo-inositol and phospholipid metabolism in cultured fibroblasts from patients with ataxia telangiectasia. *Biochim Biophys Acta,* 1999, 1437, 287-300.

[79] Gueven, N; Luff, J; Peng, C; Hosokawa, K; Bottle, SE and Lavin, MF. Dramatic extension of tumor latency and correction of neurobehavioral phenotype in Atm-mutant mice with a nitroxide antioxidant. *Free Radic Biol Med,* 2006, 41, 992-1000.

[80] Caldecott, KW. XRCC1 and DNA strand break repair. *DNA Repair,* 2003, 2, 955-969.

[81] Lai, CH; Chun, HH; Nahas, SA; Mitui, M; Gamo, KM; Du, L, et al. Correction of ATM gene function by aminoglycoside-induced read-through of premature termination codons. *Proc Natl Acad Sci USA,* 2004, 101, 15676-15681.

[82] Du, L; Damoiseaux, R; Nahas, S; Gao, K; Hu, H; Pollard, JM, et al. Nonaminoglycoside compounds induce readthrough of nonsense mutations. *J Exp Med,* 2009, 206, 2285-2297.

[83] Migliore, L and Copped•, F. Environmental-induced oxidative stress in neurodegenerative disorders and aging. *Mutat Res,* 2009, 674, 73-84.

[84] Crawford, TO; Mandir, AS; Lefton-Greif, MA; Goodman, SN; Goodman, BK; Sengul, H, et al. Quantitative neurologic assessment of ataxia-telangiectasia. *Neurology,* 2000, 54, 1505-1509.

[85] Buoni, S; Zanolli, R; Sorrentino, L and Fois, A. Betamethasone and Improvement of Neurological Symptoms in Ataxia-Telangiectasia. *Arch Neurol,* 2006, 63, 1479-1482.

[86] Broccoletti, T; Del Giudice, E; Amorosi, S; Russo, I; Di Bonito, M; Imperati, A, et al. Steroid-induced improvement of neurological signs in ataxia-telangiectasia patients. *Eur J Neurol,* 2008, 15, 223-228.

[87] Broccoletti, T; Del Giudice, E; Cirillo, E; Vigliano, I; Giardino, G; Ginocchio, VM, et al. Efficacy of Very-low-dose betamethasone on neurological symptoms in ataxia-telangiectasia. *Eur J Neurol,* 2011, 18, 564-570.

[88] Russo, I; Cosentino, C; Del Giudice, E; Broccoletti, T; Amorosi, S; Cirillo, E, et al. In ataxia-teleangiectasia betamethasone response is inversely correlated to cerebellar atrophy and directly to antioxidative capacity. *Eur J Neurol,* 2009, 16, 755-759.

[89] Bruscoli, S; Di Virgilio, R; Donato, V; Velardi, E; Marchetti, C; Migliorati, G, et al. Genomic and non-genomic effects of different glucocorticoids on mouse thymocyte apoptosis. *Eur J Pharmacol,* 2006, 529, 63-70.

[90] Stahn, C; Lowenberg, M; Hommes, DW and Buttgereit, F. Molecular mechanisms of glucocorticoid action and selective glucocorticoid receptor agonists. *Mol Cell Endocrinol,* 2007, 275, 71-78.

[91] D'Adamio, F; Zollo, O; Moraca, R; Ayroldi, E; Bruscoli, S; Bartoli, A, et al. A New Dexamethasone-Induced Gene of the Leucine Zipper Family Protects T Lymphocytes from TCR/CD3-Activated Cell Death. *Immunity,* 1997, 7, 803-812.

[92] Riccardi, C; Bruscoli, S and Migliorati, G. Molecular mechanisms of immunomodulatory activity of glucocorticoids. *Pharmacol Res,* 2002, 45, 361-368.

[93] Shimmer, BP and Parker, KL. Adrenocorticotropic hormone, adrenocortical sterioids and their synthetic analogs, Inhibitors of the synthesis and actions of adrenocortical hormones. In: Hardmon, JG and Limbird, LE. *Goodman and GillmanÕs Pharmacologic basis of therapeutics.* New York: McGraw-Hill; 2001; 1649-1677.

[94] Lefton-Greif, MA; Crawford, TO; Winkelstein, JA; Loughlin, GM; Koerner, CB; Zahurak, M, et al. Oropharyngeal dysphagia and aspiration in patients with ataxia-telangiectasia. *J Pediatr,* 2000, 136, 225-231.

[95] Canman, CE; Lim, DS; Cimprich, KA; Taya, Y; Tamai, K; Sakaguchi, K, et al. Activation of the ATM kinase by ionizing radiation and phosphorylation of p53. *Science,* 1998, 281, 1677-1679.

[96] McKinnon, PJ. ATM and ataxia telangiectasia. *EMBO Rep,* 2004, 5, 772-776.

[97] Ziv, S; Brenner, O; Amariglio, N; Smorodinsky, NI; Galron, R; Carrion, DV, et al. Impaired genomic stability and increased oxidative stress exacerbate different features of Ataxia-telangiectasia. *Hum Mol Genet,* 2005, 14, 2929-2943.

[98] Chen, P; Peng, C; Luff, J; Spring, K; Watters, D; Bottle, S, et al. Oxidative Stress Is Responsible for Deficient Survival and Dendritogenesis in Purkinje Neurons from ataxia-telangiectasia mutated mutant mice. *J Neurosci,* 2003, 36, 11453-11460.

In: Ataxia: Causes, Symptoms and Treatment
Editor: Sung Hoi Hong

ISBN: 978-1-61942-867-6
© 2012 Nova Science Publishers, Inc.

Chapter 3

THE NEUROBIOLOGY OF EPISODIC ATAXIA TYPE 1, A SHAKER-LIKE K⁺ CHANNEL DISORDER

*D'Adamo Maria Cristina[1], Imbrici Paola[1],
Giuseppe Di Giovanni[2] and Pessia Mauro[1]*
[1]Section of Human Physiology,
University of Perugia School of Medicine, Perugia, Italy
[2]Department of Physiology and Biochemistry,
University of Malta, Msida, Malta

ABSTRACT

Episodic ataxia type 1 (EA1) is a potassium channelopathy (CP) characterized by constant myokymia and dramatic episodes of spastic contractions of the skeletal muscles of the head, arms, and legs with loss of both motor coordination and balance. During attacks some individuals may experience vertigo, blurred vision, diplopia, nausea, headache, diaphoresis, clumsiness, stiffening of the body, dysarthric speech, and difficulty in breathing. These episodes may last seconds to minutes, and can be precipitated by anxiety, emotional stress, fatigue, startle response or sudden postural changes (*kinesigenic stimulation*). Epilepsy is overrepresented in cases of EA1. Other symptoms include delayed motor development, cognitive disability, choreoathetosis, and carpal spasm. EA1 onset is in childhood or early adolescence. It is inherited in an autosomal dominant manner and genetic analysis of several EA1 families has lead to the discovery of a number of point mutations in the voltage-dependent potassium channel gene *KCNA1* (Kv1.1), on chromosome 12p13. To date *KCNA1* is the only gene known to be associated with EA1. Functional studies have shown that these mutations impair Kv1.1 channel function with variable effects on channel assembly, trafficking and kinetics. Despite solid evidence obtained on the molecular mechanisms underlying EA1, how these cause dysfunctions within the central and peripheral nervous systems circuitries remains for the most part obscure. Without doubt, EA1 research is important for the identification of signaling pathways involved in this disease and also to find novel pharmacological interventions. More broadly, however, this research may serve as a paradigm for studying related disorders, help in the understanding of the functional properties of the proteins involved and shed new light on the physiological workings of the human body.

INTRODUCTION

Ion channels are membrane proteins that allow the selected and concerted movement of ions across cell membrane that is otherwise relatively impermeable to ions. These proteins are expressed in virtually every cell type, where they play key physiological roles. Thus, it is not surprising that ion channels dysfunction causes disease in animals and humans.

The term *channelopathy* (CP) was coined less than two decades ago to identify ion channel diseases. To date, a large group of channelopathies have been identified and new ones are continuously being discovered; therefore, they represent a heavy burden on society.

Many of them are caused by inherited genetic mutations and result in a very diverse class of diseases ranging from ataxia, epilepsy, migraine, psychiatric disorders to dysfunction of the skeletal muscle, kidney and endocrinology system. This chapter aims to provide a comprehensive and up to date account of our present understanding of episodic ataxia type 1, an autosomal dominant K^+ channel disease. It will also address the challenges involved in pinning down the mechanisms which underlie this neurological CP and a new direction for better therapeutic approaches will be considered. Additionally, the main features of related ataxia disorders will be concisely illustrated.

STRUCTURE AND FUNCTION OF SHAKER-LIKE K^+ CHANNELS

Potassium channels are encoded by more than 70 genes and therefore they are the largest group of ion channels found in virtually all cells of the human body. To understand how mutations in K^+ channels give rise to diseases requires at least a basic understanding of the molecular structure, biophysical properties, expression pattern and physiological role played by these proteins. In addition, to fully appreciate the functional studies performed from mutated Kv1.1 channels and how they alter CNS circuitries, a brief description of the experimental approaches used to study *channelopathies* (CPs) has been included for the benefit of those unfamiliar with these topics.

Voltage-gated potassium channels (Kv) were first cloned from the *Shaker* mutant of *Drosophila* in 1987 (Tempel *et al.*, 1987). These fruit flies display a shaking phenotype induced by ether, as the relevant K^+ channel gene is mutated. Therefore, they represent an animal model of a neuromuscular *CP* (Kaplan and Trout, 1969; Jan *et al.*, 1977; Tanouye and Ferrus 1985). The human Kv1.1 orthologue is encoded by *KCNA1* gene. Since the first cloning, several other Kv channel genes have been identified from many different species. Based on sequence relatedness, Kv channels have been classified in subfamilies by using the abbreviation *Kvy.x* (Gutman and Chandy, 1993). According to this standardized nomenclature *Shaker*-related channels have been classified in the subfamily *Kv1.x* and each member numbered Kv1.1 through Kv1.8 (Figure 1). The same criteria have been used to classify channels related to the subfamilies *Shab* (Kv2.1 and Kv2.2), *Shaw* (Kv3.1 to 3.4) and *Shal* (Kv4.1 to Kv4.3).

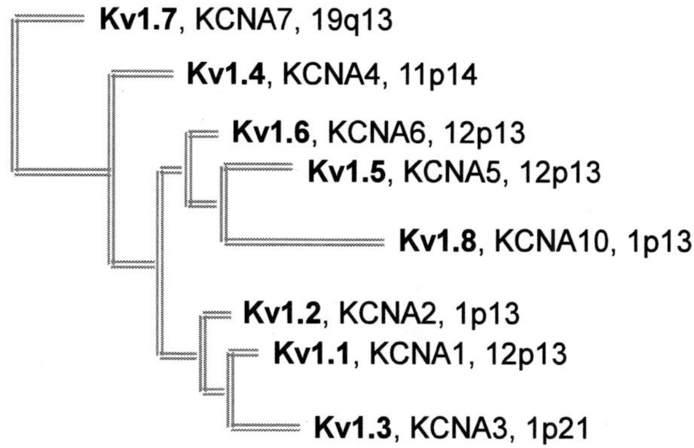

Figure 1. Phylogenetic tree for the Kv1 family.

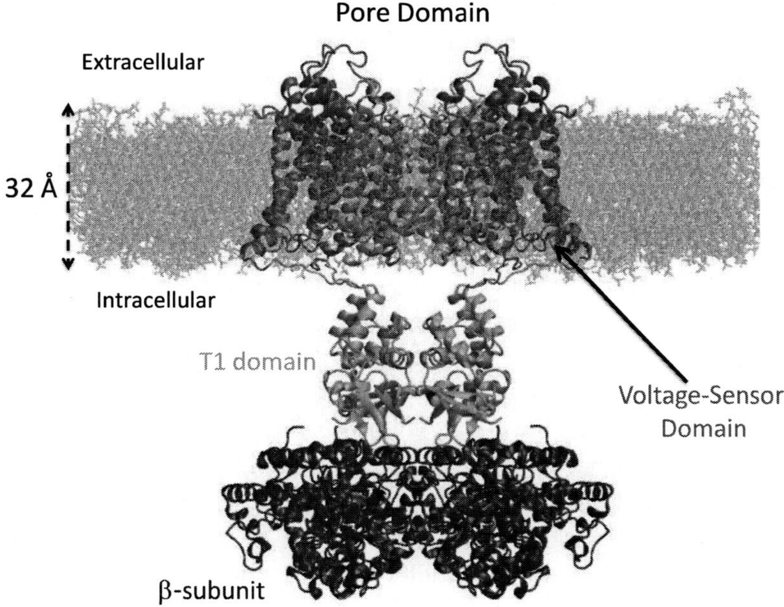

Figure 2. Architecture of a voltage-gated K+ channel. 3-Dimensional image illustrating the structure of the Kv1.2/2.1 chimera. The secondary structure elements are shown as ribbons and are colored red (voltage sensing domains), grey (ion conducting pore), green (T1 domains) and purple (accessory ⍰⍰-subunits). Only two monomers (facing each other) of the tetramer have been depicted for clarity. The lipids of the membrane bilayer are shown as light blue colored sticks.

The predicted 496-amino acid of the Kv1.1 protein contains six hydrophobic segments with the N and C-termini residing inside the cell. The predicted topology and structural features of a K^+ channel subunit are similar to each of the four voltage-gated sodium channel domains. The S5-S6 loop (*H5 region*) contributes to the ion-conducting pore. The GYG residues, residing within this loop, control the K^+ selectivity of the channel. Kv channels are composed of four homologous pore-forming subunits. Four subunits are assembled and targeted to the plasma membrane to form a functional tetrameric channel. Towards the end of the 90's, the crystal structure of KcsA, an inwardly-rectifying potassium channel from *Streptomyces lividans,* was first described by X-ray crystallography (Doyle *et al.,* 1998).

The architecture of this channel resembled an inverted tepee formed by four subunits. More recently, the entire crystal structure of a voltage-gated K^+ potassium channel has been described (Figure 2; Jiang *et al.*, 2003a; Jiang *et al.*, 2003b). Potassium channels are the most diverse class of ion channels. Indeed, they may exist as homomers, whenever four identical α-subunits are assembled. However, different types of α-subunits may heteropolymerize to form channels with properties that are different from the parental homomeric channels (Ruppersberg *et al.*, 1990; Isacoff *et al.*, 1990). This phenomenon greatly enhances potassium channel diversity. Notable examples are the heteromeric channels Kv1.1/Kv1.2 or Kv1.1/Kv1.4 that have been localized in several structures within the nervous system (Wang *et al.*, 1993; Sheng *et al.*, 1994; Wang *et al.*, 1994; D'Adamo *et al.*, 1999). The need for such a large number of potassium channels remains unclear.

Voltage-dependent Na^+, K^+ and Ca^{++} channels are generally closed at the resting membrane potential of nerve cells, which is approximately –60, –70 mV. However, the transmembrane potential of neurons undergoes continuous changes that are caused by incoming stimuli. Depolarizing steps trigger the opening of voltage-gated channels, whereas, membrane repolarization closes these channels (Figure 3).

The S4 segment of each Kv1.1 subunit is composed of regularly spaced positively charged arginines and lysines and comprises the main voltage-sensor region that opens the channel by undergoing a conformational rearrangement upon membrane depolarization. The description of the entire crystal structure of a voltage-gated K^+ potassium channel allowed MacKinnon proposed a new model by which the voltage-sensors operate. Although controversial, it appears that the S4 segment does not rotate as a *sliding helix*, but it moves back and forth like a paddling motion. Indeed, this mechanism was named "*the paddle model*" of voltage sensing (Jiang *et al.*, 2003a; Jiang *et al.*, 2003b).

The inactivation of delayed-rectifier potassium channels is a physiologically relevant process as it controls the firing properties of neurons and their response to input stimuli (Aldrich *et al.*, 1979). Kv channels show two principal types of inactivation, namely the N- and C-type. The fast *N-type* or *A-type* inactivation is caused by a "ball-and-chain" mechanism of pore occlusion operated by the first 20 amino acids located in the N-terminus of *Shaker* channels (Hoshi *et al.*, 1990; Zagotta *et al.*, 1990).

Fast inactivation, however, may be conferred to non-inactivating channels by auxiliary subunits such as Kvβ1.1 and Kvβ1.2 (Retting *et al.*, 1994). Four β subunits make up the ion channel complex.

The fast N-type inactivation mechanism has been elucidated by using crystallographic data. The new model shows that the inactivation particle works its way through one of the four lateral vestibules that provide the access to the central pore. Then, the flexible ball domain reaches its final binding site by sneaking into the central cavity located below the selectivity filter. The blocking process is now complete and the potassium flux terminates (Zhou *et al.*, 2001). Some Kv channels are characterised by a slower process of inactivation (*e.g.* Kv1.1, Kv1.2), which has been named *C-type* and *P-type* (Figure 3), depending on the structural determinants associated with this process that are located at the C-termini of each subunit.

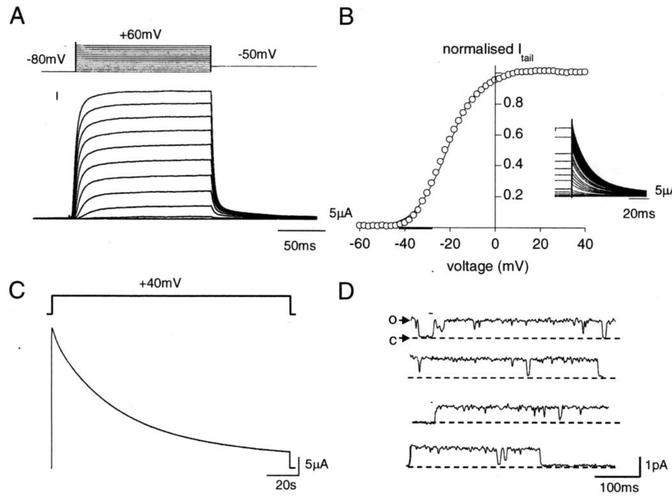

Figure 3. Heterologous expression of Kv1.1 channels. (A) Current family recorded from oocytes expressing Kv1.1 channels by means of two-electrode voltage-clamp (TEVC). The pulse protocol is indicated on top. Outward currents were evoked by 200 ms depolarizing commands from a holding potential of –80 mV. The mean amplitude of the current recorded at +40-+60 mV is commonly used to estimate the surface expression of the mutated channel in comparison to that of wild-type channels. Moreover, the activation and deactivation kinetics of the channel are determined by fitting exponential functions to current traces recorded at different voltages. (B) Current-voltage relationship for Kv1.1 channels obtained by plotting the normalized peak tail currents as a function of the pre-pulse potentials (from -60 mV to +40 mV, 3 mV increments).The solid lines represent the fit of the data points with the Boltzmann function: $NI = 1/\{1 + \exp[(V - V1/2)/k]\}$ from which the half-activation voltage (V1/2) and slope factor k for Kv1.1 channels are calculated. The inset on the right hand side shows representative tail currents recorded at -50 mV. (C) To determine the C-type inactivation kinetics of Kv1.1 channels a test pulse to +60 mV for 3.5 min is delivered to oocytes recorded under TEVC configuration. The decaying phase of the current is caused by the slow process of channel inactivation and the relevant rate constant can be calculated by fitting the current trace with exponential function. (D) Representative single-channel currents for Kv1.1 channels recorded in the inside-out configuration of the patch-clamp. The openings were evoked by 200 ms depolarizing voltage commands to +20 mV from a holding potential of -80 mV (open state level: O; closed state level: C). The slope conductance of Kv1.1 channels is ~10pS.

The molecular mechanism of this process involves conformational modification of the extracellular mouth of the pore and, particularly, a constriction of the selectivity filter (Grissmer and Cahalan, 1989; Hoshi *et al.*, 1991; Baukrowitz and Yellen, 1995; Molina *et al.*, 1997; López-Barneo *et al.*, 1993; Pardo *et al.*, 1992; Stühmer *et al.*, 1989b). During intense neuronal activity the C-type inactivation of Kv channels can accumulate, modifying both the firing rate and the shape of the action potential (Aldrich *et al.*, 1979).

At a single channel level, membrane depolarization elicits channel openings and closings (a process named *gating*) and are visible as upwards and downwards deflection of the current, respectively (Figure 3). The analysis of the time spent by the channels in the open and closed conformations allows for the determination of the mean open and closed times, respectively. Channel openings occur stochastically; therefore, the overall channel activity is assessed by determining the probability of opening (P_o), defined as the fraction of the time spent by the channel in the open state.

PHYSIOLOGICAL ROLE OF K_V CHANNELS

Kv1 family members exhibit diverse expression patterns in the central and peripheral nervous system (PNS) and are found tightly clustered within distinct neuronal compartments (*for review see* Trimmer and Rhodes 2004). Knowledge of such precise targeting has important implications for defining the roles played by individual Kv channels in regulating neuronal function and in pathophysiology. Kv channels shorten the duration of action potentials, modulate the release of neurotransmitters, and control the excitability, electrical properties and firing pattern of central and peripheral neurons (Hille, 2001; Pessia 2004). Dysfunctions in the circuits of the cortex, hippocampus, cerebellum and of peripheral nervous system have been postulated to play a role in EA1. Thus, to understand the current opinions on the pathological mechanisms underlying this disease a review of the relevant evidence obtained on the neurophysiological role of Kv1 channels in the following structures: cortex, hippocampus, cerebellum and PNS will follow.

Cortex. Kv1.1, Kv1.2 and Kv1.4 are the most abundant subunits expressed in the central nervous system and they are predominantly localized on axons and terminals. Biochemical and electrophysiological evidence indicates that these subunits are co-assembled to form heteromeric channels. Fast-spiking cells (FS cells) are a prominent subtype of neocortical GABA*ergic* interneurons that form synapses to the perisomatic region of target cells. These cells are critical regulators of cortical inhibition. A spatially delimited expression of Kv1 channels at the cell axon initial segment has been observed in FS cells (Goldberg *et al.*, 2008). These channels exert a dampening mechanism on their axon initial segment and powerfully regulate action potential threshold in order to allow FS cells to respond preferentially to large inputs (Goldberg *et al.*, 2008). Dysfunction of neocortical FS cells has been shown to lead to epilepsy (Lau *et al.*, 2000; Ogiwara *et al.*, 2007). Epilepsy is overrepresented in EA1 (Zuberi *et al.*, 1999; Liguori *et al.*, 2001) and deletion of Kv1.1 in mice produces spontaneous seizures (Smart et al., 1998). Mutations in Kv1.1-associated proteins leucine-rich glioma inactivated gene1 (*Lgi1*) and contactin-associated protein-like 2 (*Caspr2*) have also been shown to cause human epilepsy syndromes (Schulte *et al.*, 2006; Strauss *et al.*, 2006). Deletion of a host of genes known to be expressed by FS cells leads to epilepsy in mice, including Kv3.2 (Lau et al., 2000) and *SCN1A* (Na$_V$1.1; Ogiwara *et al.*, 2007). Hence, FS cell dysfunction may also contribute to the cellular basis by which Kv1.1 mutations cause epilepsy in humans but future work is required to confirm this hypothesis.

Hippocampus

The hippocampus is a major brain region, belonging to the limbic system, which plays an important role in the consolidation of information and in spatial memory. This area is often the focus of epileptic seizures. In the hippocampus, *Kv1.1, Kv1.2 Kv1.4* are found in Schaffer collateral axons and are highly expressed in axons and terminals of the medial perforant path in the middle third of the molecular layer of the dentate gyrus. In CA3, Kv1.1, Kv1.4 and, *Kvβ1.1* subunits are expressed in mossy fibre boutons (*swellings of mossy fibre axons*) that form *en passant* synapses with pyramidal neurons. This macromolecular channel complex regulates the activity-dependent spike broadening of hippocampal mossy fibre boutons and, as a consequence, the amount of neurotransmitter released during high-frequency stimuli (Geiger and Jonas, 2000). Kv1.1 gene deletion alters the hippocampal excitability. Mice lacking these channels display frequent spontaneous seizures throughout adult life, although, the intrinsic passive properties of CA3 pyramidal cells are normal. Antidromic action potentials are recruited at lower thresholds in Kv1.1 null slices and mossy fiber stimulation triggers synaptically mediated long-latency epileptiform burst discharges. This data indicates that loss of Kv1.1 results in increased excitability in the CA3 recurrent axon collateral system, perhaps contributing to the limbic and tonic–clonic components of the observed epileptic phenotype (Smart *et al.*, 1998).

Cerebellum

The cerebellum plays an important role in motor control and it is also involved in some cognitive functions. Kv1.1 and Kv1.2 are expressed at the cerebellar Pinceau, a structure composed of a number of basket cell terminals that embrace the Purkinje axon hillock and proximal axon segment (McNamara *et al.*, 1993; Wang *et al.*, 1993; Wang *et al.*, 1994; Laube *et al.*, 1996). A basket cell makes synaptic contact with several Purkinje cells. Patch-clamp recordings from cerebellar Purkinje cells have revealed that α-DTX, a selective blocker of Kv1.1 and Kv1.2 potassium channels from basket cell presynaptic terminals, increases both the amplitude and frequency of spontaneous IPSCs mediated by $GABA_A$ receptor activation (Southan and Robertson, 1998). These findings suggest that Kv1.1 and Kv1.2 heteromeric channels at basket cell terminals modulate their excitability and, as a consequence, the release of the neurotransmitter γ-aminobutyric acid (GABA) onto Purkinje cells. Therefore, Kv1.1/Kv1.2 channels, by modulating the release of GABA onto the axon hillock of Purkinje cells, control their ability to generate action potentials and, as a consequence, regulate the entire cerebellar output directed to the rest of the brain.

Sciatic Nerve

The myelinated axon of the peripheral nervous system is subdivided into several specialized domains. They include, in order, the node of Ranvier, paranode, juxtaparanode and internode. The juxtaparanodal region of myelinated axons express a macromolecular membrane complex composed of *Kv1.1, Kv1.2,* their accessory subunit *Kvβl.2* (Vacher *et al.*, 2008; Wang *et al.*, 1993; Poliak *et al.*, 1999). This macromolecular complex has been found also at the level of the axons branching to the CNS and PNS (Tsaur *et al.*,1992; Wang *et al.*, 1994). The role of Kv1.1 channels in neuromuscular transmission has been investigated by using transgenic mice (Zhou *et al.*, 1998, 1999, 2001). *Kv1.1* ablation causes repetitive neuronal activity in mouse phrenic nerve that appear to result from both spontaneous and stimulus-evoked nerve-backfiring at preterminal axon transition zones, where axons change from myelinated to non-myelinated (Smart *et al.*, 1998; Vabnick *et al.*, 1999; Zhou *et al.*, 1998, 1999). These studies pointed out that juxtaparanodal *Kv1.1* channels are critical regulators of axonal excitability.

BIOTECHNOLOGY FOR STUDYING ION CHANNELS

John Gurdon originally showed that mature oocytes dissected from *Xenopus laevis*, a fully aquatic amphibian species native of Africa (Figure 4), are able to faithfully and efficiently translate foreign genetic information. At the beginning of 1980s, Eric Barnard and colleagues showed that *Xenopus* oocytes express ion channels on their plasma membrane after a microinjection of exogenous mRNAs into their cytoplasm (Sumikawa *et al.*, 1981). Therefore, they became a useful tool for molecular neurobiology research and for the heterologous expression of ion channels. For instance, the injection of mRNA encoding for Kv1.1 into these cells normally results in functional channels after 1-5 days of incubation at 16°C (Figure 4). Other expression systems commonly used for studying ion channels include, cell lines and neurons in culture. Human Embryonic Kidney 293 cells (HEK 293) and Chinese hamster ovary cells (CHO) are cell lines which are very easy to grow and which transfect very readily; therefore, they have been widely-used in cell biology research for many years.

The *voltage-clamp* technique was developed by *Marmont and Cole* and improved by *Hodgkin and Huxley* who successfully dissected the sodium and potassium ionic currents underlying an action potential using this method. Since *Xenopus* oocytes may be as large as 1 mm in diameter, two microelectrodes can be easily inserted into the cell, one to record the potential across the membrane and the other to pass the current. By using this configuration known as *two-electrode voltage-clamp*, Kv1.1 channels in the membrane can be activated by depolarizing voltage commands to form a holding potential of -80 mV (Figure 3).

To maintain the potential clamped at a desired value (*e.g.* +40 mV), the amplifier injects current that is equal in amplitude and opposite in sign to that flowing through the whole of the cell membrane (*whole-cell current*). Therefore, by properly converting this signal the amplifier measures the amount of ionic current flowing through all the channels in the membrane at a given potential. In 1976, *Erwin Neher* and *Bert Sakmann* developed the *patch-clamp* technique that allowed for the recording of the ionic current flowing through a single channel for the first time (Neher and Sakmann, 1976; Hamill *et al.*, 1981; Figure 3). Single channel currents can be recorded by using different patch-clamp configurations, such as *cell-attached* (the glass pipette is sealed to the membrane of an intact cell), *inside-out* (the membrane patch is detached and its intracellular side is exposed to the bath solution) and *outside-out* (the extracellular side of the membrane patch is exposed to the bath solution).

These configurations permit the study of the activity of a single channel in physiological conditions (*cell-attached*) or after changing the composition of the intracellular (*inside-out*) or extracellular (*outside-out*) solutions. The potential and the ionic current flowing across the entire membrane of the cell can be recorded by using the *whole-cell* configuration of the patch-clamp. The detailed analysis of the recordings performed from cells expressing wild-type or mutated channels allows for the identification of the molecular defects underlying a specific *CP*.

The possibility of recording the electrical activity of neurons in whole-cell configuration promoted the widespread use of brain slices, in vitro. Sections of brain tissue were first used during the1920s for metabolic studies. Only during the 1950s did electrophysiologists begin to record the membrane potential of neurons from brain sections using microelectrodes.

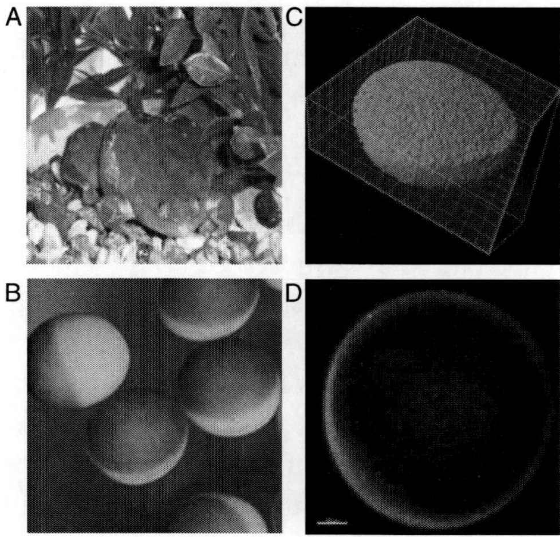

Figure 4. Xenopus laevis oocytes. (A) Picture showing a Xenopus laevis, an amphibian species native of Africa and belonging to the family of Pipidae. Often, they are erroneously called "frogs". Thousands of oocytes (B) might be collected from the ovaries of a female Xenopus. These cells may be as large as 1mm in diameter and display morphological polarity, consisting of a yellowish vegetal pole and an animal pole, which appears dark due to the presence of pigment vesicles. Such polarity is very evident in mature oocytes (stage IV-VI) which are the ones able to faithfully and efficiently translate foreign genetic information. (C) 3D reconstruction of the fluorescence surface profile of an oocyte expressing the Kv1.1-GFP (green fluorescent protein) construct, by means of confocal microscopy. (D) Fluorescence intensity, acquired at the equator, of the corresponding oocyte shown on top. This experimental procedure has been used to further investigate the surface expression pattern of ion channels.

It was soon evident that such slices provided new avenues for the study of many synaptic phenomena, including the processes involved in synaptic plasticity, and for the evaluation of the role of native ion channels and receptor subtypes in neurotransmission. The thin slice technique was developed to allow visualization of individual cells in slices less than 250μm while the thick slice technique is used in experiments where connectivity and maintenance of normal dendritic structure are crucial for study. The advent of homologous recombination has allowed for the generation of animal models of CPs, including knock-in mice, that has further boosted the exploitation of brain slices in the study of the neurological defects underlying these disorders.

EPISODIC ATAXIA TYPE 1:

Clinical Findings

EA1 [OMIM 160120] was clearly described during the mid 1970s, by Van Dyke and colleagues (Van Dyke et al., 1975). It is a CP characterized by constant myokymia and dramatic episodes of spastic contractions of the skeletal muscles of the head, arms, and legs with loss of both motor coordination and balance. During attacks some individuals may experience vertigo, blurred vision, diplopia, nausea, headache, diaphoresis, clumsiness, stiffening of the body and dysarthric speech. The duration of the attacks is brief, lasting seconds to minutes, although prolonged attacks of 5 to 12 hours have been described (Lee *et al.,* 2004). Some individuals experience severe ataxia more than 15 times per day, whereas others experience attacks less than once a month (Van Dyke et al., 1975). The first symptoms typically manifest during childhood (first or second decade of life). A specific traumatic physical or emotional event may determine the onset and worsening of the disease (Imbrici *et al.,* 2008). Attacks may be brought on by stimuli including fever, startle response, abrupt movements, vestibular caloric stimulation, emotional stress, anxiety, repeat knee bends, exercise, ingestion of caffeine, and riding a *merry-go-round.* Attacks may occur, for example, when the individual has had to suddenly alter course to avoid falling or potential collision. High temperatures that occur after a hot bath or during use of a hairdryer may also precipitate attacks (Eunson *et al.,* 2000). Whether or not interictal ataxia develops in individuals with EA1 has not been clearly reported, to date. Myokymia manifests clinically during and between attacks as fine twitching of groups of muscles and intermittent cramps and stiffness. Usually, it is evident as a fine rippling in perioral or periorbital muscles and by lateral finger movements when the hands are held in a relaxed, prone position. Episodes of intense myokymic activity during attacks without either ataxia or other neurological deficits are rarely observed. Myokymic activity is continuous. The exposure of the forearm to warm or cold temperatures may increase or decrease, respectively, the spontaneous activity recorded from a hand muscle. In some individual's myokymic activity on the EMG becomes apparent after the application of regional ischemia. Noteworthy, *Brunt and Van Weerden* observed an increase in spontaneous activity and in bursts frequency in EA1 individuals, during the first few minutes of limb ischemia, induced by an inflated sphygmomanometer. In some instances, after 5-10 min of ischemia the spontaneous discharges disappeared. By contrast, following ischemia (1-5 min) they reported a recruitment of new and large multiplets and enlargement of pre-existing complexes with extra spikes. This excess of activity began 0.5-1 min after reversal of ischemia, reached a maximum at 2-5 min and gradually declined over 10-15 min. Based on this and other evidence they proposed that these abnormal EMG responses originated peripherally (Brunt and Van Weerden 1990).

The severity of some symptoms may either improve or worsen with age. Since the first description of EA1 by Van Dyke and co-workers and the identification and characterization of mutations in the *KCNA1* gene, the phenotypic spectrum of EA1 has widened considerably. Delayed motor development, choreoathetosis, carpal spasm, clenching of the fists, and isolated neuromyotonia have been reported. Some affected individuals may also display cognitive dysfunctions that include severe receptive and expressive language delay, inability to learn to ride a bicycle, and the need to join life skill programs or attend schools for children with mild to moderate learning difficulties (Zuberi *et al.,* 1999; Demos *et al.,* 2009). Moderate muscle hypertrophy with generalized increase in muscle tone and bilateral calf hypertrophy are observed in some individuals. Neuromuscular findings secondary to the increased tone include unusual hypercontracted posture, abdominal wall muscle contraction, elbow, hip, and knee contractures and shortened Achilles tendons that may result in tiptoeing walking. Some individuals display attacks of difficulty in breathing, which can occur during ataxic episodes or as isolated episodes of an inability to inhale without wheezing (Shook *et al.,* 2008). Skeletal deformities such as scoliosis, kyphoscoliosis, high arched palate, and minor craniofacial dysmorphism have been described (Kinali *et al.,* 2004; Klein *et al.,* 2004). It is now apparent that phenotypic differences exist not only between families, but also between individuals of the same family. Tonic-clonic and partial seizures, an isolated episode consisting of photo-sensitive epilepsy (Imbrici *et al.,* 2008), as well as head-turning and eyes deviating to the same side, flickering eyelids, lip-smacking, apnoea, and cyanosis have been reported (Zuberi *et al.*, 1999). Abnormal electroencephalograms (EEGs) have been observed in individuals with EA1 (Van Dyke *et al.*, 1975; Zuberi *et al.*, 1999; Lee *et al.*, 2004). EEGs may be characterized by intermittent and generalized slow activity, frequently intermingled with spikes. Zuberi and colleagues described a 3-year-old boy who presented with an ictal EEG with rhythmical slow-wave activity over the right hemisphere, becoming spike-and-wave complexes that subsequently spread to the left hemisphere (Zuberi *et al.*, 1999). Neuromimaging with MRI is usually normal; however, a family with cerebellar atrophy has been reported (Demos *et al.*, 2009; Glaudemans et al., 2009). Typical EA1 symptoms were described for a large 5-generation Brazilian family in which 21 of 46 family members were affected (Glaudemans *et al.*, 2009). In addition, serum electrolyte levels measured during severe episodes of cramps and tetany in 2 affected family members revealed low serum magnesium with normal calcium and potassium concentrations. A younger brother of the proband had died in infancy from a severe attack of cramps and tetany, during which time his serum magnesium was as low as 0.28 mmol/l. Interestingly, intravenous magnesium administration in the proband ameliorated the paroxismal attack of facial myokymia, tremor, severe muscle spasms, muscular pain, cramps, muscular weakness, and intermittent tetanic contraction.

To establish the extent of disease in an individual diagnosed with EA1, the following evaluations are recommended: 1) detailed medical history of the individual; 2) neurologic examination; 3) initiate and witness attacks of ataxia by using either mild exercise or vestibular stimuli; 4) EMG to confirm the presence of myokymia, particularly if it is not visible on examination; 5) EEG to look for epilepsy (Zuberi *et al.*, 1999, Eunson *et al.*, 2000, Chen *et al.*, 2007). To confirm diagnosis in individuals displaying a complex phenotype, molecular genetic testing is mandatory.

Genetic Causes

EA1 is a disorder inherited in an autosomal dominant manner. Linkage studies in several EA1 families has lead to the discovery of a number of heterozygous point mutations in the voltage-dependent potassium channel gene KCNA1 (Kv1.1), on chromosome 12p13 (Figure 5; Browne et al., 1994; Browne et al., 1995; Comu et al., 1996; Litt et al., 1994; Imbrici et al., 2008). To date KCNA1 is the only gene known to be associated with EA1. Most individuals diagnosed with EA1 have an affected parent, although, one de novo mutation has been identified (Demos et al., 2009). More than 20 KCNA1 mutations have been identified by sequence analysis and are distributed throughout the gene (Figure 5).

Most are missense mutations, although, nonsense and small deletion mutations have also been identified (Eunson et al., 2000, Shook et al., 2008). Most individuals harboring a KCNA1 mutation exhibit features of EA1, nevertheless, penetrance is incomplete. Based on limited data, a disease prevalence of 1:500,000 has been proposed. The actual prevalence may well be considerably higher, as the disorder may remain either unrecognized in many families or incorrectly diagnosed.

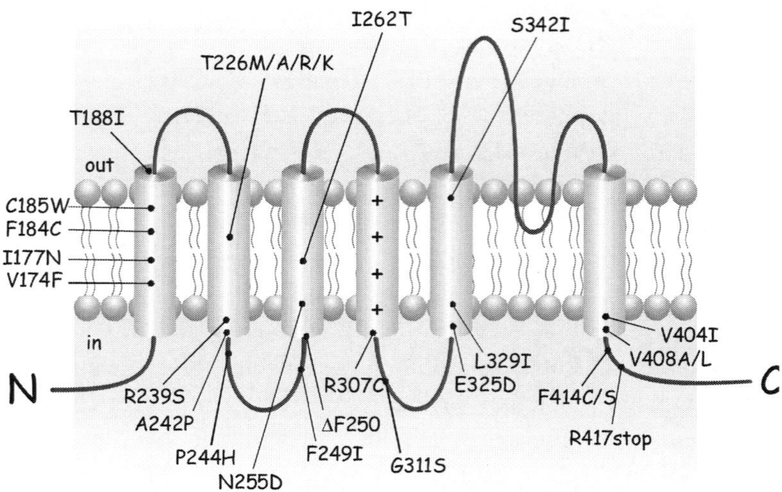

Figure 5. KCNA1 mutations identified in EA1 individuals. Cartoon showing the membrane topology of a human Kv1.1 subunit and the positions of the EA1 mutations.

The amino acid residues mutated in the Kv1.1 channel of EA1 patients, are at positions highly conserved amongst the delayed-rectifier potassium channel genes of several species from Drosophila melanogaster to humans (Browne et al., 1994). Therefore, these residues are highly conserved throughout evolution. Interestingly, four different mutations of the highly conserved threonine 226, located within the second transmembrane segment, have been identified (Rajakulendran et al., 2007). In particular, the p.Thr226Arg mutation is associated with epilepsy, infantile contractures, postural abnormalities, and skeletal deformities.

Although, the defects caused by the p.Thr226Ala, p.Thr226Arg and p.Thr226Met mutations on channel function are virtually identical, they lead to diverse phenotypes. Even identical twins harboring the same EA1 mutation displayed unexpectedly large differences in severity and frequency of attacks in a study by Graves et al, (2010). Indeed, one twin sought treatment, whereas the less severely affected twin did not require medication. These findings suggest that symptom heterogeneity among individuals harboring the same mutation reflects the interplay not only of modifier genes, but also of non- genetic factors (Graves et al., 2010). Moreover, due to such a wide interfamilial and intrafamilial phenotypic variability genotype–phenotype correlation has been extremely difficult to reliably establish (Kullmann et al., 2010).

Molecular Pathogenetic Mechanisms Underlying EA1

The molecular mechanisms underlying EA1 have been established by determining the functional properties of wild-type and several mutant channels in *Xenopus* oocytes and mammalian cell lines (Table 1; Adelman *et al.*, 1995; D'Adamo *et al.*, 1998; Zerr *et al.*, 1998; D'Adamo *et al.*, 1999; Zuberi *et al.*, 1999; Eunson *et al.*, 2000; Manganas *et al.*, 2001; Imbrici *et al.*, 2003; Cusimano *et al.*, 2004; Imbrici *et al.*, 2006; Imbrici *et al.*, 2007; Imbrici *et al.*, 2008; Imbrici *et al.*, 2009).

Table 1. Summary of the main functional defects caused by EA1 mutations

Mutation	Main functional defects compared to wild-type channels	References
V174F	Marked reduction of surface expression	Adelman et al, NEURON 1995
I177N	Reduction of surface expression with dominant negative effect, positive shift of voltage dependence	Imbrici et al, PFLUG ARCH 2003
	of activation, slower activation, faster deactivation	
F184C	Reduction of surface expression, positive shift of voltage dependence of activation, slower kinetic of	Adelman et al, NEURON 1995
	activation	
C185W		Tomlinson et al., BRAIN 2010
T226A/M	Marked reduction of surface expression, positive shift of voltage dependence of activation, slower	Zerr et al, FEBS 1998
	deactivation, slower activation	
T226R	Marked reduction of surface expression with dominant negative effect, positive shift of voltage	Zuberi et al, BRAIN 1999
	dependence of activation, slower activation, slower deactivation	
T226K	Not functional with dominant negative effect	Chen et al., NEUROGENETICS 2007
R239S	Not functional with strong dominant negative effect	Adelman et al, NEURON 1995
A242P	Marked reduction of surface expression, negative shift of voltage dependence of activation, slower	Eunson et al, ANN NEUR 2000
	activation, slower deactivation	
P244H	No differences between wild-type and mutant	Eunson et al, ANN NEUR 2000
F249I	Marked reduction of surface expression, slower deactivation	Adelman et al, NEURON 1995
ΔF250	N/A	Shook et al, MUSCLE & NERVE 2008
N255D	Not functional with dominant negative effect	Glaudemans et al, J CLIN INV 2009
I262T	N/A	Klein et al, NEUROPEDIAT 2004
R307C	Not functional with dominant negative effect, positive shift of voltage dependence of activation	Graves et al, NEUROLOGY 2010

Table 1. (Continued)

Mutation	Main functional defects compared to wild-type channels	References
G311S	Reduction of surface expression, positive shift of voltage dependence of activation, faster C-type inactivation	Zerr et al, FEBS 1998
E325D	Marked reduction of surface expression with strong dominant negative effect, 60mV positive shift of voltage dependence of activation, faster deactivation, faster activation, faster C-type inactivation	Adelman et al, NEURON 1995
L329I	N/A	Knight et al, HUM MUT 2000
S342I	N/A	Lee et al, HUM MUT 2004
V404I	Small effect on surface expression, positive shift of voltage dependence of activation, slower activation, slower deactivation	Eunson et al, ANN NEUR 2000
V408A	Faster activation and deactivation, faster C-type inactivation, faster recovery from inactivation	Adelman et al, NEURON 1995
V408L	Faster C-type inactivation	Demos et al, MOV DISORD 2009
R417stop	Not functional with dominant negative effect	Eunson et al, ANN NEUR 2000
F414C	Not functional	Imbrici et al., NEUROSCIENCE 2008
F414S	Not functional with dominant negative effect, positive shift of voltage dependence of activation	Graves et al, NEUROLOGY 2010

By studying the properties of Kv1.1 channels bearing the EA1 point mutations identified by the early genetic studies, Adelman and *co-workers* first demonstrated that EA1 subunits form channels with altered gating properties (Adelman *et al.*, 1995). In particular, they showed that V408A channels have voltage-dependence similar to that of wild-type channels, but with faster kinetics and increased C-type inactivation, while the voltage-dependence of F184C channels was shifted 20 mV positive. Individuals with EA1 are heterozygous for a *KCNA1* mutation, possessing a normal and a mutant allele, which may be equally or differently expressed. Therefore, channels composed of wild-type and mutated subunits might be formed. The heterozygous channels composed of 2 Kv1.1 wild-type and 2 mutated subunits, linked as dimers, showed gating properties intermediate between channels formed from four normal or four mutated subunits at both whole-cell and single channel level (D'Adamo *et al.*, 1998). These results indicated that the degree of impairment of the delayed rectifier function of affected neurons is related to the type and number of mutated subunits which make up the tetrameric Kv1.1 channels (D'Adamo *et al.*, 1998). Co-expression experiments have also shown that some mutant subunits exert dominant negative effects on wild-type subunits, resulting in less than half the normal current, whereas others have virtually no effect. (Zerr *et al.*, 1998; D'Adamo *et al.*, 1999, Rea *et al.*, 2002, Imbrici *et al.*, 2006, 2011; Graves *et al.*, 2010).

Overall, these studies have demonstrated that allelic variations underlying EA1 impair channel function and reduce the outward K^+ flux through the channel, although with highly variable effects on aspects of channel expression and gating. Kv1.1, Kv1.2 and Kv1.4 are the most abundant subunits expressed in the central nervous system and are assembled to form heteromeric channels composed of Kv1.1/Kv1.2 and Kv1.1/Kv1.4 subunits. The functional effects of EA1 mutations on the properties of these channel types have been thoroughly investigated. These studies demonstrated that the human Kv1.2 and Kv1.1 subunits co-assemble to form a novel channel with distinct gating properties which are remarkably altered by EA1 mutations. In particular, the V408A and E325D subunits combine with Kv1.2 to produce channels with altered kinetics of activation, deactivation, C-type inactivation and voltage-dependence (D'Adamo *et al.*, 1999). Kv1.4 co-assembles with Kv1.1 and confers fast N-type inactivating properties to resulting heteromeric channels. It has been shown that EA1 mutations which have normal surface expression, reduce the rate of inactivation by a decreased affinity for the inactivation domain while the mutations which have reduced subunit surface expression, increase the rate of N-type inactivation due to a stoichiometric increase in the number of Kv1.4 subunits (Imbrici *et al.*, 2011). Thus, subunit surface expression may affect in opposite ways distinct functional properties of the channel. Overall, these studies have also demonstrated that allelic variations in a single gene (*KCNA1*) also alter the function of other proteins that interact with Kv1.1. These mechanisms are expected to broaden the spectrum of the defects caused by even very subtle mutations.

The effects of Zn^{2+} ions on hippocampal excitability is controversial. Chelation of zinc by diethyldithiocarbamate facilitates bursting in CA3 pyramidal cells (Xu and Mitchell, 1993), while granule cell epileptiform activity is facilitated by recurrent mossy fiver-released zinc (Timofeeva and Nadler, 2006). On the other hand, lack of vesicular zinc in mossy fibers does not affect synaptic excitability of CA3 pyramidal cells in zinc transporter 3 knockout mice (Lopantsev et al., 2003).

All boutons of mossy fibers contain Zn^{2+} in the pre-synaptic vesicles. Zn^{2+} concentration in these vesicles is high and it has been estimated at approximately 300 μM (Frederickson et al., 1983). The release of Zn^{2+} into the synaptic cleft modulates the activity of selected members of ligand-gated and voltage-gated ion channels including Kv1. Indeed, we have shown that channels composed of Kv1.1/Kv1.4 and Kvβ1.1 subunits possesses a high affinity (<10 μM) and a low affinity (<0.5 mM) site for Zn^{2+} ions. The EA1 mutation F184C decreased the equilibrium dissociation constants for Zn^{2+} binding to both the high affinity and low affinity sites markedly.

This study suggested that during the vesicular release of Zn^{2+} its effects would be additional to the intrinsic gating defects caused by the mutation and likely exacerbate the symptoms by impairing the integration and transmission of signals within distinct brain areas such as the hippocampus (Imbrici et al., 2007).

These effects may also underlie the cognitive deficits observed in some individuals. Nevertheless, exactly how these defects contribute to signaling dysfunctions, which will manifest with distinct consequences in multiple neural networks in which Kv1.1 channels contain Kv1.2 or Kv1.4 subunits, is mostly unclear. The causes that trigger the paroxysms of ataxia also remain elusive, although, a phenomenon akin to *spreading acidification of the cerebellar cortex* has been suggested (Chen *et al.*, 1999; Ebner and Chen, 2003; Chen *et al.*, 2005).

Animal Models of EA1

By inserting the heterozygous p.Val408Ala mutation in one *Kv1.1* allele, a mouse model of EA1 has been generated that recapitulates the disease. In particular, a procedure that mimics stress-fear responses induced motor dysfunctions in $Kv1.1^{V408A/+}$ animals similar to EA1 (Herson *et al.*, 2003). The p.Val408Ala is a homozygous-lethal mutation that causes embryonic death between E3-E9. Conversely, heterozygous $Kv1.1^{V408A/+}$ animals are viable and displayed increased frequency and amplitude of spontaneous GABA$_A$ inhibitory post synaptic currents (IPSCs) at cerebellar basket cell–Purkinje cell synapse compared to wild-type $Kv1.1^{+/+}$ mice (Herson *et al.*, 2003). This evidence accords with previously postulated pathogenetic mechanisms of EA1 (D'Adamo *et al.*, 1999) and with a report showing that α–DTX, a blocker of *Kv1.1/Kv1.2* channels, increases both the amplitude and frequency of spontaneous IPSCs mediated by GABA release from basket cell presynaptic terminals (Southan and Robertson 1998). This evidence clearly demonstrated that p.Val408Ala mutation causes dysfunctions in a CNS circuitry that may underlie the cerebellar symptoms of the disease. Kv1.1 channels are normally present at juxtaparanodal regions of sciatic nerves but absent at both the end-plate and muscle fibers (Arroyo *et al.*, 1999; Vacher *et al.*, 2008; Zhou *et al.*, 1998). By using *in vivo* preparations of *lateral gastrocnemius* nerve–muscle from $Kv1.1^{+/+}$ and $Kv1.1^{V408A/+}$ mice, we observed that the mutant animals display spontaneous *myokymic*–like discharges consisting of repeated singlets, duplets or multiplets. This bursting activity was exacerbated by either single nerve stimulus or stresses, such as fatigue, ischemia and lower temperatures (*report submitted for publication*). The distinct expression of *Kv1.1* in axonal structures and the fact that spontaneous discharges are present despite severing the motor nerve supplying the $Kv1.1^{V408A/+}$ muscle indicates that sciatic nerve is certainly a site of origin of anomalous re-excitation. This represents a more clear indication that myokymic activity in EA1 patients originates also from hyper-excitability of the peripheral nerve endings. This conclusion is consistent with previous studies from patients and animal models of EA1. Indeed, patients manifesting EA1 symptoms, including neuromyotonia or myokymia, and harboring different *KCNA1* mutations displayed 100% higher axonal superexcitability compared to healthy controls (Tomlinson *et al.*, 2010). The possible mechanisms underlying myokymia/neuromyotonia have been investigated by using mice from which the *Kv1.1* gene was deleted. This genetic manipulation produces only small changes in the excitability of the nerve trunk. It is only when the nerve terminal is approached that the impact of the absence of *Kv1.1* channels becomes dramatic. In fact, *Kv1.1* ablation causes repetitive neuronal activity in the phrenic nerve in mouse resulting from both spontaneous and stimulus-evoked nerve-backfiring at preterminal axon transition zones, where axons change from myelinated to non-myelinated (Smart *et al.*, 1998; Zhou *et al.*, 1998; Zhou *et al.*, 1999; Vabnick *et al.*, 1999). This scenario is consistent also with computer simulations showing that lack of juxtaparanodal *Kv1.1* channels leads to reentrant excitation of nodes due to nerve backfiring at axon transition zones in myelinated nerve terminals (Zhou *et al.*, 1999). This abnormal transmission of signals observed in the phrenic nerve of Kv1.1 null mice may underlie the respiratory symptoms reported in some EA1 individuals who display attacks of difficulty in breathing, which can occur during ataxic episodes or as isolated episodes of inability to inhale without wheezing (Shook *et al.*, 2008).

Treatment of EA1

To reduce the frequency and severity of the attacks in EA1 patients *acetazolamide* (ACTZ), a carbonic-anhydrase (CA) inhibitor, has been used. The recommended starting dosage is 125 mg once a day, given orally. However, individuals with good renal function may require higher daily doses, ranging from 8 to 30 mg/kg/day in one to four divided doses. The total amount of drug prescribed should not exceed 1 gram per day. ACTZ treatment should be avoided in individuals with liver, renal, or adrenal insufficiency. Chronic treatment with ACTZ may result in side effects including paresthesias, rash, and formation of renal calculi. Several patients are not responsive to ACTZ. The mechanism by which ACTZ reduces the frequency and severity of the attacks is unclear. It has been proposed that ACTZ may act by modulating intracellular pH or HCO_3^- gradient. Interestingly, stress-induced motor dysfunctions in $Kv1.1^{V408A/+}$ animals are ameliorated by ACTZ (Herson *et al.*, 2003). Antiepileptic drugs may significantly reduce the frequency of the attacks in responsive individuals. *Diphenylhydantoin* treatment at a dose of 150-300 mg daily resulted in reasonable control of seizures in some individuals (Van Dyke *et al.*, 1975). However, the response is heterogeneous, as some individuals are particularly resistant to drugs (Eunson *et al.*, 2000). *Phenytoin* treatment at a dose of 3.7 mg/kg/day may improve muscle stiffness and motor performance (Kinali *et al.*, 2004). Nevertheless, phenytoin should be used with caution in young individuals, as it may cause permanent cerebellar dysfunction and atrophy (De Marco *et al.*, 2003).

The attack rate may be reduced by *sulthiame* 50-200 mg daily. During this treatment abortive attacks lasting a few seconds were still noticed. Paresthesias and intermitted carpal spasm were the troublesome side effects observed in patients. Finally, *carbamazepine* up to 1600 mg daily has been prescribed to ameliorate EA1 symptoms (Eunson *et al.*, 2000). However, the dose needs to be adjusted according to different factors including age, weight, the particular carbamazepine product being used, responsiveness of the individual, and other medications s/he is taking.

BRIEF OVERVIEW OF RELATED ATAXIA DISORDERS

Episodic ataxia type 2 (EA2) [OMIM 108500] is characterized by paroxysmal attacks of ataxia, vertigo, and nausea typically lasting minutes to days in duration. Stress, exertion, caffeine and alcohol may trigger attacks that can be associated with dysarthria, diplopia, tinnitus, dystonia, hemiplegia, and headache. About 50% of individuals with EA2 have migraine headaches. Onset is typically in childhood or early adolescence. MRI can demonstrate atrophy of the cerebellar vermis. EA2 is inherited in an autosomal dominant manner. The symptom that might distinguish EA2 from EA1 is interictal nystagmus. The attacks of EA2 may be prevented by treatment with acetazolamide. The locus for EA2 was mapped to chromosome 19p13 by linkage studies (Kramer *et al.*, 1995; Von Brederlow *et al.*, 1995; Teh *et al.*, 1995). The initial mutation analysis of EA2 families revealed two mutations in the *CACNL1A4* gene, which encodes for the α_{1A}-subunit of P/Q-type Ca^{++} channels ($Ca_v2.1$; Ophoff *et al.*, 1996): a basepair deletion, that resulted in a frame-shift and in the formation of a premature stop codon, and a splice-site mutation. The detailed pathophysiological mechanisms of this neurologic disease remain poorly understood (Jen, 1999).

Two other neurological diseases result from mutations in the same *CACNL1A4* gene. Spinocerebellar ataxia type 6 (SCA6) an autosomal dominant disorder characterized by ataxia, nystagmus and cerebellar degeneration. Affected individuals are eventually confined to a wheelchair. The genotypic analysis of a number of SCA6 patients revealed an expansion of CAG repeats in the *CACNL1A4* gene. The resulting Poly-Q repeat is located within the C-terminal region of the $Ca_v2.1$ channel (Zhuchenko *et al.*, 1997). The *leaner mice (Cacna1a $^{tg-la}$)* can be regarded as a mouse model of EA2. Their phenotype is characterized by severe ataxia, stiffness, retarded motor activity, neurodegeneration of the cerebellum (loss of Golgi, Purkinje and granule neurons) and typical intermittent seizures that resemble absence epilepsy. A splice site mutation has been found in the *CACNL1A* gene of learner mice resulting in a great decrease of $Ca_v2.1$ current density (Fletcher *et al.*, 1996; Dove *et al.*, 1998). The reduction in calcium currents that results from this genetic mutation appears to be a key determinant of cerebellar neurodegeneration.

Episodic ataxia type 3 (EA3) [OMIM 606552] has been described in two Caucasian families from rural North Carolina by Farmer and Mustian (1963) and Vance *et al.*, (1984). A relationship between the two kindreds is suspected but has not been established. EA3 is characterized by attacks of vertigo, diplopia, and ataxia beginning in early adulthood. In some individuals, slowly progressive cerebellar ataxia occurs. This condition does not link to loci identified with EA1, EA2, or spinocerebellar ataxia types 1, 2, 3, 4, and 5. A candidate region on chromosome 1q42 has been identified (Cader *et al.*, 2005).

Episodic ataxia type 4 (EA4) [OMIM 606554] has been described in a large Canadian Mennonite family (Steckley *et al.*, 2001). EA4 is also known as familial periodic vestibulocerebellar ataxia and is characterized by brief ACTZ-responsive attacks of vestibular ataxia, vertigo, tinnitus, and interictal myokymia. Interictal nystagmus, and ataxia were not identified. The age of onset is variable. The gene defect that underlies EA4 is unknown and it does not link to the EA1 or EA2 loci.

Episodic ataxia type 5 (EA5) [OMIM 601949] can result from a mutation in the *CACNB4* gene which encodes the beta-4 isoform of the regulatory beta subunit of voltage-activated Ca^{2+} channels. A c.311G>T (p.Cys104Phe; reference sequences NM_000726.3; NP_000717.2) mutation has been described in a French-Canadian family (Escayg *et al.*, 2000). The phenotype was characterized by recurrent episodes of vertigo and ataxia that lasted for several hours. Interictal examination showed spontaneous downbeat and gaze-evoked nystagmus and mild dysarthria and truncal ataxia. Acetazolamide prevented the attacks. EA5 is allelic with juvenile myoclonic epilepsy (JME); the semiology of seizures in EA5 is similar to JME. Episodic ataxia type 6 (EA6) [OMIM 612656] is characterized by attacks of ataxia precipitated by fever, subclinical seizures, slurred speech followed by headache, and bouts of arm jerking with concomitant confusion and alternating hemiplegia.

EA6 can result from mutations in the gene *SLC1A3*, which encodes the excitatory amino acid transporter 1 (EAAT1). In cells expressing mutated proteins, glutamate uptake is reduced, suggesting that glutamate transporter dysfunction underlies the disease (Jen *et al.*, 2005, de Vries *et al.*, 2009).

Episodic ataxia type 7 (EA7) [OMIM 611907] has been described in a 4-generation family whose affected individuals showed episodic ataxia before age 20 years (Kerber *et al.*, 2007). The disease is characterized by attacks associated with weakness, vertigo, and dysarthria lasting hours to days. Attacks may be brought about by exercise and excitement. A candidate region, termed the *EA7* locus, on chromosome 19q13 has been identified (Kerber *et al.*, 2007).

Autosomal dominant spastic ataxia (ADSA) [OMIM 108600]. Affected individuals initially show progressive leg spasticity of variable degrees followed by ataxia in the form of involuntary head jerk, dysarthria, dysphagia, and ocular movement abnormalities. The age at onset was from early childhood to early twenties. Linkage studies identified a locus on 12p13, termed *SAX1* (Meijer et al., 2002). Familial paroxysmal kinesigenic dyskinesia (PKD) [OMIM 128200; 611031] is characterized by attacks lasting a few seconds to hours of dystonia, choreoathetosis, and ballism that are sometimes preceded by an aura and precipitated by sudden movements, cold, hyperventilation, and mental tension. Attacks can be as frequent as 100 per day to as few as one per month and the age of onset is typically in childhood (Bruno *et al.*, 2004). Familial PKD is inherited in an autosomal dominant manner; however, the gene/s associated with PKD have not been identified. Linkage of familial PKD to 16q11.2-q22.1 has been established in several families PKD (Tomita *et al.*, 1999, Bennett *et al.*, 2000, Valente *et al.*, 2000).

Familial paroxysmal non-kinesigenic dyskinesia (PNKD) [OMIM 118800; 609023] is characterized by attacks of dystonia, chorea, ballismus, or athetosis provoked by alcohol, caffeine, excitement, stress, or fatigue. Attacks are not typically triggered by movement, may be accompanied by a preceding aura, last minutes to hours, and rarely occur more than once per day. Age of onset is typically in childhood or early teens. Familial PNKD is inherited in an autosomal dominant manner and the gene encoding myofibrillogenesis regulator 1 is the only gene known to be associated with this disease (Lee *et al.*, 2004, Rainier *et al.*, 2004, Chen *et al.*, 2005). A second locus for familial PNKD has been identified on chromosome 2q31 in a Canadian family of European decent (Spacey *et al.*, 2006). Isaac's syndrome (Acquired neuromyotonia, NMT) is a rare neuromuscular disorder characterized by hyperexcitability of the motor nerve that results in continuously contracting or twitching muscles (myokymia) and muscle hypertrophy. Individuals also experience cramping, increased sweating, and delayed muscle relaxation. Stiffness is most prominent in limb and trunk muscles. Symptoms are not usually triggered by exercise and occur even during sleep or when individuals are under general anesthesia. A few affected individuals report sleep disorders, anxiety, and memory loss (Morvan's syndrome). Onset is between 15 and 60 years of age. The acquired form occasionally develops in association with peripheral neuropathies or after radiation treatment. Twenty per cent of affected individuals have an associated thymoma. Antibodies to voltage-gated potassium channels are detected in approximately 40% of affected individuals (Hart *et al.*, 2002). It has been shown that antibodies bind variably to the Kv1.1 and 1.2-containing juxtaparanodes of peripheral and central myelinated axons (Kleopa *et al.*, 2006). Mutations in two other genes *KCNQ2* and *KCNQ3* that encode potassium channels were identified in families with dominantly inherited benign familial neonatal convulsions (BFNC). *KCNQ2* and *KCNQ3* encode Kv7.2 and Kv7.3, respectively, which co-assemble to form a slowly activated channel that is closed by the activation of M1 muscarinic receptors. The spectrum of the CP associated with *KCNQ2* has broadened with the identification of dominant-negative mutations that neutralize voltage-sensing residues in the S4 segment of Kv7.2. This results in a shift in activation threshold to more depolarized potentials. These mutations cause spontaneous motor-unit activity (*that manifests as myokymia*) in addition to neonatal seizures, consistent with the expression of Kv7.2 in motoneurons. Missense mutations of *KCNC3*, which encodes the Kv3.3 channel subunit, cause a dominantly inherited progressive ataxia (spinocerebellar ataxia type 13 or *SCA13*). Paroxysmal symptoms are not prominent, which is unusual for a CP. Although the channel is expressed in the cerebellum, the two identified mutations appear to have opposite effects on channel function, which precludes a simple explanation for the disease. A dominant missense mutation in the *KCNMA1* gene is associated with paroxysmal dyskinesia and epilepsy in one large kindred. This gene encodes the ubiquitous neuronal BK Ca^{2+}-activated potassium channel, which opens in response to cytoplasmic Ca^{2+} and helps to repolarize neurons after action potentials. Surprisingly, the mutation increases Ca^{2+} sensitivity and allows the channel to open at more negative potentials. It is thus another exception to the general principle that only *loss-of-function* potassium channel mutations cause seizures (Sicca *et al.*, 2011).

CONCLUSION

Although important advances have been made in understanding the pathophysiology of EA1 and other ataxia syndromes some crucial information still remains elusive. The central and peripheral neurological alterations resulting in ataxia symptoms are unclear. What determines the episodic nature of ataxia and of common paroxysomal disorders, including idiopathic epilepsy and migraine is mostly unknown. Why attacks are triggered by physiological stresses that stimulate otherwise normal responses in healthy subjects is also not understood. Finding an answer to all these puzzling questions will be the challenge of future studies. By using higher resolution technologies biophysicists are shedding new light on the molecular machinery of channel gating. The knowledge resulting from these studies is crucial to directing an exhaustive biophysical characterization of variants associated with CPs that, in turn, will allow for the full understanding of how mutations in ion channel genes cause the disease. Additionally, we need to know the normal location and function of the channel subunits and how they contribute to cell or circuit excitability. Physiologists using cutting edge biotechnologies, ion channel blockers and activators and genetically engineered mouse strains are continuously discovering novel roles played by ion channels and by the many gene products of unknown function which result from the disclosure of the human genome. This valuable knowledge combined with the detailed genetic, behavioral and electrophysiological analysis of mice carrying naturally or artificially introduced mutations in their ion channel genes is currently providing important information about the causes of several human diseases. Certainly, research on CPs is important in identifying signaling pathways and circuits involved in these diseases and in finding novel pharmacological interventions to ameliorate the symptoms.

More broadly, however, they help in understanding the functional properties of these proteins. As stated by *Shirley Bryant*, a pioneer in ion channel diseases, *"of the many mutations that have occurred over millions of years, the ones that resulted in disease must point to a functionally important part of the protein."* Accordingly, a mutation that results in overt phenotype must affect important body functions. Thus, understanding these experiments or mistakes that *Nature* has made will help to identify the physiological workings of the human body.

ACKNOWLEDGMENTS

Correspondence should be addressed to: cdadamo@unipg.it and pessia@unipg.it. This work was supported by COMPAGNIA di San Paolo (Turin) *"Programma Neuroscienze"*, Telethon (GGP11188) and Fondazione Cassa di Risparmio di Perugia.

Ricerca realizzata con il sostegno della

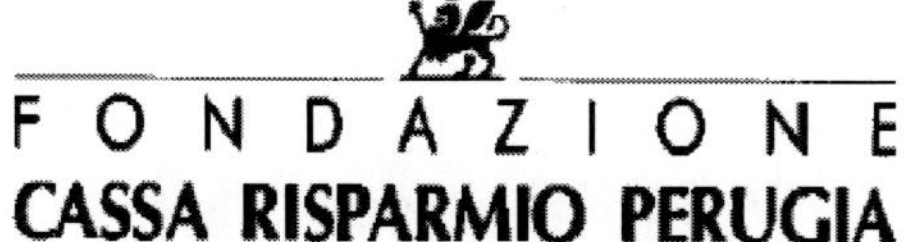

REFERENCES

Adelman JP, Bond CT, Pessia M, Maylie J. (1995) Episodic ataxia results from voltage-dependent potassium channels with altered functions. *Neuron* 15: 1449-1454.

Aldrich RW Jr, Getting PA, Thompson SH. (1979) Mechanism of frequency-dependent broadening of molluscan neurone soma spikes. *J. Physiol.* 291: 531-544.

Arroyo EJ, Xu YT, Zhou L, Messing A, Peles E, Chiu SY and Scherer SS (1999). Myelinating Schwann cells determine the internodal localization of Kv1.1, Kv1.2, Kvbeta2, and Caspr. J. Neurocytol. 28: 333-47.

Baukrowitz T, Yellen G. (1995) Modulation of K+ current by frequency and external [K+]: a tale of two inactivation mechanisms. Neuron 15: 951-960.

Bennett LB, Roach ES, Bowcock AM. (2000)A locus for paroxysmal kinesigenic dyskinesia maps to human chromosome 16. *Neurology* 54: 125–30.

Browne DL, Gancher ST, Nutt JG, Brunt ER, Smith EA, Kramer P, Litt M. (1994) Episodic ataxia/myokymia syndrome is associated with point mutations in the human potassium channel gene, KCNA1. Nat. *Genet.* 8: 136-140.

Browne DL, Brunt ER, Griggs RC, Nutt JG, Gancher ST, Smith EA, Litt M. Identification of two new KCNA1 mutations in episodic ataxia/myokymia families. *Hum. Mol. Genet.* 4: 1671–1672, 1995.

Bruno MK, Hallett M, Gwinn-Hardy K, Sorensen B, Considine E, Tucker S, Lynch DR, Mathews KD, Swoboda KJ, Harris J, Soong BW, Ashizawa T, Jankovic J, Renner D, Fu

YH, Ptacek LJ. Clinical evaluation of idiopathic paroxysmal kinesigenic dyskinesia: new diagnostic criteria. *Neurology.* 2004; 63: 2280–7.

Brunt ERP, van Weerden TW. (1990) Familial paroxysmal kinesigenic ataxia and continuous myokymia. *Brain* 113: 1361-1382.

Cader M, Steckley J, Dyment D, McLachlan R, Ebers G (2005) A genome-wide screen and linkage mapping for a large pedigree with episodic ataxia. *Neurology* 65:156–8.

Chen G, Hanson CL, Dunbar RL, Ebner TJ. (1999)Novel form of spreading acidification and depression in the cerebellar cortex demonstrated by neutral red optical imaging. J. Neurophysiol. Apr;81(4):1992-8.

Chen G, Gao W, Reinert KC, Popa LS, Hendrix CM, Ross ME, Ebner TJ. (2005) Involvement of kv1 potassium channels in spreading acidification and depression in the cerebellar cortex. J. Neurophysiol. Aug;94(2):1287-98.

Chen DH, Matsushita M, Rainier S, Meaney B, Tisch L, Feleke A, Wolff J, Lipe H, Fink J, Bird TD, Raskind WH. Presence of alanine-to-valine substitutions in myofibrillogenesis regulator 1 in paroxysmal non-kinesigenic dyskinesia: confirmation in 2 kindreds. *Arch. Neurol.* 2005; 62: 597–600.

Chen H, von Hehn C, Kaczmarek LK, Ment LR, Pober BR, Hisama FM (2007) Functional analysis of a novel potassium channel (KCNA1) mutation in hereditary myokymia. *Neurogenetics* 8:131-5.

Comu S, Giuliani M, Narayanan V. Episodic ataxia and myokymia syndrome: a new mutation of potassium channel gene Kv1.1. *Ann. Neurol.* Oct;40(4):684-7, 1996.

Cusimano A, D'Adamo MC, Pessia M (2004) An episodic ataxia type-1 mutation in the S1 segment sensitises the hKv1.1 potassium channel to extracellular Zn2+ *FEBS. Lett* 576:237-44.

D'Adamo MC, Imbrici P, Sponcichetti F, Pessia M. (1999) Mutations in the KCNA1 gene associated with episodic ataxia type-1 syndrome impair heteromeric voltage-gated K+ channel function. *FASEB J.* 13: 1335-1345.

D'Adamo MC, Liu Z, Adelman JP, Maylie J, Pessia M. (1998) Episodic ataxia type-1 mutations in the hKv1.1 cytoplasmic pore region alter the gating properties of the channel. *EMBO J.* 17: 1200-1207.

De Marco FA, Ghizoni E, Kobayashi E, Li LM, Cendes F (2003) Cerebellar volume and long-term use of phenytoin. *Seizure* 12:312-15.

Demos MK, Macri V, Farrell K, Nelson TN, Chapman K, Accili E, Armstrong L (2009) A novel KCNA1 mutation associated with global delay and persistent cerebellar dysfunction. *Mov. Disord.* 24:778-82.

de Vries B, Mamsa H, Stam AH, Wan J, Bakker SLM, Vanmolkot KRJ, Haan J, Terwindt GM, Boon EMJ, Howard BD, Frants RR, Baloh RW, Ferrari MD, Jen JC, van den Maagdenberg AMJM (2009) Episodic ataxia associated with EAAT1 mutation C186S affecting glutamate reuptake. *Arch. Neurol.* 66:97-101.

Dove LS, Abbott LC, Griffith WH. (1998) Whole-cell and single-channel analysis of P-type calcium currents in cerebellar Purkinje cells of leaner mutant mice. *J. Neurosci.* 18: 7687-7699.

Doyle DA, Morais Cabral J, Pfuetzner RA, Kuo A, Gulbis JM, Cohen SL, Chait BT, Mackinnon R. (1998) The structure of the potassium channel: molecular basis of K^{+} conduction and selectivity. *Science* 280: 69-77.

Ebner TJ, Chen G. 2003Spreading acidification and depression in the cerebellar cortex. Neuroscientist. Feb;9(1):37-45.

Escayg A, De Waard M, Lee DD, Bichet D, Wolf P, Mayer T, Johnston J, Baloh R, Sander T, Meisler MH (2000) Coding and non-coding variation of the human calcium-channel beta4-subunit gene CACNB4 in patients with idiopathic generalized epilepsy and episodic ataxia. *Am. J. Hum. Genet* 66:1531-9.

Eunson LH, Rea R, Zuberi SM, Youroukos S, Panayiotopoulos CP, Liguori R, Avoni P, McWilliam RC, Stephenson JB, Hanna MG, Kullmann DM, Spauschus A. (2000) Clinical, genetic, and expression studies of mutations in the potassium channel gene KCNA1 reveal new phenotypic variability. *Ann. Neurol.* 48: 647-656.

Farmer TW, Mustian VM (1963) Vestibulo-cerebellar ataxia: a newly defined hereditary syndrome with periodic manifestations. *Arch. Neurol.* 8:471-80.

Fletcher CF, Lutz CM, O'Sullivan TN, Shaughnessy JD Jr, Hawkes R, Frankel WN, Copeland NG, Jenkins NA. (1996) Absence epilepsy in tottering mutant mice is associated with calcium channel defects. *Cell* 87: 607-617.

Frederickson CJ. (1989) Neurobiology of zinc and zinc-containing neurons. Int. Rev. Neurobiol. 31:145-238.

Geiger JR, Jonas P (2000) Dynamic control of presynaptic Ca(2+) inflow by fast-inactivating K(+) channels in hippocampal mossy fiber boutons. *Neuron* 28:927-39.

Glaudemans B, van der Wijst J, Scola RH, Lorenzoni PJ, Heister A, van der Kemp AW, Knoers NV, Hoenderop JG, Bindels RJ (2009) A missense mutation in the Kv1.1 voltage-gated potassium channel-encoding gene KCNA1 is linked to human autosomal dominant hypomagnesemia. *J. Clin. Invest.* 119:936-42.

Goldberg EM, Clark BD, Zagha E, Nahmani M, Erisir A, Rudy B. K+ channels at the axon initial segment dampen near-threshold excitability of neocortical fast-spiking GABAergic interneurons. *Neuron.* May 8;58(3):387-400, 2008.

Graves TD, Rajakulendran S, Zuberi SM, Morris HR, Schorge S, Hanna MG, Kullmann DM. Nongenetic factors influence severity of episodic ataxia type 1 in monozygotic twins. *Neurology* 75: 367-372, 2010.

Grissmer S, Cahalan M. (1989) TEA prevents inactivation while blocking open K+ channels in human T lymphocytes. *Biophys. J.* 55: 203-206.

Gutman GA, Chandy KG. (1993) Nomenclature of mammalian voltage-dependent potassium channel genes. *Semin. Neurosci.* 5: 101-106.

Hart IK, Maddison P, Newsom-Davis J, Vincent A, Mills KR (2002) Phenotypic variants of autoimmune peripheral nerve hyperexcitability. *Brain* 125:887-95.

Hamill OP, Marty A, Neher E, Sakmann B, Sigworth FJ. (1981) Improved patch-clamp techniques for high-resolution current recording from cells and cell-free membrane patches. *Pflugers Arch.* 391: 85-100.

Herson PS, Virk M, Rustay NR, Bond CT, Crabbe JC, Adelman JP, Maylie J (2003). A mouse model of episodic ataxia type-1. *Nat. Neurosci.* 6, 378–383.

Hille B. (2001) Ionic Channels of Excitable Membranes , 3rd. Sinauer, Sunderland, MA.

Hodgkin AL, Huxley AF. (1952) A quantitative description of membrane current and its application to conduction and excitation in nerve. *J. Physiol.* 117: 500-544.

Hoshi T, Zagotta WN, Aldrich RW. (1990) Biophysical and molecular mechanisms of Shaker potassium channel inactivation. *Science* 250: 533-538.

Hoshi T, Zagotta WN, Aldrich RW. (1991) Two types of inactivation in Shaker K+ channels: effects of alterations in the carboxy-terminal region. *Neuron* 7: 547-556.

Imbrici P, Cusimano A, D'Adamo MC, De Curtis A, Pessia M (2003) Functional characterization of an episodic ataxia type-1 mutation occurring in the S1 segment of hKv1.1 channels. *Pflugers Arch.* 446:373-79.

Imbrici P, D'Adamo MC, Kullmann DM, Pessia M (2006) Episodic Ataxia Type 1 Mutations in the KCNA1 Gene Impair the Fast Inactivation Properties of the Human K$^+$ Channels Kv1.4-1.1/Kv□1.1 and Kv1.4-1.1/Kv□1.2. *Eur. J. Neurosci.* 24:3073-83.

Imbrici P, D'Adamo MC, Cusimano A, Pessia M (2007) Episodic ataxia type 1 mutation F184C alters Zn2+-induced modulation of the human K+ channel Kv1.4-Kv1.1/Kvbeta1.1. *Am. J. Physiol. Cell Physiol.* 292:C778-87

Imbrici P, Gualandi F, D'Adamo MC, Taddei Masieri M, Cudia P, De Grandis D, Mannucci R, Nicoletti I, Tucker SJ, Ferlini A, Pessia M (2008) *A Novel KCNA1 Mutation Identified in an Italian Family Affected by Episodic Ataxia Type 1. Neuroscience* 157:577-87.

Imbrici P, Grottesi A, D'Adamo MC, Mannucci R, Tucker S, Pessia M (2009) Contributions of the central hydrophobic residue in the PXP motif of Voltage-Dependent K$^+$ Channels to S6 flexibility and Gating Properties. *Channels (Austin)* 3:39-45.

Imbrici P, D'Adamo MC, Grottesi A, Biscarini A, Pessia M. (2011) Episodic ataxia type 1 mutations affect fast inactivation of K+ channels by a reduction in either subunit surface expression or affinity for inactivation domain. *Am. J. Physiol. Cell Physiol.* Jun;300(6):C1314-22.

Isacoff EY, Jan NY, Jan LY. (1990) Evidence for the formation of heteromultimeric potassium channels in Xenopus oocytes. *Nature* 345: 530-534.

Jan YN, Jan LY, Dennis MJ. (1977) Two mutations of synaptic transmission in Drosophila. Proc. R. Soc. Lond. B *Biol. Sci.* 198: 87-108.

Jen J. (1999) Calcium channelopathies in the central nervous system. Curr. Opin. Neurobiol. 9: 274-280.

Jen JC, Wan J, Palos TP, Howard BD, Baloh RW (2005) Mutation in the glutamate transporter EAAT1 causes episodic ataxia, hemiplegia, and seizures. *Neurology* 65:529-34.

Jiang Y, Lee A, Chen J, Ruta V, Cadene M, Chait BT, MacKinnon R. (2003a) X-ray structure of a voltage-dependent K+ channel. *Nature* 423: 33-41.

Jiang Y, Ruta V, Chen J, Lee A, MacKinnon R. (2003b) The principle of gating charge movement in a voltage-dependent K+ channel. *Nature* 423: 42-8.

KaplanWD, Trout WE. (1969) The behaviour of four neurological mutants of Drosophila. *Genetics* 61: 399-409.

Kerber KA, Jen JC, Lee H, Nelson SF, Baloh RW (2007) A new episodic ataxia syndrome with linkage to chromosome 19q13. *Arch. Neurol.* 64:749-52

Kinali M, Jungbluth H, Eunson LH, Sewry CA, Manzur AY, Mercuri E, Hanna MG and Muntoni F (2004). Expanding the phenotype of potassium channelopathy: severe neuromyotonia and skeletal deformities without prominent episodic ataxia. *Neuromuscul. Disord.* 14, 689–693.

Klein A, Boltshauser E, Jen J, Baloh RW (2004) Episodic ataxia type 1 with distal weakness: a novel manifestation of a potassium channelopathy. *Neuropediatrics* 35:147-9.

Kleopa KA, Elman LB, Lang B, Vincent A, Scherer SS (2006) Neuromyotonia and limbic encephalitis sera target mature Shaker-type K+ channels: subunit specificity correlates with clinical manifestations. *Brain* 129:1570-84.

Kramer PL, Yue Q, Gancher ST, Nutt JG, Baloh R, Smith E, Browne D, Bussey K, Lovrien K, Nelson S, Litt M. (1995) A locus for the nystagmus-associated form of episodic ataxia maps to an 11cM region on chromosome 19p. *Am. J. Hum. Genet.* 57: 182-185.

Kullmann DM (2010). Neurological channelopathies. Ann Rev Neurosci 33, 151-72. Llano I, Tan YP and Caputo C (1997). Spatial heterogeneity of intracellular Ca2+ signals in axons of basket cells from rat cerebellar slices. J. Physiol. 502, 509-19.

Lau D, Vega-Saenz de Miera EC, Contreras D, Ozaita A, Harvey M, Chow A, Noebels JL, Paylor R, Morgan JI, Leonard CS, Rudy B. (2000) Impaired fast-spiking, suppressed cortical inhibition, and increased susceptibility to seizures in mice lacking Kv3.2 K+ channel proteins. J. Neurosci. 15;20(24):9071-85.

Laube G, Roper J, Pitt JC, Sewing S, Kistner U, Garner CC, Pongs O, Veh RW. (1996) Ultrastructural localization of Shaker-related potassium channel subunits and synapse-associated protein 90 to separate-like junctions in rat cerebellar Pinceaux. *Brain Res. Mol. Brain Res.* 42: 51-61.

Lee HY, Xu Y, Huang Y, Ahn AH, Auburger GW, Pandolfo M, Kwiecinski H, Grimes DA, Lang AE, Nielsen JE, Averyanov Y, Servidei S, Friedman A, Van Bogaert P, Abramowicz MJ, Bruno MK, Sorensen BF, Tang L, Fu YH, Ptacek LJ. The gene for paroxysmal non-kinesigenic dyskinesia encodes an enzyme in a stress response pathway. *Hum. Mol. Genet.* 2004; 13: 3161–70.

Liguori A, Napoli A, Sindona G. (2001) Electron transfer vs. proton transfer within radical-cation clusters of guanosine and deoxyguanosine with substituted naphthalenes and sinapinic acid. J. Am. Soc. Mass. Spectrom. 12(2):176-9.

Litt M, Kramer P, Browne D, Gancher S, Brunt ER, Root D, Phromchotikul T, Dubay CJ, Nutt J. (1994) A gene for episodic ataxia/myokymia maps to chromosome 12p13. *Am. J. Hum. Genet.* 55: 702-709.

Liu Y, Holmgren M, Jurman ME, Yellen G. (1997) Gated access to the pore of a voltage-dependent K+ channel. *Neuron* 19: 175-184.

Lopantsev V, Wenzel HJ, Cole TB, Palmiter RD, Schwartzkroin PA. (2003) Lack of vesicular zinc in mossy fibers does not affect synaptic excitability of CA3 pyramidal cells in zinc transporter 3 knockout mice. *Neuroscience.*;116(1):237-48.

Lopez-Barneo J, Hoshi T, Heinemann SH, Aldrich RW. (1993) Effects of external cations and mutations in the pore region on C-type inactivation of Shaker potassium channels. *Receptors Channels* 1: 61-71.

Manganas LN, Akhtar S, Antonucci DE, Campomanes CR, Dolly JO, Trimmer JS. (2001) Episodic ataxia type-1 mutations in the Kv1.1 potassium channel display distinct folding and intracellular trafficking properties. *J. Biol. Chem.* 276: 49427-49434.

McNamara NM, Muniz ZM, Wilkin GP, Dolly JO. (1993) Prominent location of a K+ channel containing the alpha subunit Kv 1.2 in the basket cell nerve terminals of rat cerebellum. *Neuroscience.* Dec;57(4):1039-45.

Meijer IA, Hand CK, Grewal KK, Stefanelli MG, Ives EJ, Rouleau GA (2002) A locus for autosomal dominant hereditary spastic ataxia, SAX1, maps to chromosome 12p13. *Am. J. Hum. Genet.* 70:763-9.

Molina A, Castellano AG, Lopez Barneo J. (1997) Pore mutations in Shaker K+ channels distinguish between the sites of tetraethylammonium blockade and C-type inactivation. *J. Physiol.* (Lond.) 499: 361-367.

Neher E, Sakmann B. (1976) Single-channel currents recorded from membrane of denervated frog muscle fibres. *Nature* 260: 779-802.

Ogiwara I, Miyamoto H, Morita N, Atapour N, Mazaki E, Inoue I, Takeuchi T, Itohara S, Yanagawa Y, Obata K, Furuichi T, Hensch TK, Yamakawa K. (2007) Na(v)1.1 localizes to axons of parvalbumin-positive inhibitory interneurons: a circuit basis for epileptic seizures in mice carrying an Scn1a gene mutation. *J. Neurosci.* 30;27(22):5903-14.

Ophoff RA, Terwindt GM, Vergouwe MN, van Eijk R, Oefner PJ, Hoffman SMG, Lamerdin JE, Mohrenweiser HW, Bulman DE, Ferrari M, Haan J, Lindhout D, van Ommen GB, Hofker MH, Ferrari MD, Frants RR. (1996) Familial hemiplegic migraine and episodic ataxia type-2 are caused by mutations in the Ca^{2+} channel gene CACNL1A4. *Cell* 87: 543-552.

Pardo LA, Heinemann SH, Terlau H, Ludewig U, Lorra C, Pongs O, Stuhmer W. (1992) Extracellular K+ specifically modulates a rat brain K+ channel. *Proc. Natl. Acad. Sci. USA* 89: 2466-2470.

Pessia M (2004) Ion Channels and Electrical Activity. In: Wayne Davies R, Morris BJ (eds) *Molecular Biology of the Neuron*, Oxford University Press, pp 103-37.

Pessia M, Hanna M (2010) Episodic Ataxia type 1. In GeneReviews [Internet], ed. Pagon RA, Bird TC, Dolan CR, Stephens K. University of Washington, Seattle; 2010.

Poliak S, Gollan L, Martinez R, Custer A, Einheber S, Salzer JL, Trimmer JS, Shrager P, Peles E. (1999) Caspr2, a new member of the neurexin superfamily, is localized at the juxtaparanodes of myelinated axons and associates with K^+ channels. *Neuron* 24: 1037-1047.

Rainier S, Thomas D, Tokarz D, Ming L, Bui M, Plein E, Zhao X, Lemons R, Albin R, Delaney C, Alvarado D, Fink JK. Myofibrillogenesis regulator 1 gene mutations cause paroxysmal dystonic choreoathetosis. *Arch. Neurol.* 2004; 61: 1025–9.

Rajakulendran S, Schorge S, Kullmann DM, Hanna MG (2007) Episodic ataxia type 1: a neuronal potassium channelopathy. *Neurotherapeutics* 2:258-66.

Rea R, Spauschus A, Eunson LH, Hanna MG, Kullmann DM. (2002) Variable K(+) channel subunit dysfunction in inherited mutations of KCNA1. *J. Physiol.* 538: 5-23.

Retting J, Heinemann SH, Wunder F, Lorra C, Parcej DN, Dolly JO, Pongs O. (1994) Inactivation properties of voltage-gated K+ channels altered by presence of beta-subunit. *Nature* 369: 289-294.

Ruppersberg JP, Schroter KH, Sakmann B, Stocker M, Sewing S, Pongs O. (1990) Heteromultimeric channels formed by rat brain potassium-channel proteins. *Nature* 345: 535-537.

Sheng M, Tsaur ML, Jan YN, Jan LY. (1994) Contrasting subcellular localization of the Kv1.2 K+ channel subunit in different neurons of rat brain. *J. Neurosci.* 14: 2408-2417.

Schulte, U., Thumfart, J.O., Klocker, N., Sailer, C.A., Bildl, W., Biniossek, M., Dehn, D., Deller, T., Eble, S., Abbass, K., Wangler, T., Knaus, H.G. and Fakler, B. (2006) The epilepsy-linked lgi1 protein assembles into presynaptic kv1 channels and inhibits inactivation by kvbeta1. *Neuron* 49, 697-706.

Shook SJ, Mamsa H, Jen JC, Baloh RW, Zhou L (2008) Novel mutation in KCNA1 causes episodic ataxia with paroxysmal dyspnea. *Muscle Nerve* 37:399-402.

Sicca F, Imbrici P, D'Adamo MC, Moro F, Bonatti F, Brovedani P, Grottesi A, Guerrini R, Masi G, Santorelli FM, Pessia M. (2011) Autism with seizures and intellectual disability: possible causative role of gain-of-function of the inwardly-rectifying K+ channel Kir4.1. *Neurobiol. Dis.* 43:239-47.

Smart SL, Lopantsev V, Zhang CL, Robbins CA, Wang H, Chiu SY, Schwartzkroin PA, Messing A, Tempel BL. (1998) Deletion of the Kv1.1 potassium channel causes epilepsy in mice. *Neuron* 20: 809-819.

Southan AP, Robertson B. (1998) Patch-clamp recordings form cerebellar basket cell bodies and their presynaptic terminals reveal an asymmetric distribution of voltage-gated potassium channels. *J. Neurosci.* 18: 948-955.

Spacey SD, Adams PJ, Lam PC, Materek LA, Stoessl AJ, Snutch TP, Hsiung GY. (2006) Genetic heterogeneity in paroxysmal nonkinesigenic dyskinesia. *Neurology.*; 66: 1588–90.

Steckley JL, Ebers GC, Cader MZ, McLachlan RS (2001) An autosomal dominant disorder with episodic ataxia, vertigo, and tinnitus. *Neurology* 57:1499–502.

Strauss KA, Puffenberger EG, Huentelman MJ, Gottlieb S, Dobrin SE, Parod JM, Stephan DA, Morton DH. (2006) Recessive symptomatic focal epilepsy and mutant contactin-associated protein-like 2. N. Engl. J. Med. 30;354(13):1370-7.

Stuhmer W, Ruppersberg JP, Schroter KH, Sakmann B, Stocker M, Giese KP, Perschke A, Baumann A, Pongs O. (1989b) Molecular basis of functional diversity of voltage-gated potassium channels in mammalian brain. *EMBO J.* 8: 3235-3244.

Sumikawa K, Houghton M, Emtage JS, Richards BM, Barnard EA. (1981) Active multi-subunit ACh receptor assembled by translation of heterologous mRNA in Xenopus oocytes. *Nature* 292: 862-864.

Tanouye MA, Ferrus A. (1985) Action potentials in normal and Shaker mutant drosophila. *J. Neurogenet.* 2: 253-271.

Teh BT, Silburn P, Lindblad K, Betz R, Boyle R, Schalling M, Larsson C. (1995) Familial periodic cerebellar ataxia withouth myokymia maps to a 19-cM region on 19p13. *Am. J. Hum. Genet.* 56: 1443-1449.

Tempel BL, Papazian DM, Schwarz TL, Jan YN, Jan LY. (1987) Sequence of a probable potassium channel component encoded at Shaker locus of Drosophila. *Science* 237: 770-775.

Temple e Vacher 2008.

Timofeeva O, Nadler JV. (2006)Facilitation of granule cell epileptiform activity by mossy fiber-released zinc in the pilocarpine model of temporal lobe epilepsy. *Brain Res.* 17;1078(1):227-34.

Tomita H, Nagamitsu S, Wakui K, Fukushima Y, Yamada K, Sadamatsu M, Masui A, Konishi T, Matsuishi T, Aihara M, Shimizu K, Hashimoto K, Mineta M, Matsushima M, Tsujita T, Saito M, Tanaka H, Tsuji S, Takagi T, Nakamura Y, Nanko S, Kato N, Nakane Y, Niikawa N. Paroxysmal kinesigenic choreoathetosis locus maps to chromosome 16p11.2-q12.1. *Am. J. Hum. Genet.* 1999; 65: 1688–97.

Tomlinson ES, Veronica Tan S, Kullmann DM, Griggs RC, Burke D, Hanna MG and Bostock H (2010). Nerve excitability studies characterize KV1.1 fast potassium channel dysfunction in patients with episodic ataxia type 1. *Brain* 133, 3530–3540.

Trimmer JS, Rhodes KJ. Localization of voltage-gated ion channels in mammalian brain. *Annu. Rev. Physiol.* 66: 477-519, 2004.

Tsaur ML, Sheng M, Lowenstein DH, Jan YN, Jan LY. (1992) Differential expression of K+ channel mRNAs in the rat brain and down-regulation in the hippocampus following seizures.Neuron 8(6):1055-67.

Vabnick I, Trimmer JS, Schwarz TL, Levinson SR, Risal D and Shrager P (1999). Dynamic potassium channel distributions during axonal development prevent aberrant firing patterns. J. Neurosci. 19, 747-58.

Valente EM, Spacey SD, Wali GM, Bhatia KP, Dixon PH, Wood NW, Davis MB. A second paroxysmal kinesigenic choreoathetosis locus (EKD2) mapping on 16q13-q22.1 indicates a family of genes which give rise to paroxysmal disorders on human chromosome 16. *Brain.* 2000; 123(Pt 10): 2040–5.

VanDyke DH, Griggs RC, Murphy MJ, Goldstein MN. (1975) Hereditary myokymia and periodic ataxia. *J. Neurol. Sci.* 25: 109-118.

Vassilev PM, Scheuer T, Catterall WA. (1988) Identification of an intracellular peptide segment involved in sodium channel inactivation. *Science* 241: 1658-1661.

Vacher H, Mohapatra DP and Trimmer JS (2008). Localization and targeting of voltage-dependent ion channels in mammalian central neurons. Physiol. Rev. 88, 1407-47.

Vance JM, Pericak-Vance MA, Payne CS, et al (1984) Linkage and genetic analysis in adult onset periodic vestibulo-cerebellar ataxia: report of a new family. *Am. J. Hum. Genet.* 36:78S.

Von Brederlow B, Hahn AF, Koopman WJ, Ebers GC, Bulman DE. (1995) Mapping the gene for acetazolamide responsive hereditary paryoxysmal cerebellar ataxia to chromosome 19p. *Hum. Mol. Genet.* 4: 279-284.

Wang H, Kunkel DD, Martin TM, Schwartzkroin PA, Tempel BL. (1993) Heteromultimeric K^+ channels in terminal and juxtaparanodal regions of neurons. *Nature* 365: 75-79.

Wang H, Kunkel DD, Schwartzkroin PA, Tempel BL. (1994) Localization of Kv1.1 and Kv1.2, two K+ channel proteins, to synaptic terminals, somata, and dendrites in the mouse brain. *J. Neurosci.* 14: 4588-4599.

Xu H, Mitchell CL. (1993) Chelation of zinc by diethyldithiocarbamate facilitates bursting induced by mixed antidromic plus orthodromic activation of mossy fibers in hippocampal slices. Brain Res. 8;624(1-2):162-70.

Zagotta WN, Hoshi T, Aldrich RW. (1990) Restoration of inactivation in mutants of Shaker potassium channels by a peptide derived from ShB. *Science* 250: 568-571.

Zerr P, Adelman JP, Maylie J. (1998b) Characterization of three episodic ataxia mutations in the human Kv1.1 potassium channel. *FEBS Lett.* 431: 461-464.

Zhou L, Messing A, Chiu SY (1999). Determinants of excitability at transition zones in Kv1.1-deficient myelinated nerves. J. Neurosci. 19: 5768-81.

Zhou L, Zhang CL, Messing A, Chiu SY (1998) Temperature-sensitive neuromuscular transmission in Kv1.1 null mice: role of potassium channels under the myelin sheath in young nerves. *J. Neurosci.* 18: 7200-7215.

Zhou L and Chiu SY (2001) Computer Model for Action Potential Propagation Through Branch Point in Myelinated Nerves. *J. Neurophysiol.* 85:197-210.

Zhuchenko O, Bailey J, Bonnen P, Ashizawa T, Stockton DW, Amos C, Dobyns WB, Subramony SH, Zoghbi HY, Lee CC. (1997) Autosomal dominant cerebellar ataxia

(SCA6) associated with small polyglutamine expansions in the alpha 1A-voltage-dependent calcium channel. *Nat. Genet.* 15: 62-69.

Zuberi SM, Eunson LH, Spauschus A, De Silva R, Tolmie J, Wood NW, McWilliam RC, Stephenson JP, Kullmann DM, Hanna MG (1999) A novel mutation in the human voltage-gated potassium channel gene (Kv1.1) associates with episodic ataxia type 1 and sometimes with partial epilepsy. *Brain* 122:817-25.

Chapter 4

MITOCHONDRIAL ATAXIAS

Michelangelo Mancuso, Daniele Orsucci and Gabriele Siciliano*

Department of Neuroscience, Neurological Clinic, University of Pisa, Italy

ABSTRACT

Mitochondrial dysfunction has been implicated in the pathogenesis of Friedreich Ataxia and other hereditary ataxias. In some cases, mitochondrial DNA primary genetic abnormalities (i.e., myoclonic epilepsy with ragged red fibers syndrome [MERRF}; neuropathy, ataxia and pigmentary retinopathy syndrome [NARP]; Kearns-Sayre syndrome) or secondary mitochondrial dysfunction (i.e., due to mitochondrial polymerase *POLG1* gene mutation or coenzyme Q10 deficiency) can directly cause ataxia. In this chapter, we revise the role of mitochondrial dysfunction in hereditary ataxias, and we discuss the well-defined "mitochondrial ataxias". Mitochondrial diseases are a group of disorders caused by impairment of the mitochondrial respiratory chain. The effects of mutations which affect the respiratory chain may be multisystemic, with involvement of visual and auditory pathways, heart, central nervous system, and skeletal muscle. Genetic ataxias other from well-defined mitochondrial ataxias and Friedreich ataxia will not be extensively discussed here, but the role of mitochondrial dysfunction in some of these diseases will be briefly reviewed.

INTRODUCTION

Mitochondria evolved from the aerobic bacteria which about 1.5 billion years ago populated primordial eukaryotic cells, thus endowing the host cells with oxidative phosphorylation (much more efficient than anaerobic glycolysis) (DiMauro and Schon, 2003). The most crucial task of the mitochondrion is the generation of energy as adenosine triphosphate (ATP), by means of the electron transport chain (Figure 1). The electron

* Corresponding author: Michelangelo Mancuso, M.D., PhD Department of Neuroscience, Neurological ClinicUniversity of Pisa, Italy, Via Roma 67, 56126 Pisa, Tel. 0039-050-992440 Email mancusomichelangelo@gmail.com Fax 0039-050-554808,

transport chain, or respiratory chain, consists of five multimeric protein complexes located in the inner mitochondrial membrane (DiMauro and Schon, 2003), and also requires two electron carriers, coenzyme Q10 (or ubiquinone) and cytochrome c. Electrons are transported along the complexes to molecular oxygen (O_2), finally producing water. At the same time, protons are pumped across the mitochondrial inner membrane, from the matrix to the intermembrane space, by the complexes I, III, and IV. This process creates an electrochemical proton gradient. ATP is produced by the influx of these protons back through the complex V, or ATP synthase (the "rotary motor") (Okuno et al., 2011). This metabolic pathway is under control of both nuclear (nDNA) and mitochondrial (mtDNA) genomes (DiMauro and Schon, 2003). The mtDNA (Figure 2) encodes information for mitochondrial transfer RNAs (tRNAs), for ribosomal RNAs (rRNAs), and for a few of subunits of the respiratory chain. The rest of the mitochondrial proteins are encoded by genes in the nuclear chromosomes, and finally imported into the mitochondrion (DiMauro and Schon, 2003).

The mitochondrial electron transport chain transfers electrons from NADH or FADH through a series of electron acceptors to the final oxygen acceptor, with production of water. These biochemical reactions lead to the production of reactive oxygen species (ROS) (see Figure 1). Excessive ROS accumulation can damage biomolecules, including lipids, proteins and nucleic acids (Chan, 2006).

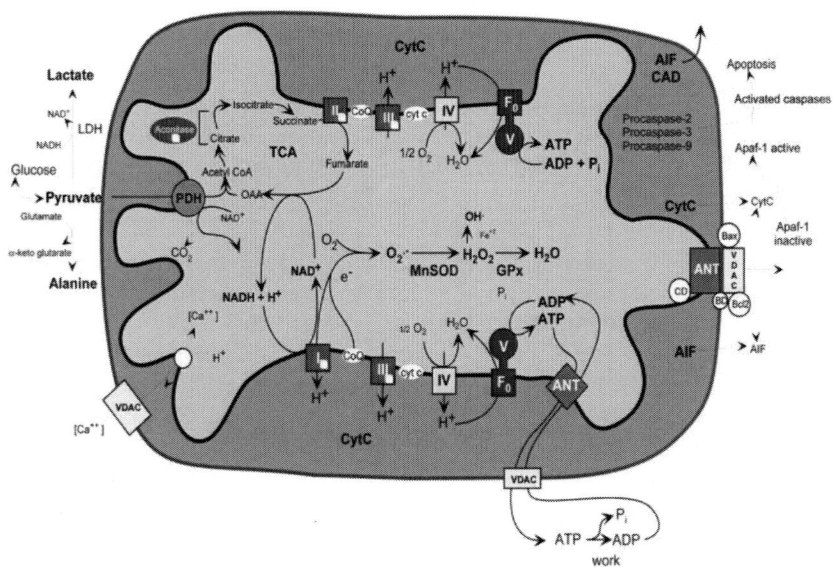

Figure 1. Mitochondrial metabolism. Schematic representation of mitochondrial biochemical pathways, representing relationship between energy production (tricarboxylic acid cycle [TCA] and electron transport chain), reactive oxygen species production (superoxide $O2^{\cdot -}$, hydroxyl radical $OH^{\cdot}$), apoptosis regulation. Electron transport chain complexes: I (NADH:ubiquinone reductase), II (succinate:ubiquinone reductase), III (ubiquinone-cyt c oxidoreductase), IV (cytochrome c oxidase), F0V (ATP synthase). ADP, adenosine 5'-diphosphate; ATP, adenosine 5'-triphosphate; AIF, apoptosis inducing factor; ANT, adenine nucleotide transporter; CAD, caspase-activated DNase; CytC, cytochrome c; GPX, glutathione peroxidase; LDH, lactic dehydrogenase; MnSOD, manganese superoxide dismutase; NAD+/NADH, oxidized/reduced nicotinamide adenine dinucleotide; OAA, oxalacetic acid; PDH, pyruvate dehydrogenase; Pi, inorganic phosphorus; VDAC, voltage-dependent anion channel. From MITOMAP: A Human Mitochondrial Genome Database, allowed reproduction (http://www.mitomap.org).

Oxidative stress can specifically lead to the degradation of mtDNA (Shokolenko et al., 2009). The steady-state concentration of oxidants is maintained at nontoxic levels by a variety of antioxidant defences and repair enzymes, but these delicate homeostasis may be disrupted by either deficient defenses or excessive ROS production (i.e., in case of respiratory chain dysfunction) (Turrens, 2003). MtDNA is sensitive to oxidative damage because of its proximity to the inner mitochondrial membrane, where oxidants are formed, and because it is not protected by histones. Because mtDNA genes encode subunits of the mitochondrial respiratory chain, oxidative base modifications to mtDNA can lead to bioenergetic dysfunctions, thus generating a vicious cycle of mitochondrial dysfunction, increased ROS production, and cell death (Chan, 2006).

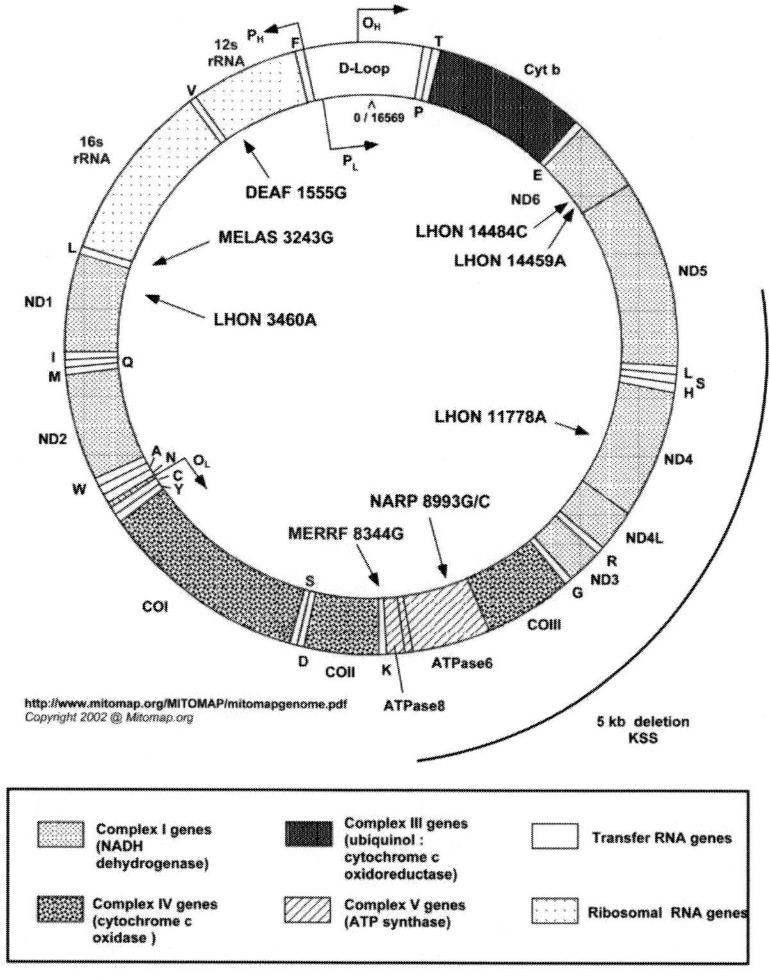

Figure 2. The mitochondrial genome. Some common mutations are represented, including the single, sporadic, large-scale deletion associated with Kearns-Sayre Syndrome (KSS) and progressive external ophthalmoplegia. DEAF, mitochondrial deafness; LHON, Leber hereditary optic neuropathy; MELAS, mitochondrial encephalomyopathy, lactic acidosis, stroke-like episodes syndrome; MERRF, myoclonic epilepsy with "ragged red" fibers; NARP, neuropathy, ataxia, pigmentary retinopathy. From MITOMAP: A Human Mitochondrial Genome Database, allowed reproduction (http://www.mitomap.org).

Mitochondrial dysfunction has tight links with neurodegeneration (Chan, 2006). In this chapter, we discuss the well-defined forms of mitochondrial disease which most frequently may manifest with cerebellar ataxia ("mitochondrial ataxias") and we discuss the role of mitochondrial dysfunction in hereditary ataxias, with special regard to Friedreich ataxia.

ATAXIA IN MITOCHONDRIAL DISORDERS

Mitochondrial diseases are a group of disorders caused by impairment of the mitochondrial respiratory chain. The effects of mutations which affect the respiratory chain may be multisystemic, with involvement of visual and auditory pathways, heart, central nervous system (CNS), and skeletal muscle. The estimated prevalence of mitochondrial disorders is 1-2 in 10000 (Schaefer et al., 2008). They are, therefore, one of the most common neurogenetic conditions.

The genetic classification of mitochondrial disorders (Table 1) distinguishes disorders due to defects in mtDNA (see Figure 2) from those due to defects in nDNA (Filosto and Mancuso, 2007). The first ones are inherited according to the rules of mitochondrial genetics (maternal inheritance, heteroplasmy and the threshold effect, mitotic segregation). Each cell contains multiple copies of mtDNA (polyplasmy), which in normal individuals are identical to one another (homoplasmy). Heteroplasmy refers to the coexistence of two populations of mtDNA, normal and mutated. Mutated mtDNA in a given tissue has to reach a minimum critical number before oxidative metabolism is impaired severely enough to cause dysfunction (threshold effect) (DiMauro and Schon, 2003). The pathogenic threshold varies from tissue to tissue according to the relative dependence of each tissue on oxidative metabolism (DiMauro and Schon, 2003). CNS, skeletal muscle, heart, endocrine glands, the retina, the renal tubule and the auditory sensory cells, frequent targets of mitochondrial disorders, have a high energy demand and, therefore, a lower threshold for a critical load of mtDNA mutation. Most mtDNA-related disorders are multisystemic (DiMauro et al., 2004). The sporadic occurrence of a mitochondrial disease, such as progressive external ophthalmoplegia (PEO), Kearns-Sayre syndrome (ophthalmoplegia associated to pigmentary retinopathy and cardiac conduction block) and Pearson syndrome (refractory sideroblastic anemia associated with pancreatic insufficiency) is suggestive for a single, sporadic, mtDNA deletion (Filosto and Mancuso, 2007).

The percentage and location of the single deletion could differ between these syndromes, and the moment when the deletion is produced probably determines the affected tissues and the phenotype, as well as the percentage and location of the deletion (Lopez-Gallardo et al., 2009). Mitochondrial disorders related to nDNA are caused by mutations in structural components or ancillary proteins of the electron transport chain, by defects of the membrane lipid milieu, of coenzyme Q10 biosynthetic genes and by defects in intergenomic signaling (associated to mtDNA depletion or multiple deletions) (DiMauro and Schon, 2003). Nuclear mutations affecting the respiratory are often autosomal recessive. Tissue involvement is less variable than in mtDNA-related disorders, and the onset is earlier (often soon after birth). Most causes of Leigh syndrome involve mutations in genes encoding subunits or assembly proteins of the electron transport chain (DiMauro et al., 2004).

Table 1. Genetic classification of mitochondrial diseases. MELAS, mitochondrial encephalomyopathy with lactic acidosis and stroke-like episodes; MERRF, myoclonic epilepsy with ragged red fibers; MNGIE, Mitochondrial neurogastrointestinal encephalomyopathy; MLASA, mitochondrial myopathy and sideroblastic anemia; NARP, neuropathy, ataxia, retinitis pigmentosa; PEO, progressive external ophthalmoplegia (Modified from Filosto and Mancuso, 2007)

Disorders of mitochondrial genome	Mitochondrial disorders caused by nuclear genes
<u>Sporadic rearrangements</u> Kearns-Sayre syndrome (KSS) Pearson syndrome Sporadic PEO Diabetes and deafness	<u>Defects of genes encoding for structural proteins of the complexes of respiratory chain</u> Leigh Syndrome Cardiomyopathy hypertrophic, histiocitoide Paraganglioma, pheochromocytomas Multisystemic syndromes
<u>Sporadic point mutations</u> PEO MELAS Exercise intolerance Isolated myopathy	<u>Defects of genes encoding factors involved in the assembling complexes of respiratory chain ("Assembly genes")</u> Leigh Syndrome Multisystemic Syndromes
<u>Maternal-inherited mtDNA point mutations</u> *Genes encoding structural proteins* Leber hereditary optic neuropathy NARP Maternal-inherited Leigh syndrome *Genes encoding tRNAs* MELAS MERRF Cardiomyopathy and myopathy PEO Isolated myopathy Diabetes and deafness Sensorineural hearing loss Hypertrophic cardiomyopathy Tubulopathy *Genes encoding rRNAs* Aminoglycosides-induced deafness Hypertrophic cardiomyopathy	<u>Defects of genes altering mtDNA stability and integrity (intergenomic communication)</u> Autosomal PEO Early-onset parkinsonism Multisystemic syndromes MNGIE mtDNA depletion syndromes <u>Coenzyme Q10 deficiency</u> Cerebellar form *COQ2, COQ8* Myopathic form *ETFDH* Encephalomyopathy Infantile multisystemic disease *PDSS1, COQ2* Leigh syndrome *PDSS2* <u>Defects of the lipid milieu</u> Barth syndrome <u>Syndromes due to defects of mitochondrial ribonucleic acid</u> MLASA <u>Defects of mitochondrial fission or fusion</u> Autosomal dominant optic atrophy (ADOA) Charcot-Marie-Tooth (CMT) 2A

The diagnostic process of mitochondrial diseases does not differ from that employed for other neuromuscular disorders, and should start from patient and family history and physical and neurologic examination (DiMauro et al., 2004). "Red flags" for mitochondrial diseases are short stature, neurosensory hearing loss, ptosis, ophthalmoplegia, axonal neuropathy, diabetes mellitus, hypertrophic cardiomyopathy, renotubular acidosis, migraine.

Diagnosis of mitochondrial diseases requires a complex approach: measurements of serum lactate, electromyography, magnetic resonance spectroscopy, muscle histology and enzimology, and genetic analysis. Recently, 1H magnetic resonance spectroscopy showed elevated cerebellar lactate in nine of eleven patients with cerebellar ataxia ascribed to mitochondrial disease (Boddaert et al., 2008).

The treatment of mitochondrial diseases is still inadequate. Apart from symptomatic treatments, therapies that have been attempted include respiratory chain cofactors, other metabolites secondarily decreased in mitochondrial disorders, antioxidants and agents acting on lactic acidosis. However, their role in the treatment of the majority of mitochondrial disorders remains unclear (Chinnery et al., 2006).

Administration of metabolites and cofactors is the mainstay of real-life therapy and is especially important in disorders due to primary deficiencies of specific compounds, such as coenzyme Q10. In the next paragraphs, specific mitochondrial diseases which more frequently may manifest with cerebellar ataxia are reviewed.

MtDNA Point Mutations

Myoclonic epilepsy with ragged red fibres (MERRF) has a variable onset and is mostly characterized by generalized seizures, myoclonus and lactic acidosis; cerebellar ataxia is also common. This syndrome has been associated with various mtDNA point mutations, the most frequent of which are A8344G and T8356C in tRNA lysine (Filosto and Mancuso, 2007). Other point mutations in the tRNA lysine (Virgilio et al., 2009), tRNA phenylalanine (Mancuso et al., 2004) and tRNA proline (Blakely et al., 2009) have been reported in patients with typical MERRF clinical picture, including ataxia. Ito and co-workers reported three MERRF patients (with A8344G mutation) in whom cerebellar ataxia was the first symptom; conventional brain magnetic resonance imaging showed atrophy of the superior cerebellar peduncles and the cerebellum in all patients and brainstem atrophy in two patients (Ito et al., 2008).

The MELAS (mitochondrial encephalomyopathy, lactic acidosis and stroke-like episode) phenotype consists of a progressive encephalomyopathy characterized by repeated stroke-like events that often involve the posterior cerebral areas, recurrent headache, exercise intolerance, seizures and lactic acidosis. Onset can be before the age of 40. Mutations most frequently associated with this condition are A3243G and T3271C in tRNA leucine (UUR) in the mitochondrial genome (Filosto and Mancuso, 2007). Ataxia may be present, but is not typical (Petruzzella et al., 2004), and cerebellar cortical degeneration of granular cell type has been reported (Tsuchiya et al., 1999).

Maternally inherited Leigh syndrome (MILS) has its onset generally during the first year of life. The patient may present with motor retardation, hypotonia, ataxia, epileptic seizures, myoclonus, neuropathy, optic atrophy, pigmentary retinopathy, lactic acidosis and psychomotor regression. It is usually associated with point mutations in the gene of APTase6 (complex V of the respiratory chain – ATP synthase), especially at nucleotide 8993. If the percentage of mutant mtDNA is <90% (between 70% and 90%), the clinical picture is more benign, late-onset and characterized by neuropathy, ataxia and pigmentary retinopathy (NARP syndrome) (Filosto and Mancuso, 2007). Marked phenotypic differences even between family members have been reported (Gelfand et al., 2011), and the mtDNA background seems to play an important role in modulating the biochemical defects and clinical outcome in NARP/MILS (D'Aurelio et al., 2010). Interestingly, rare MILS patients may show an unexpected resolution of the disease and develop in adult life a more benign NARP phenotype (Debray et al., 2007). "NARP/MILS" cells have been protected from death by alpha-ketoglutarate/aspartate, which may increase mitochondrial substrate-level phosphorylation, suggesting potential approaches based on the supplementation of alpha-ketoglutarate/aspartate to patients with impaired ATP synthase activity (Sgarbi et al., 2009). APTase6 gene mutations have been also associated with cognitive developmental delay, learning disability, and progressive ataxia (Sikorska et al., 2009). Morevover, mtDNA *ND6* gene should be also analyzed in Leigh syndrome presenting with optic atrophy, ataxia, dystonia, and epilepsy, regardless of age (Leshinsky-Silver et al., 2011).

Leber hereditary optic neuropathy, is a retrobulbar neuritis associated with pseudopapilledema, retinal blood vessel alteration, and, in some instances, cerebellar ataxia, peripheral neuropathy and cardiac conduction defects. Typically, onset is between 18 and 30 years of age with monocular loss of vision followed, within weeks or months, by the involvement of the contralateral eye. At least five pathogenic point mutations in genes encoding subunits of complex I are associated with the disease (Filosto and Mancuso, 2007).

Recently, a pathogenic mutation in the tRNA leucine (CUN) gene of mtDNA (previously only associated with myopathy and PEO) has been reported in a young woman with childhood-onset and slowly progressive encephalopathy with ataxia, cognitive impairment, and hearing loss (Coku et al., 2010). Other mtDNA point mutations have been linked to complex neurological phenotypes including ataxia; i.e. tRNA proline (Da Pozzo et al., 2009), tRNA glutamate (Pancrudo et al., 2007), tRNA tryptophan (Silvestri et al., 2000), and others tRNAs. Sequencing of the 22 tRNA mitochondrial genes (from muscle DNA) is indicated in all unusual neurological syndromes, even in the absence of clear maternal inheritance.

MtDNA Sporadic Rearrangements

Kearns-Sayre syndrome is associated with a single large-scale mtDNA deletion (see Figure 2), and is clinically characterized by pigmentary retinopathy and progressive external ophthalmoplegia. At least one of the following conditions must be associated: cardiac conduction defects, cerebellar ataxia and hyperproteinorrachia higher than 100 mg/dl. Onset is often before 20 years of age. Additional features may include growth retardation, short stature, deafness, muscle weakness, endocrinopathies, renal tubular dysfunction and hyperlactacidaemia (Filosto and Mancuso, 2007). Neuropathological studies revealed cerebellar spongiform degeneration and by immunohistochemistry a disruption of presynaptic terminals and of the terminal arborizations of Purkinje cell axons on multipolar neurons of the dentate nucleus, suggesting that a disconnection of Purkinje cells at the dentate nucleus may play a role in the pathogenesis of cerebellar ataxia in Kearns-Sayre syndrome (Tanji et al., 1999). Cerebellar ataxia may also represent a feature of "PEO plus" phenotypes due to single mtDNA deletions.

Infantile Onset Spinocerebellar Ataxia

Infantile onset spinocerebellar ataxia (IOSCA) is a severe autosomal recessively inherited neurodegenerative disorder characterized by progressive atrophy of the cerebellum, brainstem and spinal cord and sensory axonal neuropathy (Nikali et al., 2005). After analyzing all positional candidate transcripts, Nikali and co-workers identified two point mutations in the gene *C10orf2* encoding Twinkle, a mtDNA-specific helicase, underlying IOSCA. The founder IOSCA mutation, homozygous in all but one of the patients, leads to a Y508C aminoacid change in the polypeptides (Nikali et al., 2005). Interestingly, different mutations in this same gene cause autosomal dominant progressive external ophthalmoplegia (adPEO) with multiple mtDNA deletions (due to mtDNA replication pausing or stalling) (Goffart et al., 2009), and IOSCA phenotype is the first recessive one due to *C10orf2* mutations. *C10orf2* mutant variants retain helicase function under optimized in vitro conditions despite partial reductions in DNA binding affinity, nucleotide hydrolysis, or thermal stability for some mutants (Longley et al., 2010). Recessive mutations of the Twinkle helicase can also manifest as early encephalopathy with liver involvement, a phenotype reminiscent of Alpers syndrome (more commonly linked to *POLG1*) (Hakonen et al., 2007). IOSCA patients show mtDNA depletion in the brain and the liver, and IOSCA may represent a new member of the mtDNA depletion syndromes (Hakonen et al., 2008).

POLG1-Related Diseases

It is now well established that defects in mtDNA replication can lead to mitochondrial dysfunction and disease. DNA polymerase gamma (POLG) is the only DNA polymerase in human mitochondria and is essential for mtDNA replication and repair (Chan and Copeland, 2009). In addition to its 5' to 3' polymerase activity, POLG has a 3' to 5' exonuclease activity important in the repair process. Mitochondria have their own small 16.5 kb circular double-stranded DNA that encodes 22 tRNAs, 2 rRNAs and 13 polypeptides that are essential for electron transport and oxidative phosphorylation. Nuclear genes encode the other mitochondrial proteins, including the proteins involved in mtDNA replication, such as POLG subunits 1 and 2 (codified by *POLG1* and *POLG2* nuclear genes) (Chan and Copeland, 2009). *POLG1* mutations lead to uncorrect nucleotide incorporation in mtDNA (Batabyal et al., 2010). A homozygous knock-in mice expressing a proof-reading-deficient version of POLG shows a "mtDNA mutator" phenotype with increased amounts of point mutations and deleted mtDNA. This increase in somatic mtDNA mutations is associated with reduced lifespan and premature onset of aging-related phenotypes, thus providing a link between mtDNA mutations and aging in mammals (Trifunovic et al., 2004).

POLG1 mutations can cause dominant or recessive disorders, frequently associated with severe and multisystem involvement. These forms of mitochondrial disorders are associated with secondary accumulation of multiple deletions in mtDNA (Gonzalez-Vioque et al., 2006). Mutations in the *POLG1* gene have emerged as one of the most common causes of inherited mitochondrial disorders in children and adults (Wong et al., 2008). Functional genetic variants of *POLG1* are present in up to 0.5% of the general population, and pathogenic mutations have been described in most exons of the gene (Hudson and Chinnery, 2006). The most severe manifestations have been associated with mutations of the "spacer" region of *POLG1* (i.e., ataxia-myopathy syndrome) (Luoma et al., 2005). In a large study, the clinical presentation ranged from the neonatal period to late adult life, with an overlapping phenotypic spectrum from severe encephalopathy and liver failure to late-onset PEO, ataxia, myopathy and isolated muscle pain or epilepsy (Horvath et al., 2006). A high incidence of psychiatric disease and primary gonadal failure have also been documented in some families transmitting dominant *POLG1* mutations (Hudson and Chinnery, 2006). Very recently, a new nosological entity has been also suggested – "*POLG1*-related multiple sclerosis-like illness" (Echaniz-

Laguna et al., 2010; Harris et al., 2010). One form of chronic *POLG1*-encephalopathy, associated with the G1399GA and G2243C mutations, is characterized by progressive cerebral and cerebellar atrophy on imaging studies (Tzoulis et al., 2010).

The most common *POLG1* disease mutation (A467T) has been found in all of the major *POLG1*-related diseases, i.e. Alpers syndrome, ataxia–neuropathy syndromes and PEO (Chan and Copeland, 2009). The A467T mutation is generally reported as a recessive mutation, however it may give rise to a mild dominant phenotype with late-onset ptosis (Chan and Copeland, 2009). This mutation was shown to lead to a severe catalytic defect, disrupting physical association between POLG catalytic and accessory subunits, with great reduction of both polymerase and exonuclease POLG activities (Chan et al., 2005).

Moreover, mutations in *POLG1* cause a recessively inherited syndrome with episodic features and progressive ataxia (Winterthun et al., 2005). Hakonen and co-workers reported the high carrier frequency of the W748S *POLG1* substitution in control subjects in Finland, explaining the high prevalence of "mitochondrial recessive ataxia syndrome" (MIRAS) in Scandinavia (Hakonen et al., 2005). However, although A467T and W748S are a common cause of ataxia in Scandinavia, they are rare in other European regions, such as the United Kingdom and Italy (Craig et al., 2007). It is therefore likely that the high prevalence of MIRAS in Finland and Norway is due to a founder effect. W748S heterozygotes show no clinically manifesting phenotype, but subclinical sensory polyneuropathy is common (Rantamaki et al., 2007).

Recently, it has been reported that *POLG1* mutations are rather common in Central European ataxia patients, and cause ataxia with PEO (47%), and, more rarely, with psychiatric comorbidities (20%) and epilepsy (14%) (Schicks Md et al., 2010). However, *POLG1* is not a common cause of isolated epilepsy or ataxia in childhood (Isohanni et al., 2011).

OPA1-Related Diseases

POLG1 and Twinkle have been already discussed; a third cause of defect in intergenomic signaling (causing mtDNA multiple deletions) with ataxia are *OPA1* gene mutations (Hudson et al., 2008). *OPA1* is the most common cause of autosomal dominant optic atrophy. Recently, 104 patients from 45 independent families have been reported (Yu-Wai-Man et al., 2010). Extra-ocular neurological complications were common, affecting up to 20% of all mutational carriers. Bilateral sensorineural deafness beginning in late childhood and early adulthood was a prominent manifestation, followed by a combination of ataxia, myopathy, peripheral neuropathy and progressive external ophthalmoplegia from the third decade of life onwards (Yu-Wai-Man et al., 2010). Multi-system neurological disease was associated with all mutational subtypes; histochemical and molecular characterization of skeletal muscle biopsies revealed the presence of cytochrome *c* oxidase-deficient fibers and multiple mtDNA deletions in the majority of patients, even in those with isolated optic nerve involvement. However, the cytochrome *c* oxidase-deficient load was over four times higher in the multi-system patients (Yu-Wai-Man et al., 2010).

Coenzyme Q10 Deficiency

Coenzyme Q10 deficiency is a rare, autosomal recessive, heterogeneous condition which has been associated with five major syndromes: (i) encephalomyopathy (with recurrent myoglobinuria, brain involvement and ragged red fibers); (ii) severe infantile multisystemic disease; (iii) cerebellar ataxia; (iv) Leigh syndrome (growth retardation, ataxia and deafness); (v) isolated myopathy (DiMauro et al., 2007). Primary coenzyme Q10 deficiency due to mutations in ubiquinone biosynthetic genes (i.e. *COQ2, PDSS1, PDSS2, CABC1*) has been identified in patients with the infantile multisystemic and cerebellar ataxic phenotypes (Quinzii et al., 2008). In contrast, secondary coenzyme Q10 deficiency, due to mutations in genes not directly related to ubiquinone biosynthesis (i.e. *APTX, ETFDH, BRAF*), has been identified in patients with cerebellar ataxia, pure myopathy, and cardiofaciocutaneous syndrome (Quinzii et al., 2008).

Coenzyme Q10 deficiency with cerebellar ataxia has been also associated to mutation in *CABC1/COQ8/ ADCK3* gene (Lagier-Tourenne et al., 2008; Mollet et al., 2008). Recently, Gerards and co-workers reported the the first nonsense mutations in *CABC1* that most likely lead to complete absence of a functional CABC1 protein, and suggested that *CABC1* is an important candidate for mutation analysis in progressive cerebellar ataxia and atrophy on imaging studies (Gerards et al., 2010).

Some cases of the ataxic variant of coenzyme Q10 deficiency have been linked to a homozygous mutation in the aprataxin (*APTX*) gene, which causes ataxia oculomotor apraxia type 1 (Le Ber et al., 2007). However, a recent study showed that coenzyme Q10 levels were normal in muscle, fibroblasts, and plasma of five of six subjects with oculomotor apraxia type 1 (Castellotti et al., 2011). The clinical phenotype was homogeneous and it was mainly characterized by early-onset cerebellar signs, sensory neuropathy, cognitive decline, and oculomotor deficits; three cases had slightly raised alpha-fetoprotein (Castellotti et al., 2011). The relationship between aprataxin, involved in DNA repair (Crimella et al., 2011), and coenzyme Q10 deficiency, if any, is still unclear.

Coenzyme Q10 deficiency is a treatable condition, so heightened "clinical awareness" about this diagnosis is essential, especially for pediatricians and infantile neurologists. Varying degrees of coenzyme Q10 deficiency cause variable defects of ATP synthesis and oxidative stress; 10-15% and >60% residual coenzyme Q10 are not associated with significant ROS production, whereas 30-50% residual coenzyme Q10 is accompanied by increased ROS production and cell death (Quinzii et al., 2010). An early treatment with high-dose coenzyme Q10 may radically change the natural history. Patients with all forms of coenzyme Q10 deficiency have shown clinical improvement with oral coenzyme Q10 supplementation, but cerebral symptoms are only partially ameliorated (probably because of irreversible structural brain damage before treatment and because of poor penetration of coenzyme Q10 across the blood-brain barrier). Patients were given various doses of coenzyme Q10 ranging from 90 to 2000 mg daily. The small number of patients precluded any statistical analysis but improvement was undoubtedly reported (DiMauro et al., 2007). In several patients coenzyme Q10 supplementation also ameliorated the mitochondrial function (electron transport chain activities, lactic acid values, muscle coenzyme Q10 content). The beneficial effects of exogenous coenzyme Q10 require high doses and long-term administration (DiMauro et al., 2007). Interestingly, primary coenzyme Q10 deficiencies should be treated with coenzyme Q10 supplementation but not with short-tail ubiquinone analogs, such as idebenone, because short-tail ubiquinone analogs cannot replace coenzyme Q10 in the mitochondrial respiratory chain under conditions of coenzyme Q10 depletion (Lopez et al., 2010).

FRIEDREICH ATAXIA

Friedreich ataxia, the most common autosomal recessive ataxia in Caucasian population, is due to mutations in the *FXN* gene, mostly an expanded GAA triplet repeat in the intron 1 (Campuzano et al., 1996; Fogel and Perlman, 2007; Pandolfo, 2008a; Shishkin et al., 2009). Age at onset is 5-25 years. Cerebellar/sensory ataxia is the cardinal symptom. Clinical course is variable, but on average 10 to15 years after onset, patients lose the ability to walk, stand, and sit without support (Pandolfo, 2008a). Age at diagnosis, which may incorporate other genetic and environmental factors, may be more important than GAA length in predicting cardiomyopathy, scoliosis, and disease progression (La Pean et al., 2008).

Sensory neurons in the dorsal root ganglia are initially lost, with secondary degeneration of the spinocerebellar and pyramidal tracts, as well as of the dorsal columns (Fogel and Perlman, 2007). For this reason, Friedreich ataxia is characterized by progressive gait and limb ataxia, dysarthria, loss of vibration and proprioceptive sense, areflexia, abnormal eye movements, and pyramidal signs. Other tracts may be involved (i.e., auditory, optic etc.). During the disease course, hypertrophic cardiomyopathy may develop (Kipps et al., 2009; Raman et al., 2011). Diabetes, scoliosis, and pes cavus are other possible manifestations of Friedreich ataxia, as well as restless legs syndrome (Frauscher et al., 2011). Very rarely, myopathy with mitochondrial features may also represent part of the phenotype (Gallagher et al., 2002).

The genetic abnormality results in the deficiency of frataxin (Campuzano et al., 1997), a protein targeted to the mitochondrion (Schmucker et al., 2008). A physical interaction between human frataxin and succinate dehydrogenase (complex II of the respiratory chain) has been described (Gonzalez-Cabo et al., 2005), and frataxin appears to be an activator of oxidative phosphorylation (Ristow et al., 2000). Although the exact physiological function of frataxin is not known, its involvement in iron–sulphur cluster biogenesis has been suggested (Levi and Rovida, 2009). A combined deficiency of a Krebs-cycle enzyme, aconitase, and three mitochondrial respiratory-chain complexes has been reported in endomyocardial biopsy samples from patients with Friedreich ataxia (Rustin et al., 1999). All four enzymes share iron-sulphur cluster-containing proteins that are damaged by iron overload through generation of oxygen free radicals (Rustin et al., 1999). Frataxin iron-binding capacity is quite robust (Correia et al., 2010). Current evidence suggests that loss of frataxin impairs mitochondrial iron handling and respiratory chain function and contributes to increased oxidative stress and cellular damage (Fogel and Perlman, 2007). Furthermore, increased mitochondrial iron uptake coupled with decreased utilization and release may lead to mitochondrial iron-loading (Huang et al., 2009; Richardson et al., 2010).

Pathology in the frataxin-deficient nervous system may involve decreased mitochondrial membrane potential and ATP production, with failure of mitochondrial axonal transport (Shidara and Hollenbeck, 2010). Oxidative damage within the mitochondria seems to have a key role in the disease phenotype (Gakh et al., 2006). Using phosphorus magnetic resonance spectroscopy, Lodi and co-workers (Lodi et al., 1999) reported a maximum rate of muscle mitochondrial ATP production below the normal range in all the twelwe studied patients and a strong negative correlation between mitochondrial ATP production and the number of GAA repeats in the smaller allele, suggesting that Friedreich ataxia is a "nuclear-encoded mitochondrial disorder".

However, other studies did not confirm the idea of Friedreich ataxia as a neurodegenerative disease associated with oxidative damage (Seznec et al., 2005), and further studies are still needed. Furthermore, profound changes in frataxin-targeted mitochondrial proteins or mitochondrial function or an increase of apoptosis in peripheral blood cells have not been observed, suggesting that functional mitochondrial defects are not readily apparent under resting conditions in peripheral cells (Selak et al., 2011).

Mitochondrial Therapies for Friedreich Ataxia

Treatment options have been mostly directed at antioxidant protection against mitochondrial damage (Kearney et al., 2009). Ubiquinones have been shown to protect mitochondria from oxidative damage, but only a small proportion of externally administered ubiquinone is taken up by mitochondria (Cocheme et al., 2007). Jauslin and co-workers compared the efficacy of mitochondria-targeted and untargeted antioxidants derived from coenzyme Q10 and from vitamin E at preventing oxidative stress-induced cell death in fibroblasts from patients with Friedreich ataxia (Jauslin et al., 2003). Conjugation of the lipophilic triphenylphosphonium cation to a ubiquinone moiety has produced a compound, MitoQ, which accumulates selectively into mitochondria (Cocheme et al., 2007). MitoQ was 800-fold more potent than the untargeted analogue idebenone (Jauslin et al., 2003). The mitochondria-targeted antioxidant MitoVit E was 350-fold more potent than the water soluble analog (Jauslin et al., 2003). Therefore, targeted antioxidants may have some therapeutic potential, but have not been investigated in patients with Friedreich ataxia to date.

Idebenone was cytoprotective in fibroblasts from patients with Friedreich ataxia (Jauslin et al., 2002). A dose-escalation trial found that idebenone was efficacious in a frataxin-deficient mouse (Seznec et al., 2004). Low-dose idebenone (10 and 30 mg/kg per day) showed no benefit, whereas high-dose idebenone (90 mg/kg per day) delayed the cardiac disease onset, progression and death of frataxin deficient animals by 1 week (Seznec et al., 2004; Seznec et al., 2005).

High doses of idebenone are safe and well-tolerated in patients with Friedreich ataxia (Di Prospero et al., 2007b). Schulz and co-workers (Schulz et al., 2000) measured concentrations of 8-hydroxy-2'-deoxyguanosine (8OH2'dG), a marker of oxidative DNA damage, in urine and of dihydroxybenzoic acid (DHBA), a marker of hydroxyl radical attack, in plasma of 33 patients with Friedreich ataxia. Oral treatment with 5 mg/kg/day of idebenone for 8 weeks significantly decreased urinary 8OH2'dG concentrations (Schulz et al., 2000).

Idebenone is a promising drug for treatment of Friedreich ataxia (Cooper and Schapira, 2007). Early trials (Rustin et al., 2002) have demonstrated that low-dose idebenone (5 mg/kg per day) could reduce cardiac hypertrophy (Hausse et al., 2002), with no influence upon clinical progression of the neurological disease (Mariotti et al., 2003; Rustin et al., 2002).

More recently, a randomized, placebo-controlled trial has been conducted on 48 patients (Di Prospero et al., 2007a). Treatment with higher doses of idebenone (up to 45 mg/kg) was generally well tolerated and associated with improvement also in neurological function and activities of daily living. The degree of improvement correlated with the dose of idebenone, suggesting that higher doses may be needed to have a beneficial effect on neurological function (Di Prospero et al., 2007a). However, the disease stage and patient age at which idebenone treatment is initiated may be important factors in the effectiveness of the therapy (Pineda et al., 2008). Other studies did not confirm these positive findings (Drinkard et al., 2010; Lagedrost et al., 2011; Lynch et al., 2010), and further research is still needed. Recently, a randomized, double-blind, placebo-controlled trial was performed on seventy ambulatory pediatric patients (age, 8-18 years); idebenone did not significantly alter neurological function during the 6-month study (Lynch et al., 2010). Larger studies of longer duration may be needed to assess the therapeutic potential of drug candidates on neurological function in Friedreich ataxia (Lynch et al., 2010).

Hart and co-workers (Hart et al., 2005) performed an open-labeled pilot trial over 47 months with a combined coenzyme Q10 (400 mg/d) and vitamin E (2100 IU/d) therapy, and reported some improvement in cardiac and skeletal muscle mitochondrial bioenergetics (as assessed using phosphorus magnetic resonance spectroscopy). These results must be interpreted with caution because of limited patient numbers and the absence of a placebo group.

Another pilot study investigated the potential for high dose coenzyme Q10/vitamin E therapy (Cooper et al., 2008). Fifty patients were randomly divided into high or low dose coenzyme Q10/vitamin E groups. During the trial coenzyme Q10 and vitamin E levels significantly increased in both groups. Serum coenzyme Q10 level resulted to be the best predictor of a positive clinical response to coenzyme Q10/vitamin E therapy (Cooper et al., 2008). However, because of the lack of controlled studies, the variable doses used and the association with other antioxidant medications, vitamin E has not been appropriately tested in Friedreich ataxia, and no conclusions can yet be drawn about its safety and efficacy in this disorder (Pandolfo, 2008b).

L-carnitine and creatine are natural compounds that may enhance cellular energy transduction (Orsucci et al., 2009). A placebo-controlled triple-phase crossover trial of L-carnitine (3 g/d) and creatine (6.75 g/d) has been performed in 16 patients with Friedreich ataxia (Schols et al., 2005). Ataxia rating scale and echocardiographic parameters remained unchanged (Schols et al., 2005) .

In conclusion, available evidence suggests that patients with Friedreich ataxia should be treated with idebenone, because it is well tolerated and may reduce cardiac hypertrophy and, at higher doses (up to 45 mg/kg), also improve neurological function. The first phase II trial of idebenone has shown dose-dependent effects on neurological scale scores in children and adolescents with Friedreich ataxia (Di Prospero et al., 2007a). Large trials are needed to investigate whether all patients with Friedreich ataxia can benefit from idebenone treatment, regardless of age and disease stage (Schulz et al., 2009).

Frataxin is at the center of mitochondrial iron-sulfur cluster biosynthesis (Stemmler et al., 2010), and iron chelators may represent a new therapeutical approach for patients with Friedreich ataxia, on the basis that oxidative cell damage that occurs in these patients is due to the increasing deposits of mitochondrial iron pools. Very recently, Velasco-Sánchez and co-workers evaluated the effects of a combined therapy with idebenone (20 mg/kg/day) and low oral doses of the iron chelator deferiprone (20 mg/kg/day) on the neurological signs and cardiac function parameters, with an 11-month open-label study involving twenty patients

(Velasco-Sanchez et al., 2011). Some clinical improvement in posture and gait scores, as well as in kinetic function, was reported. Echocardiography data showed a significant reduction of the interventricular septum thickness and in the left ventricular mass index (Velasco-Sanchez et al., 2011). Combined therapy was well tolerated with mild side effects, apart from the risk of neutropenia and progressive reduction of plasma iron parameters (Velasco-Sanchez et al., 2011). However, to date, pharmacological approaches (i.e., erythropoietin, iron chelators) other than idebenone and symptomatic therapies are not routinely indicated in patients with Friedreich ataxia (Mancuso et al., 2010).

MITOCHONDRIA AND OTHER GENETIC ATAXIAS

Genetic ataxias other from well-defined "mitochondrial ataxias" and Friedreich ataxia will not be extensively discussed here, and only the role of mitochondrial dysfunction in some of these diseases will be briefly mentioned.

Dominant Spino-Cerebellar Ataxias

In many instances, the phenotype of cerebellar ataxias with autosomal dominant transmission is not restricted to cerebellar dysfunction but includes complex multisystemic neurological deficits. The designation "spinocerebellar ataxias" (SCAs) indicates the involvement of at least two systems: the spinal cord and the cerebellum (Durr, 2010). SCAs are progressive neurodegenerative diseases with cerebellar ataxia, resulting in unsteady gait, clumsiness, and dysarthria. The cerebellar syndrome may be associated with other neurological signs such as pyramidal or extrapyramidal signs, ophthalmoplegia, and cognitive impairment. Onset is usually during the third or fourth decade of life, but can occur in childhood or old age (Durr, 2010). Atrophy of the cerebellum and brainstem are most often the prominent features. Interestingly, fatigue may also represent a severe and disabling symptom in adult patients with SCA, even early in the course of disease (Brusse et al., 2011), but the significance of this observation is still unclear.

Eleven of the 18 known genes are caused by protein polyglutamine expansion (i.e., SCA1, SCA2, SCA3, SCA6, SCA7, SCA17, and dentatorubro-pallidoluysian atrophy [DRPLA]). In general terms, polyglutamine expanded proteins have been reported to stimulate cellular ROS levels and significantly reduce the mitochondrial electrochemical gradient, inducing DNA damage (Bertoni et al., 2011). The remaining SCAs are caused by non-coding expansions, mutations or large rearrangements in genes with different functions, including mitochondrial activity (SCA28/AFG3L2) (Durr, 2010).

Polyglutamine expansion SCAs which have been somehow linked to mitochondrial dysfunction are SCA2 (gene *ATXN2*), SCA3 (*ATXN3*), SCA6 (*CACNA1A*), SCA7 (*ATXN7*), DRPLA (*ATN1*). In SCA3 (Machado-Joseph disease) impaired skeletal muscle energy metabolism has been reported by phosphorus magnetic resonance spectroscopy studies (Yabe et al., 2011), and oxidative mtDNA damage may have some role in this disease (Yu et al., 2009); normal and pathological ataxin-3 proteins were reported to localized in the cytoplasm and in the nucleus, as expected, but also in the mitochondria (Pozzi et al., 2008).

Mitochondrial dysfunction is clinically evident in SCA7, in which cone-rod dystrophy and hearing impairment have been associated with activation of the mitochondria-mediated apoptotic cascade (Wang et al., 2006).

Other forms which may be linked to mitochondrial dysfunction are the "non-coding expansion" SCA12 (*PPP2R2B*) and the "conventional mutation" SCA28 (*AFG3L2*) (Durr, 2010). SCA12 may be linked to mitochondrial fission dysfunction (Dagda et al., 2008). SCA28 can account for about 1.5% of European autosomal dominant cerebellar ataxias (Cagnoli et al., 2010). Along with paraplegin, which causes recessive spastic paraplegia, *AFG3L2* is a component of the conserved m-AAA metalloprotease complex involved in the maintenance of the mitochondrial proteome (Di Bella et al., 2010). Di Bella and co-workers identified heterozygous missense mutations in five unrelated families and found that *AFG3L2* is highly and selectively expressed in human cerebellar Purkinje cells. m-AAA-deficient yeast cells expressing human mutated AFG3L2 homocomplex show respiratory deficiency, proteolytic impairment and deficiency of respiratory chain complex IV (Di Bella et al., 2010). Structure homology modeling indicated that the mutations may affect *AFG3L2* substrate handling. Respiratory chain dysfunction and increased ROS production may lead to dark degeneration of Purkinje cells and cerebellar dysfunction in SCA 28 (Maltecca et al., 2009).

X-Linked Ataxias

Fragile X-associated tremor/ataxia syndrome (FXTAS) is a late-onset neurodegenerative disorder that affects individuals who are carriers of premutation expansions (55-200 CGG repeats) in the 5' untranslated region of the *FMR1* (fragile X mental retardation 1) gene. Ross-Inta and coworkers evaluated the role of mitochondrial dysfunction in FXTAS, and reported decreased NAD- and FAD-linked oxygen uptake rates and uncoupling between electron transport and synthesis of ATP in fibroblasts from premutation carriers, as well as a lower expression of mitochondrial proteins preceding both in age and in CGG repeats the appearance of overt clinical involvement (Ross-Inta et al., 2010). Mitochondrial dysfunction may be related to altered zinc transport disrupting mitochondrial protein processing/import (Napoli et al., 2011). Detection of mitochondrial dysfunction may open up additional treatment options for this disorder, but further studies are needed.

X-linked sideroblastic anemia and ataxia (XLSA/A) is a recessive disorder characterized by an infantile to early childhood onset of non-progressive cerebellar ataxia and mild anemia with hypochromia and microcytosis. A gene encoding an ATP-binding cassette (*ABC7*) transporter, mapped to Xq13, has been linked to this disease (Allikmets et al., 1999). ABC7 localizes to the mitochondrial inner membrane and is involved in iron homeostasis (Allikmets et al., 1999).

CONCLUSION

It is important to consider a possible diagnosis of mitochondrial disease in ataxic patients with other "mitochondrial features", and especially with features of *POLG1*-related mitochondrial encephalomyopathies (i.e. PEO, myopathy, isolated muscle pain, dysphagia, neuropathy, psychiatric disorders, hypogonadism, epilepsy, parkinsonism) (Orsucci et al., 2011). The lack of signs of mitochondrial dysfunction in the muscle biopsy does not exclude a *POLG1*-related disease (Milone and Massie, 2010). Moreover, mtDNA studies (from muscle DNA) are indicated in all unusual neurological syndromes.

Large, multicenter studies are strongly needed to better characterize the phenotype and natural history of rare neurogenetic conditions, including mitochondrial disorders and hereditary ataxias, in order to identify some countermeasures (i.e. pharmacological, physical, or others) capable of benefit patients with these chronic, still incurable disorders.

REFERENCES

Allikmets, R., Raskind, W. H., Hutchinson, A., Schueck, N. D., Dean, M. and Koeller, D. M. (1999). Mutation of a putative mitochondrial iron transporter gene (ABC7) in X-linked sideroblastic anemia and ataxia (XLSA/A). *Hum. Mol. Genet.* 8, 743-749.

Batabyal, D., McKenzie, J. L. and Johnson, K. A. (2010). Role of histidine-932 of the human mitochondrial DNA polymerase in nucleotide discrimination and inherited disease. *J. Biol. Chem.*

Bertoni, A., Giuliano, P., Galgani, M., Rotoli, D., Ulianich, L., Adornetto, A., Santillo, M. R., Porcellini, A. and Avvedimento, V. E. (2011). Early and late events induced by polyQ-expanded proteins: identification of a common pathogenic property of polYQ-expanded proteins. *J. Biol. Chem.* 286, 4727-4741.

Blakely, E. L., Trip, S. A., Swalwell, H., He, L., Wren, D. R., Rich, P., Turnbull, D. M., Omer, S. E. and Taylor, R. W. (2009). A new mitochondrial transfer RNAPro gene mutation associated with myoclonic epilepsy with ragged-red fibers and other neurological features. *Arch. Neurol.* 66, 399-402.

Blok, M. J., van den Bosch, B. J., Jongen, E., Hendrickx, A., de Die-Smulders, C. E., Hoogendijk, J. E., Brusse, E., de Visser, M., Poll-The, B. T., Bierau, J., de Coo, I. F. and Smeets, H. J. (2009). The unfolding clinical spectrum of POLG mutations. *J. Med. Genet.* 46, 776-785.

Boddaert, N., Romano, S., Funalot, B., Rio, M., Sarzi, E., Lebre, A. S., Bahi-Buisson, N., Valayannopoulos, V., Desguerre, I., Seidenwurm, D., Brunelle, F., Brami-Zylberberg, F., Rotig, A., Munnich, A. and de Lonlay, P. (2008). 1H MRS spectroscopy evidence of cerebellar high lactate in mitochondrial respiratory chain deficiency. *Mol. Genet. Metab.* 93, 85-88.

Brusse, E., Brusse-Keizer, M. G., Duivenvoorden, H. J. and van Swieten, J. C. (2011). Fatigue in spinocerebellar ataxia: patient self-assessment of an early and disabling symptom. *Neurology* 76, 953-959.

Cagnoli, C., Stevanin, G., Brussino, A., Barberis, M., Mancini, C., Margolis, R. L., Holmes, S. E., Nobili, M., Forlani, S., Padovan, S., Pappi, P., Zaros, C., Leber, I., Ribai, P., Pugliese, L., Assalto, C., Brice, A., Migone, N., Durr, A. and Brusco, A. (2010). Missense mutations in the AFG3L2 proteolytic domain account for approximately 1.5% of European autosomal dominant cerebellar ataxias. *Hum. Mutat.* 31, 1117-1124.

Campuzano, V., Montermini, L., Lutz, Y., Cova, L., Hindelang, C., Jiralerspong, S., Trottier, Y., Kish, S. J., Faucheux, B., Trouillas, P., Authier, F. J., Durr, A., Mandel, J. L.,

Vescovi, A., Pandolfo, M. and Koenig, M. (1997). Frataxin is reduced in Friedreich ataxia patients and is associated with mitochondrial membranes. *Hum. Mol. Genet.* 6, 1771-1780.

Campuzano, V., Montermini, L., Molto, M. D., Pianese, L., Cossee, M., Cavalcanti, F., Monros, E., Rodius, F., Duclos, F., Monticelli, A., Zara, F., Canizares, J., Koutnikova, H., Bidichandani, S. I., Gellera, C., Brice, A., Trouillas, P., De Michele, G., Filla, A., De Frutos, R., Palau, F., Patel, P. I., Di Donato, S., Mandel, J. L., Cocozza, S., Koenig, M. and Pandolfo, M. (1996). Friedreich's ataxia: autosomal recessive disease caused by an intronic GAA triplet repeat expansion. *Science* 271, 1423-1427.

Castellotti, B., Mariotti, C., Rimoldi, M., Fancellu, R., Plumari, M., Caimi, S., Uziel, G., Nardocci, N., Moroni, I., Zorzi, G., Pareyson, D., Di Bella, D., Di Donato, S., Taroni, F. and Gellera, C. (2011). Ataxia with oculomotor apraxia type1 (AOA1): novel and recurrent aprataxin mutations, coenzyme Q10 analyses, and clinical findings in Italian patients. *Neurogenetics.*

Chan, D. C. (2006). Mitochondria: dynamic organelles in disease, aging, and development. *Cell* 125, 1241-1252.

Chan, S. S. and Copeland, W. C. (2009). DNA polymerase gamma and mitochondrial disease: understanding the consequence of POLG mutations. *Biochim. Biophys. Acta.* 1787, 312-319.

Chan, S. S., Longley, M. J. and Copeland, W. C. (2005). The common A467T mutation in the human mitochondrial DNA polymerase (POLG) compromises catalytic efficiency and interaction with the accessory subunit. *J. Biol. Chem.* 280, 31341-31346.

Chinnery, P., Majamaa, K., Turnbull, D. and Thorburn, D. (2006). Treatment for mitochondrial disorders. *Cochrane Database Syst. Rev.* CD004426.

Cocheme, H. M., Kelso, G. F., James, A. M., Ross, M. F., Trnka, J., Mahendiran, T., Asin-Cayuela, J., Blaikie, F. H., Manas, A. R., Porteous, C. M., Adlam, V. J., Smith, R. A. and Murphy, M. P. (2007). Mitochondrial targeting of quinones: therapeutic implications. *Mitochondrion 7 Suppl,* S94-102.

Coku, J., Shanske, S., Mehrazin, M., Tanji, K., Naini, A., Emmanuele, V., Patterson, M., Hirano, M. and DiMauro, S. (2010). Slowly progressive encephalopathy with hearing loss due to a mutation in the mtDNA tRNA(Leu(CUN)) gene. *J. Neurol. Sci.* 290, 166-168.

Cooper, J. M. and Schapira, A. H. (2007). Friedreich's ataxia: coenzyme Q10 and vitamin E therapy. *Mitochondrion 7 Suppl,* S127-135.

Cooper, J. M., Korlipara, L. V., Hart, P. E., Bradley, J. L. and Schapira, A. H. (2008). Coenzyme Q10 and vitamin E deficiency in Friedreich's ataxia: predictor of efficacy of vitamin E and coenzyme Q10 therapy. *Eur. J. Neurol.* 15, 1371-1379.

Correia, A. R., Wang, T., Craig, E. A. and Gomes, C. M. (2010). Iron-binding activity in yeast frataxin entails a trade off with stability in the alpha1/beta1 acidic ridge region. *Biochem. J.* 426, 197-203.

Craig, K., Ferrari, G., Tiangyou, W., Hudson, G., Gellera, C., Zeviani, M. and Chinnery, P. F. (2007). The A467T and W748S POLG substitutions are a rare cause of adult-onset ataxia in Europe. *Brain* 130, E69; author reply E70.

Crimella, C., Cantoni, O., Guidarelli, A., Vantaggiato, C., Martinuzzi, A., Fiorani, M., Azzolini, C., Orso, G., Bresolin, N. and Bassi, M. T. (2011). A novel nonsense mutation in the APTX gene associated with delayed DNA single-strand break removal fails to enhance sensitivity to different genotoxic agents. *Hum. Mutat.* 32, E2118-2133.

D'Aurelio, M., Vives-Bauza, C., Davidson, M. M. and Manfredi, G. (2010). Mitochondrial DNA background modifies the bioenergetics of NARP/MILS ATP6 mutant cells. *Hum. Mol. Genet.* 19, 374-386.

Da Pozzo, P., Cardaioli, E., Malfatti, E., Gallus, G. N., Malandrini, A., Gaudiano, C., Berti, G., Invernizzi, F., Zeviani, M. and Federico, A. (2009). A novel mutation in the mitochondrial tRNA(Pro) gene associated with late-onset ataxia, retinitis pigmentosa, deafness, leukoencephalopathy and complex I deficiency. *Eur. J. Hum. Genet.* 17, 1092-1096.

Dagda, R. K., Merrill, R. A., Cribbs, J. T., Chen, Y., Hell, J. W., Usachev, Y. M. and Strack, S. (2008). The spinocerebellar ataxia 12 gene product and protein phosphatase 2A regulatory subunit Bbeta2 antagonizes neuronal survival by promoting mitochondrial fission. *J. Biol. Chem.* 283, 36241-36248.

Debray, F. G., Lambert, M., Lortie, A., Vanasse, M. and Mitchell, G. A. (2007). Long-term outcome of Leigh syndrome caused by the NARP-T8993C mtDNA mutation. *Am. J. Med. Genet.* A 143A, 2046-2051.

Di Bella, D., Lazzaro, F., Brusco, A., Plumari, M., Battaglia, G., Pastore, A., Finardi, A., Cagnoli, C., Tempia, F., Frontali, M., Veneziano, L., Sacco, T., Boda, E., Brussino, A., Bonn, F., Castellotti, B., Baratta, S., Mariotti, C., Gellera, C., Fracasso, V., Magri, S., Langer, T., Plevani, P., Di Donato, S., Muzi-Falconi, M. and Taroni, F. (2010). Mutations in the mitochondrial protease gene AFG3L2 cause dominant hereditary ataxia SCA28. *Nat. Genet.* 42, 313-321.

Di Prospero, N. A., Baker, A., Jeffries, N. and Fischbeck, K. H. (2007a). Neurological effects of high-dose idebenone in patients with Friedreich's ataxia: a randomised, placebo-controlled trial. *Lancet Neurol.* 6, 878-886.

Di Prospero, N. A., Sumner, C. J., Penzak, S. R., Ravina, B., Fischbeck, K. H. and Taylor, J. P. (2007b). Safety, tolerability, and pharmacokinetics of high-dose idebenone in patients with Friedreich ataxia. *Arch. Neurol.* 64, 803-808.

DiMauro, S. and Schon, E. A. (2003). Mitochondrial respiratory-chain diseases. *N Engl J Med* 348, 2656-2668.

DiMauro, S., Tay, S. and Mancuso, M. (2004). Mitochondrial encephalomyopathies: diagnostic approach. *Ann. N.Y.Acad. Sci.* 1011, 217-231.

DiMauro, S., Quinzii, C. M. and Hirano, M. (2007). Mutations in coenzyme Q10 biosynthetic genes. *J. Clin. Invest.* 117, 587-589.

Drinkard, B. E., Keyser, R. E., Paul, S. M., Arena, R., Plehn, J. F., Yanovski, J. A. and Di Prospero, N. A. (2010). Exercise capacity and idebenone intervention in children and adolescents with Friedreich ataxia. *Arch. Phys. Med. Rehabil.* 91, 1044-1050.

Duncan, A. J., Bitner-Glindzicz, M., Meunier, B., Costello, H., Hargreaves, I. P., Lopez, L. C., Hirano, M., Quinzii, C. M., Sadowski, M. I., Hardy, J., Singleton, A., Clayton, P. T. and Rahman, S. (2009). A nonsense mutation in COQ9 causes autosomal-recessive neonatal-onset primary coenzyme Q10 deficiency: a potentially treatable form of mitochondrial disease. *Am. J. Hum. Genet* 84, 558-566.

Durr, A. (2010). Autosomal dominant cerebellar ataxias: polyglutamine expansions and beyond. *Lancet Neurol.* 9, 885-894.

Echaniz-Laguna, A., Chassagne, M., de Seze, J., Mohr, M., Clerc-Renaud, P., Tranchant, C. and Mousson de Camaret, B. (2010). POLG1 variations presenting as multiple sclerosis. *Arch Neurol* 67, 1140-1143.

Filosto, M. and Mancuso, M. (2007). Mitochondrial diseases: a nosological update. *Acta Neurol. Scand.* 115, 211-221.

Fogel, B. L. and Perlman, S. (2007). Clinical features and molecular genetics of autosomal recessive cerebellar ataxias. *Lancet Neurol* 6, 245-257.

Frauscher, B., Hering, S., Hogl, B., Gschliesser, V., Ulmer, H., Poewe, W. and Boesch, S. M. (2011). Restless legs syndrome in Friedreich ataxia: a polysomnographic study. *Mov. Disord.* 26, 302-306.

Gakh, O., Park, S., Liu, G., Macomber, L., Imlay, J. A., Ferreira, G. C. and Isaya, G. (2006). Mitochondrial iron detoxification is a primary function of frataxin that limits oxidative damage and preserves cell longevity. *Hum Mol. Genet.* 15, 467-479.

Gallagher, C. L., Waclawik, A. J., Beinlich, B. R., Harding, C. O., Pauli, R. M., Poirer, J., Pandolfo, M. and Salamat, M. S. (2002). Friedreich's ataxia associated with mitochondrial myopathy: clinicopathologic report. *J. Child. Neurol.* 17, 453-456.

Gelfand, J. M., Duncan, J. L., Racine, C. A., Gillum, L. A., Chin, C. T., Zhang, Y., Zhang, Q., Wong, L. J., Roorda, A. and Green, A. J. (2011). Heterogeneous patterns of tissue injury in NARP syndrome. *J. Neurol.* 258, 440-448.

Gempel, K., Topaloglu, H., Talim, B., Schneiderat, P., Schoser, B. G., Hans, V. H., Palmafy, B., Kale, G., Tokatli, A., Quinzii, C., Hirano, M., Naini, A., DiMauro, S., Prokisch, H., Lochmuller, H. and Horvath, R. (2007). The myopathic form of coenzyme Q10 deficiency is caused by mutations in the electron-transferring-flavoprotein dehydrogenase (ETFDH) gene. *Brain* 130, 2037-2044.

Gerards, M., van den Bosch, B., Calis, C., Schoonderwoerd, K., van Engelen, K., Tijssen, M., de Coo, R., van der Kooi, A. and Smeets, H. (2010). Nonsense mutations in CABC1/ADCK3 cause progressive cerebellar ataxia and atrophy. *Mitochondrion* 10, 510-515.

Goffart, S., Cooper, H. M., Tyynismaa, H., Wanrooij, S., Suomalainen, A. and Spelbrink, J. N. (2009). Twinkle mutations associated with autosomal dominant progressive external ophthalmoplegia lead to impaired helicase function and in vivo mtDNA replication stalling. *Hum. Mol. Genet.* 18, 328-340.

Gonzalez-Cabo, P., Vazquez-Manrique, R. P., Garcia-Gimeno, M. A., Sanz, P. and Palau, F. (2005). Frataxin interacts functionally with mitochondrial electron transport chain proteins. *Hum. Mol. Genet.* 14, 2091-2098.

Gonzalez-Vioque, E., Blazquez, A., Fernandez-Moreira, D., Bornstein, B., Bautista, J., Arpa, J., Navarro, C., Campos, Y., Fernandez-Moreno, M. A., Garesse, R., Arenas, J. and Martin, M. A. (2006). Association of novel POLG mutations and multiple mitochondrial DNA deletions with variable clinical phenotypes in a Spanish population. *Arch. Neurol.* 63, 107-111.

Hakonen, A. H., Isohanni, P., Paetau, A., Herva, R., Suomalainen, A. and Lonnqvist, T. (2007). Recessive Twinkle mutations in early onset encephalopathy with mtDNA depletion. *Brain* 130, 3032-3040.

Hakonen, A. H., Goffart, S., Marjavaara, S., Paetau, A., Cooper, H., Mattila, K., Lampinen, M., Sajantila, A., Lonnqvist, T., Spelbrink, J. N. and Suomalainen, A. (2008). Infantile-onset spinocerebellar ataxia and mitochondrial recessive ataxia syndrome are associated with neuronal complex I defect and mtDNA depletion. *Hum. Mol. Genet.* 17, 3822-3835.

Hakonen, A. H., Heiskanen, S., Juvonen, V., Lappalainen, I., Luoma, P. T., Rantamaki, M., Goethem, G. V., Lofgren, A., Hackman, P., Paetau, A., Kaakkola, S., Majamaa, K., Varilo, T., Udd, B., Kaariainen, H., Bindoff, L. A. and Suomalainen, A. (2005). Mitochondrial DNA polymerase W748S mutation: a common cause of autosomal recessive ataxia with ancient European origin. *Am. J. Hum. Genet.* 77, 430-441.

Harris, M. O., Walsh, L. E., Hattab, E. M. and Golomb, M. R. (2010). Is it ADEM, POLG, or both? *Arch. Neurol.* 67, 493-496.

Hart, P. E., Lodi, R., Rajagopalan, B., Bradley, J. L., Crilley, J. G., Turner, C., Blamire, A. M., Manners, D., Styles, P., Schapira, A. H. and Cooper, J. M. (2005). Antioxidant treatment of patients with Friedreich ataxia: four-year follow-up. *Arch. Neurol.* 62, 621-626.

Hausse, A. O., Aggoun, Y., Bonnet, D., Sidi, D., Munnich, A., Rotig, A. and Rustin, P. (2002). Idebenone and reduced cardiac hypertrophy in Friedreich's ataxia. *Heart* 87, 346-349.

Horvath, R., Hudson, G., Ferrari, G., Futterer, N., Ahola, S., Lamantea, E., Prokisch, H., Lochmuller, H., McFarland, R., Ramesh, V., Klopstock, T., Freisinger, P., Salvi, F., Mayr, J. A., Santer, R., Tesarova, M., Zeman, J., Udd, B., Taylor, R. W., Turnbull, D., Hanna, M., Fialho, D., Suomalainen, A., Zeviani, M. and Chinnery, P. F. (2006). Phenotypic spectrum associated with mutations of the mitochondrial polymerase gamma gene. *Brain* 129, 1674-1684.

Huang, M. L., Becker, E. M., Whitnall, M., Rahmanto, Y. S., Ponka, P. and Richardson, D. R. (2009). Elucidation of the mechanism of mitochondrial iron loading in Friedreich's ataxia by analysis of a mouse mutant. *Proc. Natl. Acad. Sci. USA* 106, 16381-16386.

Hudson, G. and Chinnery, P. F. (2006). Mitochondrial DNA polymerase-gamma and human disease. *Hum. Mol. Genet.* 15 Spec No 2, R244-252.

Hudson, G., Amati-Bonneau, P., Blakely, E. L., Stewart, J. D., He, L., Schaefer, A. M., Griffiths, P. G., Ahlqvist, K., Suomalainen, A., Reynier, P., McFarland, R., Turnbull, D. M., Chinnery, P. F. and Taylor, R. W. (2008). Mutation of OPA1 causes dominant optic atrophy with external ophthalmoplegia, ataxia, deafness and multiple mitochondrial DNA deletions: a novel disorder of mtDNA maintenance. *Brain* 131, 329-337.

Isohanni, P., Hakonen, A. H., Euro, L., Paetau, I., Linnankivi, T., Liukkonen, E., Wallden, T., Luostarinen, L., Valanne, L., Paetau, A., Uusimaa, J., Lonnqvist, T., Suomalainen, A. and Pihko, H. (2011). POLG1 manifestations in childhood. *Neurology* 76, 811-815.

Ito, S., Shirai, W., Asahina, M. and Hattori, T. (2008). Clinical and brain MR imaging features focusing on the brain stem and cerebellum in patients with myoclonic epilepsy with ragged-red fibers due to mitochondrial A8344G mutation. *AJNR Am. J. Neuroradiol.* 29, 392-395.

Jauslin, M. L., Wirth, T., Meier, T. and Schoumacher, F. (2002). A cellular model for Friedreich Ataxia reveals small-molecule glutathione peroxidase mimetics as novel treatment strategy. *Hum. Mol. Genet.* 11, 3055-3063.

Jauslin, M. L., Meier, T., Smith, R. A. and Murphy, M. P. (2003). Mitochondria-targeted antioxidants protect Friedreich Ataxia fibroblasts from endogenous oxidative stress more effectively than untargeted antioxidants. *FASEB J.* 17, 1972-1974.

Kearney, M., Orrell, R. W., Fahey, M. and Pandolfo, M. (2009). Antioxidants and other pharmacological treatments for Friedreich ataxia. *Cochrane Database Syst. Rev.* CD007791.

Kipps, A., Alexander, M., Colan, S. D., Gauvreau, K., Smoot, L., Crawford, L., Darras, B. T. and Blume, E. D. (2009). The longitudinal course of cardiomyopathy in Friedreich's ataxia during childhood. *Pediatr. Cardiol.* 30, 306-310.

La Pean, A., Jeffries, N., Grow, C., Ravina, B. and Di Prospero, N. A. (2008). Predictors of progression in patients with Friedreich ataxia. *Mov. Disord.* 23, 2026-2032.

Lagedrost, S. J., Sutton, M. S., Cohen, M. S., Satou, G. M., Kaufman, B. D., Perlman, S. L., Rummey, C., Meier, T. and Lynch, D. R. (2011). Idebenone in Friedreich ataxia cardiomyopathy-results from a 6-month phase III study (IONIA). *Am. Heart J.* 161, 639-645 e631.

Lagier-Tourenne, C., Tazir, M., Lopez, L. C., Quinzii, C. M., Assoum, M., Drouot, N., Busso, C., Makri, S., Ali-Pacha, L., Benhassine, T., Anheim, M., Lynch, D. R., Thibault, C., Plewniak, F., Bianchetti, L., Tranchant, C., Poch, O., DiMauro, S., Mandel, J. L., Barros, M. H., Hirano, M. and Koenig, M. (2008). ADCK3, an ancestral kinase, is mutated in a form of recessive ataxia associated with coenzyme Q10 deficiency. *Am. J. Hum. Genet.* 82, 661-672.

Le Ber, I., Dubourg, O., Benoist, J. F., Jardel, C., Mochel, F., Koenig, M., Brice, A., Lombes, A. and Durr, A. (2007). Muscle coenzyme Q10 deficiencies in ataxia with oculomotor apraxia 1. *Neurology* 68, 295-297.

Leshinsky-Silver, E., Shuvalov, R., Inbar, S., Cohen, S., Lev, D. and Lerman-Sagie, T. (2011). Juvenile Leigh Syndrome, Optic Atrophy, Ataxia, Dystonia, and Epilepsy due to T14487C Mutation in the mtDNA-ND6 Gene: A Mitochondrial Syndrome Presenting From Birth to Adolescence. *J. Child Neurol.* 26, 476-481.

Levi, S. and Rovida, E. (2009). The role of iron in mitochondrial function. *Biochim. Biophys. Acta* 1790, 629-636.

Lodi, R., Cooper, J. M., Bradley, J. L., Manners, D., Styles, P., Taylor, D. J. and Schapira, A. H. (1999). Deficit of in vivo mitochondrial ATP production in patients with Friedreich ataxia. *Proc. Natl. Acad. Sci. USA* 96, 11492-11495.

Longley, M. J., Humble, M. M., Sharief, F. S. and Copeland, W. C. (2010). Disease variants of the human mitochondrial DNA helicase encoded by C10orf2 differentially alter protein stability, nucleotide hydrolysis, and helicase activity. *J. Biol. Chem.* 285, 29690-29702.

Lopez-Gallardo, E., Lopez-Perez, M. J., Montoya, J. and Ruiz-Pesini, E. (2009). CPEO and KSS differ in the percentage and location of the mtDNA deletion. *Mitochondrion* 9, 314-317.

Lopez, L. C., Quinzii, C. M., Area, E., Naini, A., Rahman, S., Schuelke, M., Salviati, L., Dimauro, S. and Hirano, M. (2010). Treatment of CoQ(10) deficient fibroblasts with ubiquinone, CoQ analogs, and vitamin C: time- and compound-dependent effects. *PLoS One* 5, e11897.

Luoma, P. T., Luo, N., Loscher, W. N., Farr, C. L., Horvath, R., Wanschitz, J., Kiechl, S., Kaguni, L. S. and Suomalainen, A. (2005). Functional defects due to spacer-region mutations of human mitochondrial DNA polymerase in a family with an ataxia-myopathy syndrome. *Hum. Mol. Genet.* 14, 1907-1920.

Lynch, D. R., Perlman, S. L. and Meier, T. (2010). A phase 3, double-blind, placebo-controlled trial of idebenone in friedreich ataxia. *Arch. Neurol.* 67, 941-947.

Maltecca, F., Magnoni, R., Cerri, F., Cox, G. A., Quattrini, A. and Casari, G. (2009). Haploinsufficiency of AFG3L2, the gene responsible for spinocerebellar ataxia type 28, causes mitochondria-mediated Purkinje cell dark degeneration. *J. Neurosci.* 29, 9244-9254.

Mancuso, M., Orsucci, D., Choub, A. and Siciliano, G. (2010). Current and emerging treatment options in the management of Friedreich ataxia. *Neuropsychiatr Dis. Treat* 6, 491-499.

Mancuso, M., Filosto, M., Mootha, V. K., Rocchi, A., Pistolesi, S., Murri, L., DiMauro, S. and Siciliano, G. (2004). A novel mitochondrial tRNAPhe mutation causes MERRF syndrome. *Neurology* 62, 2119-2121.

Mariotti, C., Solari, A., Torta, D., Marano, L., Fiorentini, C. and Di Donato, S. (2003). Idebenone treatment in Friedreich patients: one-year-long randomized placebo-controlled trial. *Neurology* 60, 1676-1679.

Milone, M. and Massie, R. (2010). Polymerase gamma 1 mutations: clinical correlations. *Neurologist* 16, 84-91.

Mollet, J., Delahodde, A., Serre, V., Chretien, D., Schlemmer, D., Lombes, A., Boddaert, N., Desguerre, I., de Lonlay, P., de Baulny, H. O., Munnich, A. and Rotig, A. (2008). CABC1 gene mutations cause ubiquinone deficiency with cerebellar ataxia and seizures. *Am. J. Hum. Genet.* 82, 623-630.

Napoli, E., Ross-Inta, C., Wong, S., Omanska-Klusek, A., Barrow, C., Iwahashi, C., Garcia-Arocena, D., Sakaguchi, D., Berry-Kravis, E., Hagerman, R., Hagerman, P. J. and Giulivi, C. (2011). Altered Zinc Transport Disrupts Mitochondrial Protein Processing/Import in Fragile X-Associated Tremor/Ataxia Syndrome. *Hum. Mol. Genet.*

Nikali, K., Suomalainen, A., Saharinen, J., Kuokkanen, M., Spelbrink, J. N., Lonnqvist, T. and Peltonen, L. (2005). Infantile onset spinocerebellar ataxia is caused by recessive mutations in mitochondrial proteins Twinkle and Twinky. *Hum. Mol. Genet.* 14, 2981-2990.

Okuno, D., Iino, R. and Noji, H. (2011). Rotation and Structure of FoF1-ATP synthase. *J. Biochem.*

Orsucci, D., Filosto, M., Siciliano, G. and Mancuso, M. (2009). Electron transfer mediators and other metabolites and cofactors in the treatment of mitochondrial dysfunction. *Nutr. Rev.* 67, 427-438.

Orsucci, D., Caldarazzo Ienco, E., Mancuso, M. and Siciliano, G. (2011). POLG1-Related and other "Mitochondrial Parkinsonisms": an Overview. *J. Mol. Neurosci.* 44, 17-24.

Pancrudo, J., Shanske, S., Bonilla, E., Daras, M., Akman, H. O., Krishna, S., Malkin, E. and DiMauro, S. (2007). Mitochondrial encephalomyopathy due to a novel mutation in the tRNAGlu of mitochondrial DNA. *J. Child. Neurol.* 22, 858-862.

Pandolfo, M. (2008a). Friedreich ataxia. *Arch. Neurol.* 65, 1296-1303.

Pandolfo, M. (2008b). Drug Insight: antioxidant therapy in inherited ataxias. *Nat. Clin. Pract. Neurol.* 4, 86-96.

Petruzzella, V., Zoccolella, S., Amati, A., Torraco, A., Lamberti, P., Carnicella, F., Serlenga, L. and Papa, S. (2004). Cerebellar ataxia as atypical manifestation of the 3243A>G MELAS mutation. *Clin. Genet.* 65, 64-65.

Pineda, M., Arpa, J., Montero, R., Aracil, A., Dominguez, F., Galvan, M., Mas, A., Martorell, L., Sierra, C., Brandi, N., Garcia-Arumi, E., Rissech, M., Velasco, D., Costa, J. A. and Artuch, R. (2008). Idebenone treatment in paediatric and adult patients with Friedreich ataxia: long-term follow-up. *Eur. J. Paediatr. Neurol.* 12, 470-475.

Pozzi, C., Valtorta, M., Tedeschi, G., Galbusera, E., Pastori, V., Bigi, A., Nonnis, S., Grassi, E. and Fusi, P. (2008). Study of subcellular localization and proteolysis of ataxin-3. *Neurobiol. Dis.* 30, 190-200.

Quinzii, C. M., Lopez, L. C., Naini, A., DiMauro, S. and Hirano, M. (2008). Human CoQ10 deficiencies. *Biofactors* 32, 113-118.

Quinzii, C. M., Lopez, L. C., Gilkerson, R. W., Dorado, B., Coku, J., Naini, A. B., Lagier-Tourenne, C., Schuelke, M., Salviati, L., Carrozzo, R., Santorelli, F., Rahman, S., Tazir, M., Koenig, M., DiMauro, S. and Hirano, M. (2010). Reactive oxygen species, oxidative stress, and cell death correlate with level of CoQ10 deficiency. *FASEB J.* 24, 3733-3743.

Raman, S. V., Phatak, K., Hoyle, J. C., Pennell, M. L., McCarthy, B., Tran, T., Prior, T. W., Olesik, J. W., Lutton, A., Rankin, C., Kissel, J. T. and Al-Dahhak, R. (2011). Impaired myocardial perfusion reserve and fibrosis in Friedreich ataxia: a mitochondrial cardiomyopathy with metabolic syndrome. *Eur. Heart. J.* 32, 561-567.

Rantamaki, M., Luoma, P., Virta, J. J., Rinne, J. O., Paetau, A., Suomalainen, A. and Udd, B. (2007). Do carriers of POLG mutation W748S have disease manifestations? *Clin. Genet.* 72, 532-537.

Richardson, D. R., Huang, M. L., Whitnall, M., Becker, E. M., Ponka, P. and Rahmanto, Y. S. (2010). The ins and outs of mitochondrial iron-loading: the metabolic defect in Friedreich's ataxia. *J. Mol. Med.* 88, 323-329.

Ristow, M., Pfister, M. F., Yee, A. J., Schubert, M., Michael, L., Zhang, C. Y., Ueki, K., Michael, M. D., 2nd, Lowell, B. B. and Kahn, C. R. (2000). Frataxin activates mitochondrial energy conversion and oxidative phosphorylation. *Proc. Natl. Acad. Sci. USA* 97, 12239-12243.

Ross-Inta, C., Omanska-Klusek, A., Wong, S., Barrow, C., Garcia-Arocena, D., Iwahashi, C., Berry-Kravis, E., Hagerman, R. J., Hagerman, P. J. and Giulivi, C. (2010). Evidence of mitochondrial dysfunction in fragile X-associated tremor/ataxia syndrome. *Biochem. J.* 429, 545-552.

Rustin, P., Rotig, A., Munnich, A. and Sidi, D. (2002). Heart hypertrophy and function are improved by idebenone in Friedreich's ataxia. *Free Radic. Res.* 36, 467-469.

Rustin, P., von Kleist-Retzow, J. C., Chantrel-Groussard, K., Sidi, D., Munnich, A. and Rotig, A. (1999). Effect of idebenone on cardiomyopathy in Friedreich's ataxia: a preliminary study. *Lancet* 354, 477-479.

Schaefer, A. M., McFarland, R., Blakely, E. L., He, L., Whittaker, R. G., Taylor, R. W., Chinnery, P. F. and Turnbull, D. M. (2008). Prevalence of mitochondrial DNA disease in adults. *Ann. Neurol.* 63, 35-39.

Schicks Md, J., Synofzik Md, M., Schulte, C. and Schols Md, L. (2010). POLG, but not PEO1, is a frequent cause of cerebellar ataxia in Central Europe. *Mov. Disord.*

Schmucker, S., Argentini, M., Carelle-Calmels, N., Martelli, A. and Puccio, H. (2008). The in vivo mitochondrial two-step maturation of human frataxin. *Hum. Mol. Genet.* 17, 3521-3531.

Schols, L., Zange, J., Abele, M., Schillings, M., Skipka, G., Kuntz-Hehner, S., van Beekvelt, M. C., Colier, W. N., Muller, K., Klockgether, T., Przuntek, H. and Vorgerd, M. (2005).

L-carnitine and creatine in Friedreich's ataxia. A randomized, placebo-controlled crossover trial. *J. Neural. Transm.* 112, 789-796.

Schulz, J. B., Boesch, S., Burk, K., Durr, A., Giunti, P., Mariotti, C., Pousset, F., Schols, L., Vankan, P. and Pandolfo, M. (2009). Diagnosis and treatment of Friedreich ataxia: a European perspective. *Nat. Rev. Neurol.* 5, 222-234.

Schulz, J. B., Dehmer, T., Schols, L., Mende, H., Hardt, C., Vorgerd, M., Burk, K., Matson, W., Dichgans, J., Beal, M. F. and Bogdanov, M. B. (2000). Oxidative stress in patients with Friedreich ataxia. *Neurology* 55, 1719-1721.

Selak, M. A., Lyver, E., Micklow, E., Deutsch, E. C., Onder, O., Selamoglu, N., Yager, C., Knight, S., Carroll, M., Daldal, F., Dancis, A., Lynch, D. R. and Sarry, J. E. (2011). Blood cells from Friedreich ataxia patients harbor frataxin deficiency without a loss of mitochondrial function. *Mitochondrion* 11, 342-350.

Seznec, H., Simon, D., Monassier, L., Criqui-Filipe, P., Gansmuller, A., Rustin, P., Koenig, M. and Puccio, H. (2004). Idebenone delays the onset of cardiac functional alteration without correction of Fe-S enzymes deficit in a mouse model for Friedreich ataxia. *Hum. Mol. Genet.* 13, 1017-1024.

Seznec, H., Simon, D., Bouton, C., Reutenauer, L., Hertzog, A., Golik, P., Procaccio, V., Patel, M., Drapier, J. C., Koenig, M. and Puccio, H. (2005). Friedreich ataxia: the oxidative stress paradox. *Hum. Mol. Genet.* 14, 463-474.

Sgarbi, G., Casalena, G. A., Baracca, A., Lenaz, G., DiMauro, S. and Solaini, G. (2009). Human NARP mitochondrial mutation metabolism corrected with alpha-ketoglutarate/aspartate: a potential new therapy. *Arch. Neurol.* 66, 951-957.

Shidara, Y. and Hollenbeck, P. J. (2010). Defects in mitochondrial axonal transport and membrane potential without increased reactive oxygen species production in a Drosophila model of Friedreich ataxia. *J. Neurosci.* 30, 11369-11378.

Shishkin, A. A., Voineagu, I., Matera, R., Cherng, N., Chernet, B. T., Krasilnikova, M. M., Narayanan, V., Lobachev, K. S. and Mirkin, S. M. (2009). Large-scale expansions of Friedreich's ataxia GAA repeats in yeast. *Mol. Cell* 35, 82-92.

Shokolenko, I., Venediktova, N., Bochkareva, A., Wilson, G. L. and Alexeyev, M. F. (2009). Oxidative stress induces degradation of mitochondrial DNA. *Nucleic. Acids. Res.* 37, 2539-2548.

Sikorska, M., Sandhu, J. K., Simon, D. K., Pathiraja, V., Sodja, C., Li, Y., Ribecco-Lutkiewicz, M., Lanthier, P., Borowy-Borowski, H., Upton, A., Raha, S., Pulst, S. M. and Tarnopolsky, M. A. (2009). Identification of ataxia-associated mtDNA mutations (m.4052T>C and m.9035T>C) and evaluation of their pathogenicity in transmitochondrial cybrids. *Muscle Nerve* 40, 381-394.

Silvestri, G., Mongini, T., Odoardi, F., Modoni, A., deRosa, G., Doriguzzi, C., Palmucci, L., Tonali, P. and Servidei, S. (2000). A new mtDNA mutation associated with a progressive encephalopathy and cytochrome c oxidase deficiency. *Neurology* 54, 1693-1696.

Stemmler, T. L., Lesuisse, E., Pain, D. and Dancis, A. (2010). Frataxin and mitochondrial FeS cluster biogenesis. *J. Biol. Chem.* 285, 26737-26743.

Tanji, K., DiMauro, S. and Bonilla, E. (1999). Disconnection of cerebellar Purkinje cells in Kearns-Sayre syndrome. *J. Neurol. Sci.* 166, 64-70.

Trifunovic, A., Wredenberg, A., Falkenberg, M., Spelbrink, J. N., Rovio, A. T., Bruder, C. E., Bohlooly, Y. M., Gidlof, S., Oldfors, A., Wibom, R., Tornell, J., Jacobs, H. T. and

Larsson, N. G. (2004). Premature ageing in mice expressing defective mitochondrial DNA polymerase. *Nature* 429, 417-423.

Tsuchiya, K., Miyazaki, H., Akabane, H., Yamamoto, M., Kondo, H., Mizusawa, H. and Ikeda, K. (1999). MELAS with prominent white matter gliosis and atrophy of the cerebellar granular layer: a clinical, genetic, and pathological study. *Acta Neuropathol.* 97, 520-524.

Turrens, J. F. (2003). Mitochondrial formation of reactive oxygen species. *J. Physiol.* 552, 335-344.

Tzoulis, C., Neckelmann, G., Mork, S. J., Engelsen, B. E., Viscomi, C., Moen, G., Ersland, L., Zeviani, M. and Bindoff, L. A. (2010). Localized cerebral energy failure in DNA polymerase gamma-associated encephalopathy syndromes. *Brain* 133, 1428-1437.

Velasco-Sanchez, D., Aracil, A., Montero, R., Mas, A., Jimenez, L., O'Callaghan, M., Tondo, M., Capdevila, A., Blanch, J., Artuch, R. and Pineda, M. (2011). Combined therapy with idebenone and deferiprone in patients with Friedreich's ataxia. *Cerebellum* 10, 1-8.

Virgilio, R., Ronchi, D., Bordoni, A., Fassone, E., Bonato, S., Donadoni, C., Torgano, G., Moggio, M., Corti, S., Bresolin, N. and Comi, G. P. (2009). Mitochondrial DNA G8363A mutation in the tRNA Lys gene: clinical, biochemical and pathological study. *J. Neurol. Sci.* 281, 85-92.

Wang, H. L., Yeh, T. H., Chou, A. H., Kuo, Y. L., Luo, L. J., He, C. Y., Huang, P. C. and Li, A. H. (2006). Polyglutamine-expanded ataxin-7 activates mitochondrial apoptotic pathway of cerebellar neurons by upregulating Bax and downregulating Bcl-x(L). *Cell Signal* 18, 541-552.

Winterthun, S., Ferrari, G., He, L., Taylor, R. W., Zeviani, M., Turnbull, D. M., Engelsen, B. A., Moen, G. and Bindoff, L. A. (2005). Autosomal recessive mitochondrial ataxic syndrome due to mitochondrial polymerase gamma mutations. *Neurology* 64, 1204-1208.

Wong, L. J., Naviaux, R. K., Brunetti-Pierri, N., Zhang, Q., Schmitt, E. S., Truong, C., Milone, M., Cohen, B. H., Wical, B., Ganesh, J., Basinger, A. A., Burton, B. K., Swoboda, K., Gilbert, D. L., Vanderver, A., Saneto, R. P., Maranda, B., Arnold, G., Abdenur, J. E., Waters, P. J. and Copeland, W. C. (2008). Molecular and clinical genetics of mitochondrial diseases due to POLG mutations. *Hum. Mutat.* 29, E150-172.

Yabe, I., Tha, K. K., Yokota, T., Sato, K., Soma, H., Takei, A., Terae, S., Okita, K. and Sasaki, H. (2011). Estimation of skeletal muscle energy metabolism in Machado-Joseph disease using (31)P-MR spectroscopy. *Mov. Disord.* 26, 165-168.

Yu-Wai-Man, P., Griffiths, P. G., Gorman, G. S., Lourenco, C. M., Wright, A. F., Auer-Grumbach, M., Toscano, A., Musumeci, O., Valentino, M. L., Caporali, L., Lamperti, C., Tallaksen, C. M., Duffey, P., Miller, J., Whittaker, R. G., Baker, M. R., Jackson, M. J., Clarke, M. P., Dhillon, B., Czermin, B., Stewart, J. D., Hudson, G., Reynier, P., Bonneau, D., Marques, W., Jr., Lenaers, G., McFarland, R., Taylor, R. W., Turnbull, D. M., Votruba, M., Zeviani, M., Carelli, V., Bindoff, L. A., Horvath, R., Amati-Bonneau, P. and Chinnery, P. F. (2010). Multi-system neurological disease is common in patients with OPA1 mutations. *Brain* 133, 771-786.

Yu, Y. C., Kuo, C. L., Cheng, W. L., Liu, C. S. and Hsieh, M. (2009). Decreased antioxidant enzyme activity and increased mitochondrial DNA damage in cellular models of Machado-Joseph disease. *J. Neurosci. Res.* 87, 1884-1891.

In: Ataxia: Causes, Symptoms and Treatment
Editor: Sung Hoi Hong

ISBN: 978-1-61942-867-6
© 2012 Nova Science Publishers, Inc.

Chapter 5

EPIDEMIC SEASONAL ATAXIC SYNDROME: EPIDEMIOLOGY, CLINICAL PRESENTATION, ETIOLOGICAL MECHANISMS AND THERAPY

*Bola Adamolekun**
Department of Neurology,
University of Tennessee Health Science Center
Memphis, TN, US

ABSTRACT

Epidemics of an acute ataxic syndrome occur annually in the rainy season in parts of West Africa, characterized by cerebellar ataxia, ocular abnormalities and impairment of consciousness, The onset of symptoms is usually shortly after a meal. The epidemics have been called the seasonal ataxic syndrome. Detailed epidemiological and dietary studies have indicated that the seasonal ataxic syndrome is a thiamine deficiency state similar to Wernicke's encephalopathy, occurring in poor, undernourished individuals who are mildly thiamine-deficient because of subsistence on a monotonous diet of cassava (*manihot esculenta*) meals. These individuals then suffer an acute exacerbation of thiamine deficiency from heat-stable thiaminases present in the *Anaphe venata* larvae, an invariable component of the last meals eaten prior to symptom onset. The annual period of availability of the *Anaphe* larvae coincides with the seasonal occurrence of the seasonal ataxic syndrome. This syndrome is the only thiamine-deficiency state known to be caused by thiaminases in insects. The epidemiology, clinical presentation, etiological mechanisms, therapy and control of the seasonal ataxic syndrome will be discussed in this chapter.

---

* Address for correspondence: B. Adamolekun, MD, FWACP, Department of Neurology University of Tennessee Health Science Center, 855 Monroe Avenue, Memphis TN 38163, USA, Phone: 901-4484916, Fax: 901-4487440, E-mail: badamole@uthsc.edu

INTRODUCTION

For several decades, epidemics of an acute ataxic syndromehave occurred annually in the rainy season between July and September, in parts of western Nigeria. First described in the medical literature in 1958 [1]· the syndrome was characterized by acute onset of cerebellar ataxia, gaze abnormalities and varying levels of impaired consciousness; occurring shortly after a meal [1-3].The syndrome was highly prevalent among the *Ijeshas,* living around Ilesha, a town in Western Nigeria from where the syndrome was first described [1], hence the old pseudonym *"Ilesha shakes"*[4].The current name *seasonal ataxic syndrome* was introduced by Adamolekun in 1992[5]. Epidemics of the seasonal ataxic syndrome (SAS) have been described from other towns in Western Nigeria, including Ibadan [2], Ile-Ife [3] and Ikare [6]. Epidemics have also been reported from the Benin Republic [7], a country geographically contiguous with Western Nigeria.

ETIOLOGY

For about half a century after its original description in the literature [1], the seasonal ataxic syndrome remained an annually recurring enigmatic disease of unknown etiology. Etiological hypotheses proposed included the following:

Viral Hypothesis

A viral etiologic hypothesis was initially suggested for the seasonal ataxic syndrome.Coakham [8] suggested that the syndrome was an arbovirus encephalitis involving the brainstem, while Wright and Morley [1] called the syndrome *"encephalitis tremens"* because they thought it was a form of viral encephalitis.

However, the viral hypothesis lacked convincing proof. There were no conjugal cases or clustering patterns that would be compatible with a transmissible infective agent. Subsequent cerebrospinal fluid analysis, serological tests [1]and viral studies [4] failed to show any evidence of a viral infection.

Toxins in Food

There had been suspicions that a toxin in food may be responsible for the clinical presentations of the syndrome, but no food item had been found to be common to all patients presenting with the disease. A toxin from seasonally harvested new yams (*Dioscorea spp*) was suggested as a cause by Osuntokun in 1972 [2]. Yams are a common staple food in western Nigeria whose harvest period coincided with the period of seasonal occurrence of the syndrome. However, yam consumption was found in only 23% of seasonal ataxia patients in one study [6]. In another study, dietary recall of foods consumed by patients during the previous 24 hours was compared with the foods eaten by a random group of unaffected controls. In both groups, two-thirds had eaten yam [9].

Hypothesis of Thiamine Deficiency

An etiological hypothesis of acute thiamine deficiency was proposed by this author in 1992 [5]. That hypothesis was based on the observation of the similarity of the clinical presentation of the seasonal ataxic syndrome to the triad of cerebellar ataxia, gaze paresis and encephalopathy well known to occur in patients with Wernicke's encephalopathy.

The hypothesis [5] suggested that the seasonal ataxic syndrome was an acute thiamine deficiency state, occurring in poor, undernourished individuals who were marginally thiamine-deficient because of subsistence on a monotonous diet of high carbohydrate tropical meals with minimal protein and micronutrient supplementation. These individuals were postulated to then suffer an acute exacerbation of thiamine deficiency from thiaminases or anti-thiamine factors present in seasonal foods, precipitating a Wernicke's encephalopathy and its attendant clinical features.

CLINICAL PRESENTATION OF SAS IS COMPATIBLE WITH WERNICKE'S ENCEPHALOPATHY

Epidemiological studies of the seasonal ataxic syndrome [3, 6] have indeed confirmed that the syndrome occurred exclusively in individuals in the low socio-economic strata, subsisting on monotonous diets of high carbohydrate meals with minimal protein supplementation. The patients with seasonal ataxic syndrome (SAS) havea wide age scatter, with occurrence inweaned children and adults [2, 3, 6]. The SAS has a male to female ratio of 1.5 to 1, [6]remarkably similar to the male to female ratio of 1.7 to 1 described by Victor (1976)in patients with Wernicke's encephalopathy[10].

Symptom onset is within hours of the main evening meal, with patients abruptly developing nausea, vomiting, tremors and gait imbalance. The clinical signs are those of cerebellar ataxia in all patients, gaze paresis in 9% and nystagmus in 27%. There was impairment of consciousness in 33% of patients [1, 6]. The clinical features of cerebellar ataxia, ocular abnormalities and impairment of consciousness seen in the SAS are compatible with those of Wernicke's encephalopathy (WE). Of note, in the cases of WE described by Harper et al[11], only 16% displayed the full clinical triad.

In tropical thiamine deficiency, Wernicke's encephalopathy is very rare. Only 0.17% of 32,000 British prisoners of war in Singapore who received a diet of polished rice developed Wernicke's encephalopathy [12]. Its rarity as a manifestation of tropical thiamine deficiency makes the annual occurrence of epidemic Wernicke's encephalopathy in patients with SAS particularly remarkable. There has been no other report of epidemic Wernicke's encephalopathy in the tropics.

MECHANISM OF THIAMINE DEFICIENCY IN SEASONAL ATAXIC SYNDROME

1.   Cassava Diet Causes Marginal Thiamine Deficiency

The diet of communities in the endemic areas for seasonal ataxic syndrome (SAS) is dominated by cassava (*manihot esculenta*), which is the major source of calories for the impoverished, low income people exclusively affected by the disease. Neurologically normal, low income Nigerians on Cassava diet have been shown to be thiamine - deficient compared to more affluent controls [13]. This is partly the result of inadequate dietary thiamine intake in patients subsisting on a monotonous diet of cassava derivatives (processed cassava flour contains negligibly small amounts of thiamine).A nutritional survey in western Nigeria, where SAS is prevalent confirmed a deficiency of thiamine intake in the rural and urban population of all ages [14].

2.   Thiaminases cause Acute Exacerbation of Thiamine Deficiency

Results of 24-hour dietary recall in patients with SAS indicated that all patients who presented with the syndrome consumed stews containing the roasted larvae of the African silkworm (*Anaphe Venata* Butler, (Lepidoptera, Notodontidae) as part of their last meals, within hours prior to the onset of disease [15]. The larvae of African silk worms are eaten in many parts of Africa, where the consumption of the larvae is mainly by the rural, poor population who often consider it a delicacy [16]. The larvae are prepared by roasting them in hot, dry sand and are added to stews or eaten alone as a snack. An investigation of the nutritional value of the *Anaphe Venata* larvae showed that its crude protein contentis higher than that of animal proteins such as lamb and pork, and comparable to that of chicken egg [16]. The *Anaphe Venata* larvae are univoltine, molting only once a year, showing strong seasonality for the rainy season and irregular cycles of abundance. The annual period of wide availability of the larvae in the Nigerian markets coincides with the seasonal period of peak occurrence of the seasonal ataxic syndrome [15].Nishimune et al [17] have now established that the *Anaphe Venata* larvae contained significant amounts of heat-stable thiaminases, thus confirming the hypothesis presented by Adamolekun [5]concerning the etio-pathogenesis of the seasonal ataxic syndrome. Thiaminases have been described as the cause of thiamine deficiency in foxes eating raw entrails of fish [18] and in sheep that consumed thiaminase-containing plants [19].A heat stable thiaminase in a plant called Nardoo (*marsilea drummondii)* was blamed for the deaths of three expeditionists in the interior of Australia in the nineteenth century [20]. The SAS is the only thiamine-deficiency state known to be caused by thiaminases in insects.

3.   Intra-Family Variations in Susceptibility

Genetic studies have suggested that a transketolase enzyme variant may put individuals at risk for Wernicke's encephalopathy when on a diet that is marginal or deficient in thiamine [21]. It is however unlikely that genetics play a significant role in the etio-pathogenesis of the seasonal ataxic syndrome (SAS), given the well - documented occurrence of the syndrome in only one out of five family members who are exposed to the same meals [2, 3].This intra-family variation in susceptibility to SAS is quite intriguing, given the expectation that all family members would have similar nutritional status. In a controlled study evaluating the possibility that variations in susceptibility to the SAS may be dependent on variations in baseline nutritional status prior to consumption of the *anaphe venata* larvae [22], serum albumin levels were measured as an index of protein nutriturein SAS patients and compared to serum albumin levels in family members who did not succumb to the disease. The study showed that the mean serum albumin level in SAS patients was significantly lower than in family members who did not succumb to the disease.These results imply that the protein nutrition of individuals may presage susceptibility to the seasonal ataxia. Interestingly, intra-family variations in susceptibility have also been reported in tropical ataxic neuropathy, another nutritional ataxic syndrome endemic to parts of Western Nigeria [23] and now thought to be a thiamine deficiency state [24].

THERAPY AND CONTROL OF SAS

Confirmation that the seasonal ataxic syndrome is a thiamine deficiency state was obtained from the results of a double blind, placebo-controlled study which demonstrated a dramatic, statistically significant improvement in ataxic scores within 72 hours of the administration of thiamine hydrochloride in patients with the syndrome [25]. Reversal of neurological signs to normal (no intention tremor, no ataxia) occurred during the 72 hour study period in 62.5% of the patients, with the other patients achieving a normal neurological status in the immediate post-study period. Thiamine is now used as standard therapy for the syndrome.

A focused, health education campaign highlighting the role of the *Anaphe Venata* larvae in the etiology of SAS, and discouraging its consumption resulted in a 99% reduction in the hospital prevalence of SAS over three years[26] . The health education technique used in the study allowed an oral health information cascade from health workers through patients and relatives to the susceptible segments of the society. This health education campaign, if widely adopted and combined with a long-term thiamine supplementation program; may eventually result in the complete eradication of SAS in West Africa.

REFERENCES

[1]   Wright J, Morley DC. Encephalitis tremens. *Lancet* 1958; i: 871-3.

[2]   Osuntokun BO. Epidemic ataxia in Western Nigeria. *BMJ* 1972; ii: 598.

[3]   Adamolekun B, Ndububa DA. Epidemiology and clinical presentation of a seasonal ataxia in Western Nigeria. *J. Neurol. Sci.* 1994. 124: 95-98.

[4]   Pearson CA; Moore DL; David-West TS. Virus studies in "Ilesha shakes". *West Afr. Med. J. Niger. Med. Dent. Pract.* 1973; 22 (1): 20-22.

[5]   Adamolekun B. A seasonal ataxic syndrome in South Western Nigeria: An etiological hypothesis of acute thiamine deficiency. *Ethnic. Dis.* 1992. 2 (2): 185-186.

[6]   Adamolekun B, Ibikunle FR. Investigation of an epidemic of seasonal ataxia in Ikare, Western Nigeria. *Acta. Neurol. Scand.* 1994; 90 (5): 309-311.

[7]   Fayomi EB, Comlan C, Josse C, Zohoun T. Cerebellar ataxia in a Beninian Village. *African Newsletter*: 1996; 6: 78-9.

[8]   Coakham H. Rapid irregular movement of eyes and limbs. *Br. Med J* 1972: 2 (5804); 45-6.

[9]   Pearson CA. Cerebellar ataxia. *African Newsletter*: 1997; 7: 20.

[10] Victor M. The Wernicke Korsakoff syndrome. In: Vinken PJ, Bruyn GW (Eds). *Handbook of Clinical Neurology* 28 (II). North Holland Publishing Company, Amsterdam (1976), pp 243-270.

[11] Harper CG, Giles M, Finlay Jones R. Clinical signs in the Wernicke-Korsakoff complex: A retrospective analysis of 13 cases diagnosed at necropsy. *J. Neurol. Neurosurg. Psychiatry* 1986; 49: 341-5.

[12] Djoenardi W, Noterman S.: Experimental and clinical Beriberi in East Java. *Voeding* 1990; 51:296-99.

[13] Osuntokun BO, Aladetoyinbo A, Bademosi O. Vitamin B nutrition in the Nigerian tropical ataxic neuropathy. *J. Neurol. Neurosurg. Psychiat.* 1985; 48: 154-156.

[14] Fashakin JB, Oyekanmi M. Evaluation of some Vitamin B complex nutriture in Ile-Ife and environs (Nigeria). J Nutr Res 1986; 56: 79-84.

[15] Adamolekun B. AnapheVenataentomophagy and seasonal ataxic syndrome in Southwest Nigeria. *Lancet* 1993. 341: 629.

[16] Ashiru MO. The food value of the larvae of AnapheVenata Butler (Lepidoptera: Notodontidae). *Ecology of Food and Nutrition,* 1988. 22: 313-320.

[17] Nishimune T, Watanabe Y, Okazaki H, Akai H. Thiamin is decomposed due to Anaphesppentomophagy in seasonal ataxia patients in Nigeria. *J. Nutrition* 2000. 130; 6: 1625-1628.

[18] Green RG, Carlson WE and Evans CA : A deficiency disease of foxes produced by feeding fish. *J. Nutr.* 1941; 21: 243-356.

[19] Ramos, J Maca C, Loste A et al. Biochemical changes in apparently normal sheep from flocks affected by polioencephalomalacia. *Vet. Res. Commun.,* 2003. Vol 27, 2: 111-24.

[20] Earl JW and McCleary BV. Mystery of the poisoned expedition. *Nature* 1994. 21; 368:683-684.

[21] Blass JP, Gibson GE. Abnormality of a thiamine-requiring enzyme in patients with Wernicke-Korsakoff syndrome. *N. Engl. J. Med.* 1977. 297: 367-770.

[22] Adamolekun B, Lawal T, Ndububa DA, Balogun MO. Serum albumin levels and intra-ethnic variations in susceptibility to a seasonal ataxia in Nigerians. *Ethn. Dis.* 1994. 4 (1): 87-90.

[23] Oluwole OSA, Onabolu AO, Link H et al. Persistence of tropical ataxic neuropathy in a Nigerian community. *J. Neurol. Neurosurg. Psychiatry.* 2000; 69: 96-101.

[24] Adamolekun B. Thiamine deficiency and the etiology of tropical ataxic neuropathy. *International Health* 2010; 2 (1): 17-21.

[25] Adamolekun B, Adamolekun WE, Sonibare AD, Sofowora G. A double-blind, placebo-controlled study of the efficacy of thiamine hydrochloride in a seasonal ataxia in Nigerians. *Neurology* 1994. 44: 549-551.

[26] Adamolekun B. An evaluation of the impact of health education on the hospital prevalence of a seasonal ataxia in Western Nigeria. *J. Epidemiol. and Community Health* 1995. 49: 489-491.

Chapter 6

CLINICAL AND GENETIC ASPECTS OF RECESSIVE ATAXIAS

Anne Noreau[1], Guy A. Rouleau[1,2] and Nicolas Dupré[3]
[1]Centre of Excellence in Neurosciences of Université de Montréal (CENUM),
Centre de Recherche du Centre Hospitalier de l'Université de Montréal (CRCHUM),
Montréal, Québec, Canada
[2]Research Center CHU Ste-Justine, and Department of Pediatrics and Biochemistry,
University of Montreal, Montréal,
Québec, Canada
[3]Faculty of Medicine, Laval University, Department of Neurological Sciences,
CHAUQ (Enfant-Jésus), Québec, Québec, Canada

ABSTRACT

The group of hereditary ataxias is represented by different modes of inheritance, such as X-linked, mitochondrial, autosomal dominant and the autosomal recessive ataxias. This chapter will provide an overview of the autosomal recessive group, by describing those that are best defined. For each disorder, the clinical manifestations will be described, allowing a better definition and recognition of the symptoms. Then, the causative gene and the mechanisms leading to the disease will be discussed. Currently available treatments and/or potential therapeutic targets will also be outlined. The most frequent recessive ataxias will be covered: Friedreich's Ataxia, Ataxia-Telangiectasia, Autosomal Recessive Spastic Ataxia of Charlevoix-Saguenay, Autosomal Recessive Cerebellar Ataxia type 1 and type 2, Ataxia with Oculomotor Apraxia type 1 and type 2 and Ataxia with Vitamin E Deficiency.

INTRODUCTION

Ataxia is defined as a lack of coordination in voluntary movements. It is not caused by muscle dysfunction but by nervous system impairments, particularly in the cerebellum, which is the key player in the coordination of voluntary movements. Since the description of

Friedreich's Ataxia (FA), a number of other ataxias have been described according to their specific clinical features. By bringing together patients with similar symptoms and doing appropriate genetic studies, it was possible to find several genes involved in these ataxias. This chapter will review the most frequent recessive ataxias, which can also be subdivided in four groups according to their molecular pathogenesis. The first group is the degenerative ataxias, which includes FA, Autosomal Recessive Spastic Ataxia of Charlevoix-Saguenay (ARSACS) and Autosomal Recessive Cerebellar Ataxia type 1 (ARCA-1). The second group is the metabolic ataxias, in which Autosomal Recessive Cerebellar Ataxia type 2 (ARCA-2) and Ataxia with Vitamin E Deficiency (AVED) will be discussed. The third group comprises ataxias with DNA repair defects, such as Ataxia Telangiectasia (A-T) and Ataxia with Oculomotor Apraxia type 1 (AOA-1) and 2 (AOA-2). For each of these groups we will provide descriptions of the clinical features, the genes involved, the molecular pathways and the current or future treatments.

THE DEGENERATIVE ATAXIAS

Friedreich's Ataxia

Described in 1863 by Nicholaus Friedreich, professor of Medicine in Heidelberg, Germany, FA (#MIM229300) is certainly the most frequent form of cerebellar ataxias. The mean age of onset is 15 years old, but can vary from 2 to 25 years of age. The first recognized abnormality is gait instability, but FA can also be characterized by other signs, such as dysarthria, sensory loss, muscle weakness, scoliosis, foot deformities, an absence of tendon reflexes and a Babinski sign. Cognitive function is preserved. Other clinical features, such as hypertrophic cardiomyopathy, cardiac conduction defects, type 2 diabetes and hearing loss, can be seen. The disease progression varies between individuals, but the mean age of death is around 38 years old, usually caused by progressive cardiomyopathy. Brain Magnetic Resonance Imaging (MRI) of patients is usually normal, except in some cases where iron deposits can be seen in the cerebellum's dentate nucleus. However, atrophy of the spinal cord is observed and, in advanced cases of FA, mild cerebellar atrophy can also be observed [1]. Nerve conduction studies demonstrated the presence of an axonal neuropathy, with small or absent sensory action potentials [1-4]. Furthermore, compound Muscle Action Potentials (C-MAPs) are either normal or show a slight reduction in amplitudes and velocities. "The Quebec Collaborative Group" [5] and Harding [6] established the essential clinical criteria for FA diagnosis. According to Harding, the essential features are: (1) autosomal recessive mode of inheritance; (2) onset before 20 years of age; (3) progressive gait and limb ataxia; (4) absent tendon reflexes in the lower extremities; and finally (5) electrophysiological evidence of axonal sensory neuropathy followed by dysarthria, areflexia, loss of distal position and vibration sense, extensor plantar responses and pyramidal weakness of the legs [6].

A locus has been mapped to chromosome 9q13 [7] mainly with families originating from Southern Italy, with French-Canadians from Quebec and with Acadians from Louisiana [7]. FA is caused by mutations in the *FRDA* gene, which encodes a protein involved in mitochondrial iron regulation. This gene, also known as *FNX* gene or X25, encompasses seven exons, spanning 95 Kb of genomic sequence, and encodes a highly conserved 220 amino acid mitochondrial protein called frataxin. Almost 96 % of patients are homozygous for an expansion in trinucleotide repeats (GAA), occurring in the first intron of the *FRDA* gene. The remaining 4% are explained by compound heterozygosity, which is a combination of this expansion and a number of different missense mutations [8, 9]. To date, no FA patients have been reported to carry homozygous point mutations, which suggests that the missense mutations might still maintain some function [10]. Normal alleles contain from 6 to 27 GAA triplet repeats, whereas disease predisposing alleles have 120 to 1,700 repeats. The most commonly found repeat sizes varies from 600 to 900 [11]. A strong correlation between the size of the smaller repeat allele (GAA) and the age of onset and disease progression was established, in which larger expansions correlate with an earlier age of onset [12]. This observation was seen in Caucasian FA patients, but not in Acadian FA patients [13]. Overexpansion of GAA triplets creates a different conformation called "sticky DNA" or "triplex" and inhibits transcription, leading to a reduced expression of frataxin mRNA levels [10, 14, 15]. Consequently, this reduced expression leads to a reduced amount of the frataxin protein [16]. In normal condition, frataxin expression levels are low in the cerebellum and in the cerebral cortex, but high in spinal cord, heart, liver, muscle and pancreatic tissues [8]. Since its complete inactivation leads to early embryonic lethality in mice, C.*elegans* and Drosophila, this protein is essential for normal embryonic development [17]. Experiments in cell systems, especially in yeast, have provided relevant information about frataxin's possible function in mitochondria. At least five hypotheses have been proposed [18]. Indeed, frataxin could play a role in iron transport, iron-sulfur cluster (ISC) biosysthesis, iron storage, antioxidation and stimulation of oxidative phosphorylation [10, 19-25].

One approach to treat FA patients is to use strategies that increase frataxin levels. This can be achieved by blocking triplex structure formation using oligodeoxyribonucleotides, which will increase transcription through the GAA repeats [26]. Compounds such as pyrrol-imidazole polyamides or pentamidine [27], histone deacetylase inhibitors (HDACi) [28] and human erythropoietin (rhuEPO) [29-31] are also known to increase frataxin transcription. Furthermore, anti-oxidants, such as parabenzoquinone derivative (Idebedone or coenzyme Q1)), were reported to possibly improve FA patients' life quality [32-34].

Autosomal Recessive Spastic Ataxia of Charlevoix-Saguenay (ARSACS)

ARSACS (MIM#270770) is a disorder initially described in Quebec and is the most commonly inherited ataxias in this province. Most of the families originate from the regions of Charlevoix and Saguenay-Lac-St-Jean, where the estimated carrier frequency is 1/22 [35]. ARSACS has also been described in other regions of the world including Europe (Italy, Spain, Holland and Belgium) [36-39], North Africa (Morocco and Tunisia) [40, 41], the Middle-East (Turkey) [42, 43] and Asia (Japan) [44].

In ARSACS, spasticity develops first, typically in the legs with abnormal gait initiation (at 12-18 months of age) [45]. The disease progresses during adolescence and the twenties, with an increase in muscle tone and in deep tendon reflexes. Speech is slurred. There is a slower motor development in ARSACS preschoolers, but no global intellectual impairment is observed. Gait is often jerky, sometimes with scissoring. Distal amyotrophy develops with time. In most cases, ankle jerks become brisk, and typically disappear around 25 years of age [45]. Others clinical signs include bilateral abnormal plantar responses and saccadic alterations of smooth ocular pursuits. Myelinated fibers around the optic disc on fundoscopy are more commonly described in Quebec ARSACS patients.

Nerve conduction studies and needle electromyography show a progressive mixed sensory-motor neuropathy [46]. C-MAPs show reduced velocities and by the end of the third decade, distal motor latencies can no longer be recorded in lower extremities [45]. On MRI, atrophy of the superior cerebellar vermis is always present, even in younger patients. Progressive cerebellar cortical atrophy progresses throughout the disease, but the inferior vermis remains thick. Brain autopsies of ARSACS patients grossly reveal atrophic superior cerebellar vermis, especially in the anterior structures, where Purkinje cells are absent. In addition, severe bilateral loss of myelin staining is seen along the spinal cord.

Due to a founder effect present in the French-Canadian population, the ARSACS gene was mapped to chromosome 13q12 [47]. Two mutations in the SACS gene were initially reported [48]. The first mutation, present in 94% of French-Canadian cases, is a deletion causing a frameshift [49]. Worldwide, over 70 different mutations have been described. The initial SACS gene was known to encompasse only one single large exon [48, 50]. After finding mutations in a group of patients harboring the same symptoms, a Japanese group identified eight new exons, all located downstream of the previously reported exon [51]. Highly expressed in human brain, especially in motor neuron and Purkinje cells, the SACS gene encodes a 4,579 amino acid protein [52]. This protein has an ubiquitin-like domain (UBL) that interacts with a proteasome, a J –domain and two domains similar to HSP90. The latter is known to be involved in different biological processes, such as protein folding, transport and cell survival [52]. To date, there is no treatment for ARSACS [50].

Autosomal Recessive Cerebellar Ataxia Type 1 (ARCA-1)

ARCA-1 (MIM#610743) is a new disease, that was described in 2007, following the study of patients affected by the same phenotype and originating from the same region of Quebec (Canada) called Beauce [53].

All affected individuals presented similar clinical characteristics that included ataxia and/or dysarthria with a middle-age onset. Associated features can be seen following onset, such as dysmetria, brisk lower extremity tendon reflexes, minor abnormalities in saccades and smooth pursuit and mild cognitive impairments [54, 55].

There is no associated peripheral neuropathy since nerve conduction studies are always normal. On MRI, a diffuse cerebellar atrophy is present (Figure 1), without cortical or brainstem atrophy [56]. Genome-wide linkage revealed a candidate interval on chromosome 6q that contained a single gene called synaptic nuclear envelope protein 1 (*SYNE1*) [53]. *SYNE1* is one of the biggest genes in the human genome: 147 exons encoding a 27,652 bp mRNA that translates an 8,797 amino acid protein. Seven mutations were identified in *SYNE-1*: four nonsense, two splice-sites and one deletion, all leading to the protein's premature truncation [53, 54]. The SYNE1 protein contains two N-terminal actin binding regions, comprising tandem-paired calponin-homology-domains, a transmembrane domain, multiple spectrin repeats, and a C-terminal KASH domain.

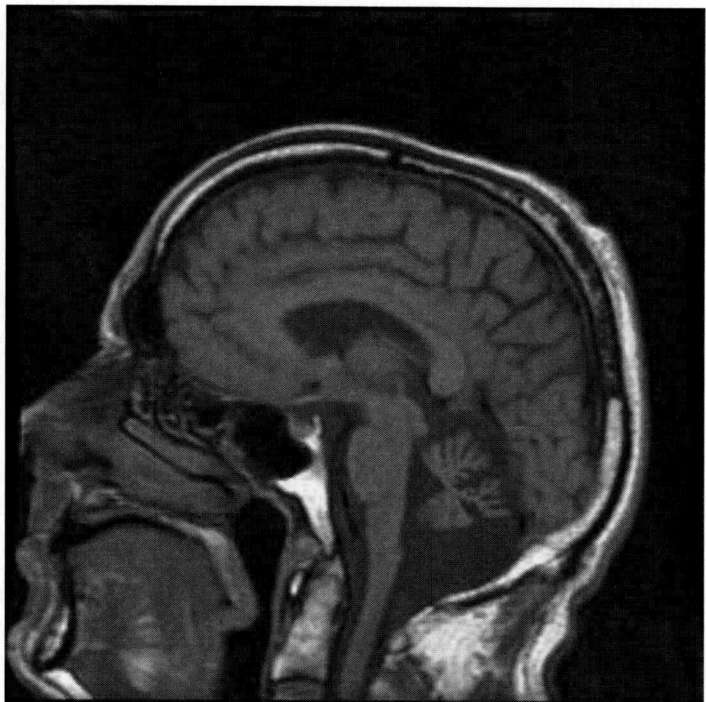

Figure 1. Legend: MRI showing mild cerebellar atrophy of ARCA-1 patient.

This protein is particularly abundant in the cerebellum. In muscles, SYNE1 is involved in anchoring specialized myonuclei under the neuromuscular junction [53]. It has been predicted that mutations in this gene would underlie a significant fraction of recessive or sporadic cases with pure cerebellar ataxia. For now, there is no cure for ARCA-1.

METABOLIC ATAXIAS

Autosomal Recessive Cerebellar Ataxia Type 2 (ARCA-2)

Described in 2003, ARCA-2 (#612016) is also known as Autosomal Recessive Spinocerebellar Ataxia type 9 (SCAR9). It is characterized by a childhood onset cerebellar atrophy [57]. This ataxia is associated with an important decrease in skeletal muscle levels of coenzyme Q10 (CoQ10). This leads to mitochondrial dysfunction, since CoQ10 is responsible for electron transfer in the mitochondrial respiratory chain [57]. Associated symptoms include seizures, developmental delays, intellectual disabilities, pyramidal signs, exercise intolerance and elevated lactate levels at rest after moderate exercise. MRI shows diffuse cerebellar atrophy. Homozygosity mapping in a large Algerian family lead to the identification of the linked region on chromosome 1q41-1q42. A homozygous mutation of the donor splice-site in intron 11, in the aarf-domain-containing-kinase 3 gene (*ADCK3* or *CABC1*), was identified as causative [58]. CoQ10 oral supplementation therapy shows mild subjective improvements and stabilization of the cerebellar ataxia [58].

Ataxia with Vitamin E Deficiency (AVED)

Ataxia with Vitamin E Deficiency (AVED) (MIM#227460) clinically resembles FA, and is characterized by sensory and cerebellar ataxia, dysarthria, hyporeflexia, a decreased vibration and positional sense, and a bilateral Babinski sign. Other additionnal features, such as glucose intolerance, cardiomyopathy, head titubation, dystonia and retinitis pigmentosa, can be observed [59]. Age of onset is generally before 20 years of age with a large variation from 2 to 52 years of age [60, 61]. The diagnosis can be made by observing the serum's low vitamin E concentration (less than 2,5mg/L), in absence of intestinal malabsorption [62]. Axonal sensory neuropathy is shown on electrophysiological studies [60]. Mutations in the tocopherol transfert protein alpha gene (*TTPA*) cause this disease [63, 64]. Located on chromosome 8q13 [65, 66], the *TTPA* gene encodes a 278 amino-acid protein, which is a cytosolic liver protein involved in tocopherol's intracellular transport. It is the most active vitamin E isomer [67, 68]. Patients with mutations in *TTPA* gene cannot add a-tocopherol in VLDLs [69]. The exact link between the pathological processes and vitamin E is not entirely clear but oxidative stress may play a major role [70] as Vitamin E is a fat-soluble antioxidant that prevents lipid oxidation in the membranes. The severity of the disease and age of onset can be modulated by the type of mutations found in *TTPA* gene. In fact, missense mutations lead to a milder and a later onset phenotype compared to truncating mutations [71]. Oral supplementation with vitamin E [72] usually stabilizes or improves the neurological symptoms [73].

DNA REPAIR DEFECT ATAXIAS

Ataxia-Telangiectasia (AT)

Ataxia-telangiectasia (AT) (MIM#208900) is the most common recessive ataxia in children under 5 years old [74]. It is characterized by ataxia and the presence of oculocutanoeous telangiectases appearing between 2 to 8 years of age. It is associated with immunodeficiency leading to recurrent infections, skin and endocrine abnormalities and predisposition to malignancies [74-76].

A large range of ophthalmological abnormalities, such as nystagmus, hypometric, strabismus and oculomotor apraxia, can be detected [77]. Other symptoms can be seen after few years like: dysarthria, dysphagia, facial hypomimia, generalized hypotonia, peripheral neuropathy, tremor, and chorea. [77]. MRI reveals cerebellar atrophy, initially more apparent in the superior vermis, which later becomes diffused [78]. AT is due to mutations in the ataxia telangiectasia gene (*ATM*) located on chromosome 11q22-q23 [79]. *ATM* gene is composed of 66 exons and encodes a protein of 3056 amino acids. *ATM* is a Ser/Thr protein kinase and is a member of the phosphoinositide 3-kinase (PI3K)-related protein kinase (PIKK) family, responsible for DNA repair during the cell cycle, which prevents the incorporation of deleterious mutations [78, 80]. Over 432 causing mutations have been found in the *ATM* gene [81].

Ataxia with Oculomotor Apraxia Type 1 (AOA-1)

Ataxia with oculomotor apraxia (AOA-1) (MIM#208920) is a disease that develops in childhood and early adolescence. It is characterized by oculomotor apraxia, areflexia, peripheral neuropathy, strabismus, chorea, dystonia. MRI reveals marked cerebellar atrophy, mild brainstem atrophy and, in advanced cases, cortical atrophy is observed [82]. Laboratory findings of patients show hypoalbuminemia, hypercholesterolemia and elevated creatine kinase levels, while serum alpha-fetoprotein levels are always normal [83, 84]. AOA-1 is caused by mutations in the aprataxin (*APTX*) gene, located on chromosome 9q33.3-q34.3 [85]. This gene encodes a 342 amino acid protein, localized in the nucleus [86-88]. This protein is involved in single-strand DNA repair, acting in the same pathway as the ATM protein [80, 89].

Ataxia with Oculomotor Apraxia Type 2 (AOA-2)

Ataxia with oculomotor apraxia type 2 (MIM#606002) has several characteristics in common with the previously described ataxia (AOA-1). Disease onset is between 10 to 25 years of age and AOA-2 is characterized by cerebellar atrophy, axonal senrorimotor neuropathy, oculomotor apraxia [90]. However, in contrast with AOA-1, AOA-2 patients show elevated serum alpha-fetoprotein levels [90]. In the majority of patients, the initial symptom is ataxia, but in some cases it is preceded by strabismus, dystonia and postural tremor. The disease progresses slowly and other features can be observed in its course, such as dystonic posture of the hands, choreic movements, head or postural tremor, extensor plantar responses or sphincter disturbances and mildly impaired cognitive functions [91]. The linked locus was found to be on the chromosome 9q33.3-q34.3 [85, 92] and the disease is due to mutations in the senataxin (*SETX*) gene [90, 93]. *SETX* encodes a large protein called senataxin. It contains a DNA-RNA helicase activity and is involved in RNA processing and DNA repair [80, 93, 94]. Patients with *SETX* mutation show an increased sensitivity to oxidative DNA damage. New roles were defined for this protein as it seems to be involved in the coordination of transcriptional events and neurotoxic damage mediation [95, 96].

CONCLUSION

Genetic studies have given us the ability to identify several genes and have helped us unravel some of the pathophysiological mechanisms underlying the recessive ataxias. Routine testing is currently available for AOA1, AOA2, AVED, and FA. In movement disorder clinics, despite extensive genetic testing, almost half of recessive ataxia cases remain undiagnosed. Therefore, there are many additional genes left to discover. It is likely that new sequencing technologies, which allow massive targeted sequencing (Exome Capture) or full genome sequencing, will play a central role in genetic studies and accelerate the gene discovery. With an ever increasing understanding of the pathogenic mechanisms underlying recessive ataxias, novel therapeutic avenues will surely be found.

REFERENCES

[1]   Alper, G; Narayanan, V. (2003). Friedreich's ataxia. *Pediatr. Neurol.*, *28*, 335-341.

[2]   Harding, AE. (1993). Clinical features and classification of inherited ataxias. *Adv. Neurol.*, *61*, 1-14.

[3]   Pandolfo, M; Montermini, L. (1998). Prenatal diagnosis of Friedreich ataxia. *Prenat. Diagn.*, *18*, 831-833.

[4]   Delatycki, MB; Williamson, R; Forrest, SM. (2000). Friedreich ataxia: an overview. *J. Med. Genet.*, *37*, 1-8.

[5]   Geoffroy, G; Barbeau, A; Breton, G; Lemieux, B; Aube, M; Leger, C; Bouchard, JP. (1976). Clinical description and roentgenologic evaluation of patients with Friedreich's ataxia. *Can. J. Neurol. Sci.*, *3*, 279-286.

[6]   Harding, A. (1981). Friedreich's ataxia: a clinical and genetic study of 90 families with an analysis of early diagnostic criteria and intrafamilial clustering of clinical features. *Brain*, *104*, 589-620.

[7]   Chamberlain, SSJ, Rowland A et al. (1988). Mapping of mutations causing Friedreich's ataxia to human chromosome 9. *Nature*, *334*, 248-250.

[8]   Campuzano, V; Montermini, L; Molto, MD; Pianese, L; Cossee, M; Cavalcanti, F; Monros, E; Rodius, F; Duclos, F; Monticelli, A; Zara, F; Canizares, J; Koutnikova, H; Bidichandani, SI; Gellera, C; Brice, A; Trouillas, P; De Michele, G; Filla, A; De Frutos, R; Palau, F; Patel, PI; Di Donato, S; Mandel, JL; Cocozza, S; Koenig, M; Pandolfo, M. (1996). Friedreich's ataxia: autosomal recessive disease caused by an intronic GAA triplet repeat expansion. *Science*, *271*, 1423-1427.

[9]   Cossee, M; Durr, A; Schmitt, M; Dahl, N; Trouillas, P; Allinson, P; Kostrzewa, M; Nivelon-Chevallier, A; Gustavson, KH; Kohlschutter, A; Muller, U; Mandel, JL; Brice, A; Koenig, M; Cavalcanti, F; Tammaro, A; De Michele, G; Filla, A; Cocozza, S; Labuda, M; Montermini, L; Poirier, J; Pandolfo, M. (1999). Friedreich's ataxia: point mutations and clinical presentation of compound heterozygotes. *Ann. Neurol.*, *45*, 200-206.

[10]   Schmucker, S; Puccio, H. (2010). Understanding the molecular mechanisms of Friedreich's ataxia to develop therapeutic approaches. *Hum. Mol. Genet.*, *19*, R103-110.

[11]   Montermini, L; Richter, A; Morgan, K; Justice, CM; Julien, D; Castellotti, B; Mercier, J; Poirier, J; Capozzoli, F; Bouchard, JP; Lemieux, B; Mathieu, J; Vanasse, M; Seni, MH; Graham, G; Andermann, F; Andermann, E; Melancon, SB; Keats, BJ; Di Donato, S; Pandolfo, M. (1997). Phenotypic variability in Friedreich ataxia: role of the associated GAA triplet repeat expansion. *Ann. Neurol.*, *41*, 675-682.

[12]   Durr, A; Cossee, M; Agid, Y; Campuzano, V; Mignard, C; Penet, C; Mandel, JL; Brice, A; Koenig, M. (1996). Clinical and genetic abnormalities in patients with Friedreich's ataxia. *N. Engl. J. Med.*, *335*, 1169-1175.

[13]   Montermini, L; Andermann, E; Labuda, M; Richter, A; Pandolfo, M; Cavalcanti, F; Pianese, L; Iodice, L; Farina, G; Monticelli, A; Turano, M; Filla, A; De Michele, G; Cocozza, S. (1997). The Friedreich ataxia GAA triplet repeat: premutation and normal alleles. *Hum. Mol. Genet.*, *6*, 1261-1266.

[14] Bidichandani, SI; Ashizawa, T; Patel, PI. (1998). The GAA triplet-repeat expansion in Friedreich ataxia interferes with transcription and may be associated with an unusual DNA structure. *Am. J. Hum. Genet., 62*, 111-121.

[15] Sakamoto, N; Chastain, PD; Parniewski, P; Ohshima, K; Pandolfo, M; Griffith, JD; Wells, RD. (1999). Sticky DNA: self-association properties of long GAA.TTC repeats in R.R.Y triplex structures from Friedreich's ataxia. *Mol. Cell, 3*, 465-475.

[16] Campuzano, V; Montermini, L; Lutz, Y; Cova, L; Hindelang, C; Jiralerspong, S; Trottier, Y; Kish, SJ; Faucheux, B; Trouillas, P; Authier, FJ; Durr, A; Mandel, JL; Vescovi, A; Pandolfo, M; Koenig, M. (1997). Frataxin is reduced in Friedreich ataxia patients and is associated with mitochondrial membranes. *Hum. Mol. Genet., 6*, 1771-1780.

[17] Puccio, H. (2009). Multicellular models of Friedreich ataxia. *J. Neurol., 256 Suppl 1*, 18-24.

[18] Puccio, H; Koenig, M. (2002). Friedreich ataxia: a paradigm for mitochondrial diseases. *Curr. Opin. Genet. Dev., 12*, 272-277.

[19] Rotig, A, de Lonlay, P., et al. (1997). Aconitase and mitochondrial iron-sulfur protein deficiency in Friedreich ataxia. *Nat.Genet., 17*, 215-217.

[20] Muhlenhoff, U, Gerber, J. et al. (2003). Components involved in assembly and dislocation or iron-sulfur clusters on the scaffold protein Isu1p. *EMBO J., 22*, 4815-4825.

[21] Martelli , A, Wattenhofer-Donze, et al. (2007). Frataxin is essential for extramitochondrial Fe-S cluster proetins in mammalian tissues. *Hum. Mol. genet., 16*, 2651-2658.

[22] Babcock, M; de Silva, D; Oaks, R; Davis-Kaplan, S; Jiralerspong, S; Montermini, L; Pandolfo, M; Kaplan, J. (1997). Regulation of mitochondrial iron accumulation by Yfh1p, a putative homolog of frataxin. *Science, 276*, 1709-1712.

[23] Foury, F; Cazzalini, O. (1997). Deletion of the yeast homologue of the human gene associated with Friedreich's ataxia elicits iron accumulation in mitochondria. *FEBS Lett., 411*, 373-377.

[24] Wong, A; Yang, J; Cavadini, P; Gellera, C; Lonnerdal, B; Taroni, F; Cortopassi, G. (1999). The Friedreich's ataxia mutation confers cellular sensitivity to oxidant stress which is rescued by chelators of iron and calcium and inhibitors of apoptosis. *Hum. Mol. Genet., 8*, 425-430.

[25] Chantrel-Groussard, K; Geromel, V; Puccio, H; Koenig, M; Munnich, A; Rotig, A; Rustin, P. (2001). Disabled early recruitment of antioxidant defenses in Friedreich's ataxia. *Hum. Mol. Genet., 10*, 2061-2067.

[26] Grabczyk, E; Usdin, K. (2000). Alleviating transcript insufficiency caused by Friedreich's ataxia triplet repeats. *Nucleic Acids Res., 28*, 4930-4937.

[27] Burnett, R; Melander, C; Puckett, JW; Son, LS; Wells, RD; Dervan, PB; Gottesfeld, JM. (2006). DNA sequence-specific polyamides alleviate transcription inhibition associated with long GAA.TTC repeats in Friedreich's ataxia. *Proc. Natl. Acad. Sci. USA, 103*, 11497-11502.

[28] Gottesfeld, JM. (2007). Small molecules affecting transcription in Friedreich ataxia. *Pharmacol. Ther., 116*, 236-248.

[29] Sturm, B; Bistrich, U; Schranzhofer, M; Sarsero, JP; Rauen, U; Scheiber-Mojdehkar, B; de Groot, H; Ioannou, P; Petrat, F. (2005). Friedreich's ataxia, no changes in

mitochondrial labile iron in human lymphoblasts and fibroblasts: a decrease in antioxidative capacity? *J. Biol. Chem.*, *280*, 6701-6708.

[30] Marmolino, D; Acquaviva, F. (2009). Friedreich's Ataxia: from the (GAA)n repeat mediated silencing to new promising molecules for therapy. *Cerebellum*, *8*, 245-259.

[31] Tsou, AY; Friedman, LS; Wilson, RB; Lynch, DR. (2009). Pharmacotherapy for Friedreich ataxia. *CNS Drugs*, *23*, 213-223.

[32] Rustin, P; Bonnet, D; Rotig, A; Munnich, A; Sidi, D. (2004). Idebenone treatment in Friedreich patients: one-year-long randomized placebo-controlled trial. *Neurology*, *62*, 524-525; author reply 525; discussion 525.

[33] Cooper, JM; Korlipara, LV; Hart, PE; Bradley, JL; Schapira, AH. (2008). Coenzyme Q10 and vitamin E deficiency in Friedreich's ataxia: predictor of efficacy of vitamin E and coenzyme Q10 therapy. *Eur J Neurol*, *15*, 1371-1379.

[34] Seznec, H; Simon, D; Monassier, L; Criqui-Filipe, P; Gansmuller, A; Rustin, P; Koenig, M; Puccio, H. (2004). Idebenone delays the onset of cardiac functional alteration without correction of Fe-S enzymes deficit in a mouse model for Friedreich ataxia. *Hum. Mol. Genet.*, *13*, 1017-1024.

[35] De Braekeleer, M; Giasson, F; Mathieu, J; Roy, M; Bouchard, JP; Morgan, K. (1993). Genetic epidemiology of autosomal recessive spastic ataxia of Charlevoix-Saguenay in northeastern Quebec. *Genet. Epidemiol.*, *10*, 17-25.

[36] Criscuolo, C; Banfi, S; Orio, M; Gasparini, P; Monticelli, A; Scarano, V; Santorelli, FM; Perretti, A; Santoro, L; De Michele, G; Filla, A. (2004). A novel mutation in SACS gene in a family from southern Italy. *Neurology*, *62*, 100-102.

[37] Criscuolo, C; Sacca, F; De Michele, G; Mancini, P; Combarros, O; Infante, J; Garcia, A; Banfi, S; Filla, A; Berciano, J. (2005). Novel mutation of SACS gene in a Spanish family with autosomal recessive spastic ataxia. *Mov. Disord.*, *20*, 1358-1361.

[38] Vermeer, S; Meijer, RP; Pijl, BJ; Timmermans, J; Cruysberg, JR; Bos, MM; Schelhaas, HJ; van de Warrenburg, BP; Knoers, NV; Scheffer, H; Kremer, B. (2008). ARSACS in the Dutch population: a frequent cause of early-onset cerebellar ataxia. *Neurogenetics*, *9*, 207-214.

[39] Ouyang, Y; Segers, K; Bouquiaux, O; Wang, FC; Janin, N; Andris, C; Shimazaki, H; Sakoe, K; Nakano, I; Takiyama, Y. (2008). Novel SACS mutation in a Belgian family with sacsin-related ataxia. *J. Neurol. Sci.*, *264*, 73-76.

[40] Lamy C, MS, Taussig D et al. . (1998). Ataxie spastique récessive de type Charlevoix-Saguenay dans une famille marocaine. . *Revue Neurologique*, *154*, 463.

[41] Mrissa, N; Belal, S; Hamida, CB; Amouri, R; Turki, I; Mrissa, R; Hamida, MB; Hentati, F. (2000). Linkage to chromosome 13q11-12 of an autosomal recessive cerebellar ataxia in a Tunisian family. *Neurology*, *54*, 1408-1414.

[42] Gucuyener, K; Ozgul, K; Paternotte, C; Erdem, H; Prud'homme, JF; Ozguc, M; Topaloglu, H. (2001). Autosomal recessive spastic ataxia of Charlevoix-Saguenay in two unrelated Turkish families. *Neuropediatrics*, *32*, 142-146.

[43] Richter, AM; Ozgul, RK; Poisson, VC; Topaloglu, H. (2004). Private SACS mutations in autosomal recessive spastic ataxia of Charlevoix-Saguenay (ARSACS) families from Turkey. *Neurogenetics*, *5*, 165-170.

[44] Ogawa, T; Takiyama, Y; Sakoe, K; Mori, K; Namekawa, M; Shimazaki, H; Nakano, I; Nishizawa, M. (2004). Identification of a SACS gene missense mutation in ARSACS. *Neurology*, *62*, 107-109.

[45] Bouchard, JP; Richter, A; Mathieu, J; Brunet, D; Hudson, TJ; Morgan, K; Melancon, SB. (1998). Autosomal recessive spastic ataxia of Charlevoix-Saguenay. *Neuromuscul. Disord., 8*, 474-479.

[46] Peyronnard, JM; Charron, L; Barbeau, A. (1979). The neuropathy of Charlevoix-Saguenay ataxia: an electrophysiological and pathological study. *Can. J. Neurol. Sci., 6*, 199-203.

[47] Richter, A; Rioux, JD; Bouchard, JP; Mercier, J; Mathieu, J; Ge, B; Poirier, J; Julien, D; Gyapay, G; Weissenbach, J; Hudson, TJ; Melancon, SB; Morgan, K. (1999). Location score and haplotype analyses of the locus for autosomal recessive spastic ataxia of Charlevoix-Saguenay, in chromosome region 13q11. *Am. J. Hum. Genet., 64*, 768-775.

[48] Engert, JC; Berube, P; Mercier, J; Dore, C; Lepage, P; Ge, B; Bouchard, JP; Mathieu, J; Melancon, SB; Schalling, M; Lander, ES; Morgan, K; Hudson, TJ; Richter, A. (2000). ARSACS, a spastic ataxia common in northeastern Quebec, is caused by mutations in a new gene encoding an 11.5-kb ORF. *Nat. Genet., 24*, 120-125.

[49] Mercier, J; Prevost, C; Engert, JC; Bouchard, JP; Mathieu, J; Richter, A. (2001). Rapid detection of the sacsin mutations causing autosomal recessive spastic ataxia of Charlevoix-Saguenay. *Genet Test, 5*, 255-259.

[50] Bouhlal, Y; Amouri, R; El Euch-Fayeche, G; Hentati, F. (2011). Autosomal recessive spastic ataxia of Charlevoix-Saguenay: An overview. *Parkinsonism. Relat. Disord., 17*, 418-422.

[51] Ouyang, Y; Sakoe, K; Shimazaki, H; Namekawa, M; Ogawa, T; Ando, Y; Kawakami, T; Kaneko, J; Hasegawa, Y; Yoshizawa, K; Amino, T; Ishikawa, K; Mizusawa, H; Nakano, I; Takiyama, Y. (2006). 16q-linked autosomal dominant cerebellar ataxia: a clinical and genetic study. *J. Neurol. Sci., 247*, 180-186.

[52] Parfitt, DA; Michael, GJ; Vermeulen, EG; Prodromou, NV; Webb, TR; Gallo, JM; Cheetham, ME; Nicoll, WS; Blatch, GL; Chapple, JP. (2009). The ataxia protein sacsin is a functional co-chaperone that protects against polyglutamine-expanded ataxin-1. *Hum. Mol. Genet., 18*, 1556-1565.

[53] Gros-Louis, F; Dupre, N; Dion, P; Fox, MA; Laurent, S; Verreault, S; Sanes, JR; Bouchard, JP; Rouleau, GA. (2007). Mutations in SYNE1 lead to a newly discovered form of autosomal recessive cerebellar ataxia. *Nat. Genet., 39*, 80-85.

[54] Dupre, N; Gros-Louis, F; Chrestian, N; Verreault, S; Brunet, D; de Verteuil, D; Brais, B; Bouchard, JP; Rouleau, GA. (2007). Clinical and genetic study of autosomal recessive cerebellar ataxia type 1. *Ann. Neurol., 62*, 93-98.

[55] Laforce, R, Jr.; Buteau, JP; Bouchard, JP; Rouleau, GA; Bouchard, RW; Dupre, N. (2010). Cognitive Impairment in ARCA-1, a Newly Discovered Pure Cerebellar Ataxia Syndrome. *Cerebellum,*

[56] Dupre N, BJ, Verreault S, Rivest D, Puymirat J, Rouleau GA. . (2002). Recessive ataxia of the Beauce,a new form of hereditary ataxia of pure cerebellar type. *Neurology, 58*, A35.

[57] Lamperti, C; Naini, A; Hirano, M; De Vivo, DC; Bertini, E; Servidei, S; Valeriani, M; Lynch, D; Banwell, B; Berg, M; Dubrovsky, T; Chiriboga, C; Angelini, C; Pegoraro, E; DiMauro, S. (2003). Cerebellar ataxia and coenzyme Q10 deficiency. *Neurology, 60*, 1206-1208.

[58] Lagier-Tourenne, C; Tazir, M; Lopez, LC; Quinzii, CM; Assoum, M; Drouot, N; Busso, C; Makri, S; Ali-Pacha, L; Benhassine, T; Anheim, M; Lynch, DR; Thibault, C; Plewniak, F; Bianchetti, L; Tranchant, C; Poch, O; DiMauro, S; Mandel, JL; Barros, MH; Hirano, M; Koenig, M. (2008). ADCK3, an ancestral kinase, is mutated in a form of recessive ataxia associated with coenzyme Q10 deficiency. *Am. J. Hum. Genet.*, *82*, 661-672.

[59] Mariotti, C; Gellera, C; Rimoldi, M; Mineri, R; Uziel, G; Zorzi, G; Pareyson, D; Piccolo, G; Gambi, D; Piacentini, S; Squitieri, F; Capra, R; Castellotti, B; Di Donato, S. (2004). Ataxia with isolated vitamin E deficiency: neurological phenotype, clinical follow-up and novel mutations in TTPA gene in Italian families. *Neurol. Sci.*, *25*, 130-137.

[60] Cavalier, L; Ouahchi, K; Kayden, HJ; Di Donato, S; Reutenauer, L; Mandel, JL; Koenig, M. (1998). Ataxia with isolated vitamin E deficiency: heterogeneity of mutations and phenotypic variability in a large number of families. *Am. J. Hum. Genet.*, *62*, 301-310.

[61] Marzouki, N; Benomar, A; Yahyaoui, M; Birouk, N; Elouazzani, M; Chkili, T; Benlemlih, M. (2005). Vitamin E deficiency ataxia with (744 del A) mutation on alpha-TTP gene: genetic and clinical peculiarities in Moroccan patients. *Eur. J. Med. Genet.*, *48*, 21-28.

[62] Palau, F; De Michele, G; Vilchez, JJ; Pandolfo, M; Monros, E; Cocozza, S; Smeyers, P; Lopez-Arlandis, J; Campanella, G; Di Donato, S; et al. (1995). Early-onset ataxia with cardiomyopathy and retained tendon reflexes maps to the Friedreich's ataxia locus on chromosome 9q. *Ann. Neurol.*, *37*, 359-362.

[63] Arita, M; Sato, Y; Miyata, A; Tanabe, T; Takahashi, E; Kayden, HJ; Arai, H; Inoue, K. (1995). Human alpha-tocopherol transfer protein: cDNA cloning, expression and chromosomal localization. *Biochem. J.*, *306 (Pt 2)*, 437-443.

[64] Hentati, A; Deng, HX; Hung, WY; Nayer, M; Ahmed, MS; He, X; Tim, R; Stumpf, DA; Siddique, T; Ahmed. (1996). Human alpha-tocopherol transfer protein: gene structure and mutations in familial vitamin E deficiency. *Ann. Neurol.*, *39*, 295-300.

[65] Ouahchi, K; Arita, M; Kayden, H; Hentati, F; Ben Hamida, M; Sokol, R; Arai, H; Inoue, K; Mandel, JL; Koenig, M. (1995). Ataxia with isolated vitamin E deficiency is caused by mutations in the alpha-tocopherol transfer protein. *Nat. Genet.*, *9*, 141-145.

[66] Yokota, T; Shiojiri, T; Gotoda, T; Arita, M; Arai, H; Ohga, T; Kanda, T; Suzuki, J; Imai, T; Matsumoto, H; Harino, S; Kiyosawa, M; Mizusawa, H; Inoue, K. (1997). Friedreich-like ataxia with retinitis pigmentosa caused by the His101Gln mutation of the alpha-tocopherol transfer protein gene. *Ann. Neurol.*, *41*, 826-832.

[67] Manor, D; Morley, S. (2007). The alpha-tocopherol transfer protein. *Vitam. Horm.*, *76*, 45-65.

[68] Zingg, JM. (2007). Vitamin E: an overview of major research directions. *Mol. Aspects Med.*, *28*, 400-422.

[69] Gabsi, S; Gouider-Khouja, N; Belal, S; Fki, M; Kefi, M; Turki, I; Ben Hamida, M; Kayden, H; Mebazaa, R; Hentati, F. (2001). Effect of vitamin E supplementation in patients with ataxia with vitamin E deficiency. *Eur. J. Neurol.*, *8*, 477-481.

[70] Kara, B; Uzumcu, A; Uyguner, O; Rosti, RO; Kocbas, A; Ozmen, M; Kayserili, H. (2008). Ataxia with vitamin E deficiency associated with deafness. *Turk. J. Pediatr.*, *50*, 471-475.

[71] Di Donato, I; Bianchi, S; Federico, A. (Ataxia with vitamin E deficiency: update of molecular diagnosis. *Neurol Sci, 31*, 511-515.

[72] Meydani, SN; Meydani, M; Blumberg, JB; Leka, LS; Pedrosa, M; Diamond, R; Schaefer, EJ. (1998). Assessment of the safety of supplementation with different amounts of vitamin E in healthy older adults. *Am. J. Clin. Nutr., 68*, 311-318.

[73] Gohil, K; Azzi, A. (2008). Reply to Drug Insight: antioxidant therapy in inherited ataxias. *Nat. Clin. Pract. Neurol., 4*, E1; author reply E2.

[74] Manto, M; Marmolino, D. (2009). Cerebellar ataxias. *Curr. Opin. Neurol., 22*, 419-429.

[75] Crawford, TO. (1998). Ataxia telangiectasia. *Semin. Pediatr. Neurol., 5*, 287-294.

[76] Smirnov, DA; Cheung, VG. (2008). ATM gene mutations result in both recessive and dominant expression phenotypes of genes and microRNAs. *Am. J. Hum. Genet., 83*, 243-253.

[77] Embirucu, EK; Martyn, ML; Schlesinger, D; Kok, F. (2009). Autosomal recessive ataxias: 20 types, and counting. *Arq. Neuropsiquiatr., 67*, 1143-1156.

[78] Chun, HH; Gatti, RA. (2004). Ataxia-telangiectasia, an evolving phenotype. *DNA Repair (Amst), 3*, 1187-1196.

[79] Gatti, RA; Berkel, I; Boder, E; Braedt, G; Charmley, P; Concannon, P; Ersoy, F; Foroud, T; Jaspers, NG; Lange, K; et al. (1988). Localization of an ataxia-telangiectasia gene to chromosome 11q22-23. *Nature, 336*, 577-580.

[80] Taylor, AM; Byrd, PJ. (2005). Molecular pathology of ataxia telangiectasia. *J. Clin. Pathol., 58*, 1009-1015.

[81] Lavin, MF. (2008). Ataxia-telangiectasia: from a rare disorder to a paradigm for cell signalling and cancer. *Nat. Rev. Mol. Cell Biol., 9*, 759-769.

[82] Ferrarini, M; Squintani, G; Cavallaro, T; Ferrari, S; Rizzuto, N; Fabrizi, GM. (2007). A novel mutation of aprataxin associated with ataxia ocular apraxia type 1: phenotypical and genotypical characterization. *J. Neurol. Sci., 260*, 219-224.

[83] Watanabe, M; Sugai, Y; Concannon, P; Koenig, M; Schmitt, M; Sato, M; Shizuka, M; Mizushima, K; Ikeda, Y; Tomidokoro, Y; Okamoto, K; Shoji, M. (1998). Familial spinocerebellar ataxia with cerebellar atrophy, peripheral neuropathy, and elevated level of serum creatine kinase, gamma-globulin, and alpha-fetoprotein. *Ann. Neurol., 44*, 265-269.

[84] Moreira, MC; Barbot, C; Tachi, N; Kozuka, N; Mendonca, P; Barros, J; Coutinho, P; Sequeiros, J; Koenig, M. (2001). Homozygosity mapping of Portuguese and Japanese forms of ataxia-oculomotor apraxia to 9p13, and evidence for genetic heterogeneity. *Am. J. Hum. Genet., 68*, 501-508.

[85] Bomont, P; Watanabe, M; Gershoni-Barush, R; Shizuka, M; Tanaka, M; Sugano, J; Guiraud-Chaumeil, C; Koenig, M. (2000). Homozygosity mapping of spinocerebellar ataxia with cerebellar atrophy and peripheral neuropathy to 9q33-34, and with hearing impairment and optic atrophy to 6p21-23. *Eur. J. Hum. Genet., 8*, 986-990.

[86] Date, H; Onodera, O; Tanaka, H; Iwabuchi, K; Uekawa, K; Igarashi, S; Koike, R; Hiroi, T; Yuasa, T; Awaya, Y; Sakai, T; Takahashi, T; Nagatomo, H; Sekijima, Y; Kawachi, I; Takiyama, Y; Nishizawa, M; Fukuhara, N; Saito, K; Sugano, S; Tsuji, S. (2001). Early-onset ataxia with ocular motor apraxia and hypoalbuminemia is caused by mutations in a new HIT superfamily gene. *Nat. Genet., 29*, 184-188.

[87] Moreira, MC; Barbot, C; Tachi, N; Kozuka, N; Uchida, E; Gibson, T; Mendonca, P; Costa, M; Barros, J; Yanagisawa, T; Watanabe, M; Ikeda, Y; Aoki, M; Nagata, T;

Coutinho, P; Sequeiros, J; Koenig, M. (2001). The gene mutated in ataxia-ocular apraxia 1 encodes the new HIT/Zn-finger protein aprataxin. *Nat. Genet.*, *29*, 189-193.

[88] Clements, PM; Breslin, C; Deeks, ED; Byrd, PJ; Ju, L; Bieganowski, P; Brenner, C; Moreira, MC; Taylor, AM; Caldecott, KW. (2004). The ataxia-oculomotor apraxia 1 gene product has a role distinct from ATM and interacts with the DNA strand break repair proteins XRCC1 and XRCC4. *DNA Repair (Amst)*, *3*, 1493-1502.

[89] Le Ber, I; Moreira, MC; Rivaud-Pechoux, S; Chamayou, C; Ochsner, F; Kuntzer, T; Tardieu, M; Said, G; Habert, MO; Demarquay, G; Tannier, C; Beis, JM; Brice, A; Koenig, M; Durr, A. (2003). Cerebellar ataxia with oculomotor apraxia type 1: clinical and genetic studies. *Brain*, *126*, 2761-2772.

[90] Moreira, MC; Klur, S; Watanabe, M; Nemeth, AH; Le Ber, I; Moniz, JC; Tranchant, C; Aubourg, P; Tazir, M; Schols, L; Pandolfo, M; Schulz, JB; Pouget, J; Calvas, P; Shizuka-Ikeda, M; Shoji, M; Tanaka, M; Izatt, L; Shaw, CE; M'Zahem, A; Dunne, E; Bomont, P; Benhassine, T; Bouslam, N; Stevanin, G; Brice, A; Guimaraes, J; Mendonca, P; Barbot, C; Coutinho, P; Sequeiros, J; Durr, A; Warter, JM; Koenig, M. (2004). Senataxin, the ortholog of a yeast RNA helicase, is mutant in ataxia-ocular apraxia 2. *Nat. Genet.*, *36*, 225-227.

[91] Le Ber, I; Bouslam, N; Rivaud-Pechoux, S; Guimaraes, J; Benomar, A; Chamayou, C; Goizet, C; Moreira, MC; Klur, S; Yahyaoui, M; Agid, Y; Koenig, M; Stevanin, G; Brice, A; Durr, A. (2004). Frequency and phenotypic spectrum of ataxia with oculomotor apraxia 2: a clinical and genetic study in 18 patients. *Brain*, *127*, 759-767.

[92] Nemeth, AH; Bochukova, E; Dunne, E; Huson, SM; Elston, J; Hannan, MA; Jackson, M; Chapman, CJ; Taylor, AM. (2000). Autosomal recessive cerebellar ataxia with oculomotor apraxia (ataxia-telangiectasia-like syndrome) is linked to chromosome 9q34. *Am. J. Hum. Genet.*, *67*, 1320-1326.

[93] Duquette, A; Roddier, K; McNabb-Baltar, J; Gosselin, I; St-Denis, A; Dicaire, MJ; Loisel, L; Labuda, D; Marchand, L; Mathieu, J; Bouchard, JP; Brais, B. (2005). Mutations in senataxin responsible for Quebec cluster of ataxia with neuropathy. *Ann. Neurol.*, *57*, 408-414.

[94] Tazir, M; Ali-Pacha, L; M'Zahem, A; Delaunoy, JP; Fritsch, M; Nouioua, S; Benhassine, T; Assami, S; Grid, D; Vallat, JM; Hamri, A; Koenig, M. (2009). Ataxia with oculomotor apraxia type 2: a clinical and genetic study of 19 patients. *J. Neurol. Sci.*, *278*, 77-81.

[95] Suraweera, A; Lim, Y; Woods, R; Birrell, GW; Nasim, T; Becherel, OJ; Lavin, MF. (2009). Functional role for senataxin, defective in ataxia oculomotor apraxia type 2, in transcriptional regulation. *Hum. Mol. Genet.*, *18*, 3384-3396.

[96] Airoldi, G; Guidarelli, A; Cantoni, O; Panzeri, C; Vantaggiato, C; Bonato, S; Grazia D'Angelo, M; Falcone, S; De Palma, C; Tonelli, A; Crimella, C; Bondioni, S; Bresolin, N; Clementi, E; Bassi, MT. (2010). Characterization of two novel SETX mutations in AOA2 patients reveals aspects of the pathophysiological role of senataxin. *Neurogenetics*, *11*, 91-100.

ISBN: 978-1-61942-867-6
© 2012 Nova Science Publishers, Inc.

Chapter 7

GENETICS AT DIFFERENT LEVELS IN MACHADO-JOSEPH DISEASE (MJD/SCA3): CAUSE, MODIFIERS AND THERAPY

Conceição Bettencourt[1,2,3] and Manuela Lima[1,2]
[1]Institute for Molecular and Cell Biology (IBMC),
University of Porto, Porto, Portugal
[2]Center of Research in Natural Resources (CIRN) and
Department of Biology, University of the Azores, Ponta Delgada, Portugal
[3]Laboratorio de Biología Molecular, Instituto de Enfermedades Neurológicas, Fundación
Socio-Sanitaria de Castilla-La Mancha, Guadalajara, Spain

ABSTRACT

Hereditary ataxias constitute a clinically and genetically heterogeneous group of rare neurological disorders that cannot be distinguished solely by clinical criteria, thus demanding a subtype confirmation by molecular diagnosis. Enclosed in this group are spinocerebellar ataxias (SCAs), which are autosomal dominant disorders. In several SCAs, the causative genes display age-dependent patterns of penetrance, implying that the *a posteriori* risk of being a carrier diminishes with aging of at-risk individuals that remain asymptomatic. Machado-Joseph disease (MJD), also known as SCA3, corresponds to the most frequent form of SCA. Similarly to other SCAs, named "polyglutamine" ataxias (*e.g.*, SCA1, SCA2, SCA6, SCA7, SCA17 and DRPLA), MJD is caused by an expansion of a CAG repeat motif in the coding region of its causative gene. In this particular case, more than 52 CAG repeats in exon 10 of the *ATXN3* gene (14q32.1) are necessary for disease expression. Despite the inverse correlation between the size of the CAG tract and the age at onset, the causative mutation only partially (50-75%) explains the observed variation in phenotype. Therefore, precise predictions of the age at onset are currently impossible. Results from recent research studies are pointing to the involvement of other factors, namely additional genetic variability related to the causative gene itself (*e.g.*, generated by alternative splicing) and/or modifier genes. The knowledge of such factors may not only enable improvements of phenotype predictions, but may also raise hypotheses of new targets for gene therapy. The present chapter will focus on MJD, using it as a paradigm to demonstrate multiple roles and usefulness of genetics for a vaster group of neurodegenerative disorders.

INTODUCTION

Hereditary ataxias (HAs) constitute a clinically and genetically heterogeneous group of rare neurological disorders, with a global prevalence of approximately 6/100,000 [1, 2]. Autosomal dominant and autosomal recessive forms represent the majority of HAs subtypes, but forms with an X-linked pattern of inheritance have also been identified [3]. Among the autosomal dominant inherited ataxias are spinocerebellar ataxias (SCAs), which constitute a heterogeneous group of typically late-onset, progressive, and often fatal neurodegenerative disorders. These are characterized by progressive cerebellar dysfunction, which may be associated with other symptoms of the central and peripheral nervous systems, in variable degrees [4-6]. Given the phenotypic overlap between subtypes of SCAs, accurate clinical diagnosis of a specific subtype is limited and sometimes impossible [7].

Although more than 30 loci of SCAs have been mapped, only 22 causative genes are known so far. Subtypes of SCAs can be classified into three major categories according to the type of their causative mutations: 1) "polyglutamine" ataxias, caused by (CAG)n repeat expansions, which encode a pure repetitive tract of the amino acid glutamine in the corresponding protein (*e.g.*, SCA1, SCA2, SCA3, SCA6, SCA7, SCA17, and DRPLA); 2) non-coding repeat ataxias, caused by expansions of repeat motifs that are located in intronic or regulatory regions of the respective disease genes (*e.g.*, SCA8, SCA10, SCA12, SCA31 and SCA36); and 3) ataxias caused by conventional mutations (namely deletion, missense, nonsense, and splice site mutations) in specific genes (*e.g.*, SCA5, SCA11, SCA14, SCA15, SCA27, SCA28, and SCA35) [4]. A relevant portion of SCAs are of unknown cause, but among those of known cause "polyglutamine" ataxias represent the largest group [8]. Within this group is Machado-Joseph disease (MJD; MIM #109150), also known as SCA3. Considered the most frequent form of SCA worldwide [7], MJD represents more than 50% of cases of SCAs in countries such as Portugal (58-74%) [9, 10] and Brazil (69-92%) [11, 12], reaching its highest prevalence values in particular populations, such as Flores Island (1/239) in the Azores (Portugal) [13, 14].

BRIEF CLINICAL CHARACTERIZATION

MJD is characterized by a complex and pleomorphic phenotype, involving predominantly the cerebellar, pyramidal, extrapyramidal, motor neuron and oculomotor systems. A clinical diagnosis is suggested in patients presenting progressive cerebellar ataxia and pyramidal signs, associated with a complex clinical presentation, which extends from extrapyramidal signs to peripheral amyotrophy [15]. External progressive ophthalmoplegia (EPO), dystonia, intention fasciculation-like movements of facial and lingual muscles, as well as bulging eyes, are minor but more specific features being, therefore, of major importance for clinical differential diagnosis of MJD [15]. The disease onset generally occurs in adulthood (mean age at onset is around 40 years), but onset extremes at 4 [16] and 70 years [17] are known.

Mean survival time with this disease rounds 21 years (ranging from 7 to 29 years) [17, 18]. The first symptoms consist mostly in gait ataxia and diplopia, which are reported as initial complaints by 92.4% and 7.6% of the patients, respectively [17].

Even within families, MJD presents clinical heterogeneity, represented not only by the high variability in the age at onset, but also by the type of neurological signs and rate of disease progression, and therefore by the resulting degree of incapacity. Coutinho and Andrade [19] observed that almost all MJD patients present cerebellar signs and EPO, associated with pyramidal signs, at variable degrees, and that distinct phenotypes could be distinguished on the basis of the presence/absence of important extrapyramidal signs, or the presence/absence of peripheral signs. According to such observations, those authors systematized the disease phenotypes into three main clinical types. Type 1 corresponds to forms with an early onset (mean of 24.3 years), a rapid progression and a more severe disease presentation, which includes marked pyramidal and extrapyramidal signs, such as dystonia, apart from cerebellar ataxia and EPO. Type 2 is characterized by an intermediate onset (mean of 40.5 years), presenting cerebellar ataxia and EPO, with or without pyramidal signs, and with possible slight extrapyramidal or peripheral signs. Type 3 has a later onset (mean of 46.8 years) and is characterized by the presence of cerebellar ataxia and EPO associated with peripheral alterations, with or without tenuous pyramidal and extrapyramidal signs [17]. These three clinical types can occasionally be present in one single family. Additionally, some authors consider rarer presentations, associated with parkinsonian features or with spastic paraplegia, as a type 4 [20] or a type 5 [21], respectively.

INHERITANCE, EMPIRICAL RISK AND CAUSATIVE MUTATION

As it is characteristic of SCAs, MJD displays an autosomal dominant pattern of inheritance. Consequently, each sibling of an affected individual, or of an asymptomatic carrier, has a 50% *a priori* risk of being itself a carrier, with both genders presenting equal probabilities of receiving/transmitting the mutated allele and expressing the disease phenotype.

The MJD gene is considered almost fully penetrant, since very few cases (2%) of obligate carriers are known to have remained asymptomatic [22]. However, MJD penetrance displays an age-dependent pattern, with the probability of being a mutation carrier, and consequently the *a posteriori* empirical risk, diminishing with age of the at-risk individuals that remain asymptomatic, and being almost null by the age of 70 [14]. A similar age-dependent penetrance pattern is observed in SCA2, for example, which presents an *a posteriori* empirical risk of approximately zero by the age of 65 [23].

The MJD locus was mapped to the long arm of chromosome 14 (14q32.1) [24]. It was then shown that an expansion of a CAG repeat motif in the coding region of the *ATXN3* gene (also known as *MJD* or *MJD1* gene), was present in all affected individuals of a pathologically confirmed MJD family. This triplet repeat expansion thus constituted MJD's causative mutation, implying the inclusion of this disease in the larger "polyglutamine" ataxias group [25].

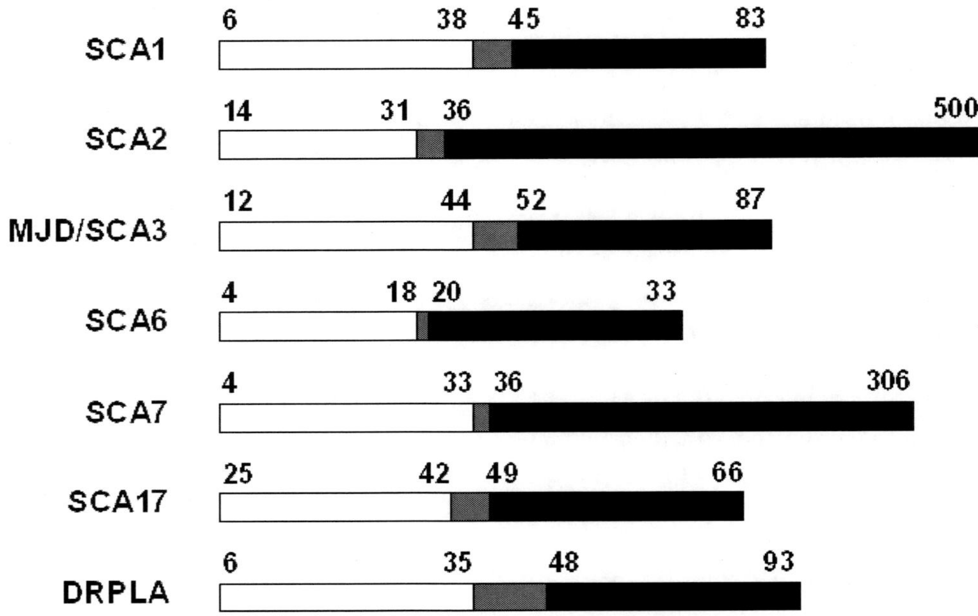

Figure 1. Schematic representation of "polyglutamine" SCAs loci. White boxes represent the size range of the CAG repeat tract in normal alleles; gray boxes represent the size range in alleles of intermediate size; black boxes represent the size range in expanded alleles.

The *ATXN3* gene was firstly described as spanning about 48 kb and containing 11 exons (with the CAG repeat tract located in exon 10) [26], but two additional exons, 6a and 9a, were identified recently [27]. This gene encodes for ataxin-3, a protein composed of 339 amino acid residues plus a variable number of glutamine residues (constituting the polyglutamine tract), with an estimated molecular weight of 40–43 kDa in normal individuals [25]. A ubiquitous expression, in neuronal and non-neuronal human tissues, of both *ATXN3* mRNA and ataxin-3 has been reported [26, 28]. In its mutated form, when the polyglutamine tract reaches the pathological threshold, ataxin-3 is thought to gain a neurotoxic function that, as a consequence, leads to selective neuronal cell death through a not fully understood process [28, 29]. Similarly to the majority of "polyglutamine" SCAs [30], normal (wild-type) alleles are polymorphic (figure 1), ranging from a few to nearly 40 repeat units (12 to 44 CAG repeats in wild-type MJD alleles), and only the presence of an expanded allele, surpassing the normal threshold, leads to expression of the disease phenotype (consistently 61 to 87 CAG repeats in expanded MJD alleles) [31]. Only a very few disease-associated alleles of intermediate size, containing between 45 and 56 CAG repeats, have been reported for MJD [32-37]. However, an allele with 51 repeats was described as apparently not associated with the disease [31], raising therefore the question whether low penetrance alleles of intermediate size, which have been reported for other "polyglutamine" (*e.g.*, SCA17 [38, 39]) and non-coding repeat ataxias (*e.g.*, SCA10 [40, 41]), may also occur in MJD. Although several cases of *de novo* mutations have been identified for SCA7 [42], this does not seem to occur in MJD, and the idea that large normal or intermediate alleles represent a reservoir for *de novo* mutations has not been supported for this disease [43].

GENOTYPE-PHENOTYPE CORRELATIONS AND GENETIC MODIFIERS

As typically occurs in the group of "polyglutamine" ataxias [44-49], an inverse correlation is found between the size of the CAG repeat tract in the expanded alleles determined in genomic DNA (and consequently the size of the polyglutamine tract) and the age at onset of MJD. The size of the CAG repeat tract in expanded alleles, however, only partially explains (50% to nearly 75%) the variation in the age of appearance of the first symptoms [50, 51]. A similar inverse correlation has also been described at the mRNA level [52]. Additionally, the size of the expanded alleles has been associated with the frequency of pseudoexophthalmos and pyramidal signs, which appear more often in patients with larger repeats [53]. Dystonic postures are also typical of patients with larger expansions [46]. On the other hand, polyneuropathy seems to be more common in patients with shorter repeats [54]. Similarly, in other subtypes of SCAs the size of the expanded alleles has also been related to particular clinical features. For example, in SCA2, myokimia, myoclonus, dystonia and fasciculations are more frequently observed in patients carrying large expansions [55], and in SCA7, the frequency of pyramidal signs, ophthalmoplegia and decreased visual acuity increases with repeat size [56]. Moreover, a gene dosage effect seems to occur in MJD, since the few molecularly confirmed cases of homozygous patients show an aggravation of the clinical phenotype, with a more severe progression and an early age at onset in subjects carrying the expanded allele in both chromosomes [16, 57, 58]. This effect is also supported by studies in animal models (*e.g.*, [59]). A similar dosage effect on severity and onset is referred for DRPLA [60] and SCA6 [61], but homozygosity for the expanded alleles may also result in atypical phenotypes, as it has been shown for SCA2 [62] and SCA17 [63], for example.

Anticipation has been reported for MJD and other "polyglutamine" ataxias, implying more severe phenotypes and/or earlier age at onset in successive generations. This is usually explained by the dynamic process of mutation underlying these diseases, which involves intergenerational instability of the repeats [30, 44]. In MJD, normal alleles are stable and are transmitted to the offspring without modifications [64], while most expanded alleles are unstable, presenting a tendency to further increase in size due to germinal instability, especially during meiosis in males [65]. Nevertheless, some authors argue that anticipation can additionally be a consequence of an observation bias (*e.g.*, [8]). Among "polyglutamine" diseases, SCA7 is the one presenting more pronounced anticipation [46].

An inverse correlation between the size of the normal *ATXN3* alleles and the age at onset of MJD has also been reported, accounting for less than 6% of onset variance [66, 67]. Similar observations of the influence of normal allele size have also been reported for SCA1 and SCA6 [48]. Apart from CAG factors, the knowledge of alternative genetic or environmental factors influencing age at onset in SCAs is very scarce [49], but some examples will be herein presented.

Familial dependence has been described as increasing the explanation of the onset variance in MJD [17, 48, 68], similarly to what happens in SCA2 [48]. The contribution of other genetic factors, namely additional intragenic variation and/or modifier genes, to the remaining MJD phenotypic variance, is thus supported by the fact that variability within families is lower than the one observed between families. The influence of environmental factors, however, cannot be totally excluded.

On what concerns intragenic variation, haplotypes, defined by intragenic single nucleotide polymorphisms (SNPs) in the *ATXN3* gene, have been suggested to influence the MJD onset variation [69]. Additionally, a large number of *ATXN3* alternative splicing variants with potential effects (either protective or increased toxicity) on the MJD phenotype were recently described [27]. Findings of a study on methylation of the *ATXN3* promoter [70] also suggested a small effect of the methylation status on the MJD onset.

Mainly due to constraints in sample size, among other aspects, it is difficult to undertake an exhaustive and whole genome search for MJD's (or for any other SCA's) modifier genes, and, therefore, only candidate-gene approaches have been attempted, so far. Jardim *et al.* [71] analyzed the relation between the size of the polymorphic CAG repeats in other"polyglutamine" ataxias loci (SCA2, SCA6, and DRPLA) and several phenotypic features of MJD. They only found an association between the length of the larger SCA2 allele (22-23 CAG repeats) and the severity of fasciculations (a minor but specific feature of MJD). No association was found with the remaining phenotypic features, namely the age at onset. A similar approach was applied on a series of SCA2 patients [72], and an association was observed between the size of large normal SCA6 alleles and an earlier SCA2 onset. Using another candidate-gene approach, it was shown that an interleukin-1 beta promoter polymorphism significantly affects the age at onset in a series of Japanese patients with SCA6 [73]. More recently, a significant association was found between the presence of the *APOE* ε2 allele and an earlier onset in MJD [74]. Nevertheless, further investigation is still warranted on this field.

GENETIC TESTING AND COUNSELING

As mentioned previously, a clinical diagnosis of a specific SCA subtype, such as MJD, may be very difficult or even impossible to establish. Especially at the disease onset, when minor but more specific signs are still missing, when family history for MJD is not known, and when the ethnic or geographic background of the patient is thought to be unusual for this disease, a clinical diagnosis may not be possible [75], and, therefore, differential diagnosis depends on the direct detection of the mutation. The identification of the causative mutation of MJD allowed its direct detection, thus enabling the molecular diagnosis for this disease [50]. Targeted analysis of the MJD mutation in the *ATXN3* gene also made possible the predictive testing (PT) for at-risk adult family members, providing them an accurate confirmation of the carrier/non-carrier status. Furthermore, the prenatal diagnosis (PND) [76], and, as a more recent alternative, the preimplantation genetic diagnosis (PGD) [77], were additionally made available.

Given the current lack of effective therapeutics for this type of disorders, the access to adequate genetic counseling (GC) is crucial to the patients and their families, in order to provide them information on the nature of the disease, the current lack of treatment, the risk for other family members as well as the availability of the molecular tests, previously mentioned. These tests (PT, PND, and PGD) should be offered within the frame of a GC program. Teams offering GC must adequately transmit the information concerning the genetic aspects of MJD, or of other SCAs, to the affected families, in order to enable them a correct comprehension of specific genetic terms (*e.g.*, pre-symptomatic carrier), which they usually have difficulties to understand [78]. Besides, adequate GC, it is also essential to evaluate and to support those families on what concerns psychological well-being [79, 80].

Regarding the interpretation of pre-symptomatic test results, several difficulties may emerge. Although *ATXN3* alleles with 52 or more CAG repeats have consistently been associated with the presence of a MJD phenotype, consequences of intermediate size alleles should be carefully interpreted. Detailed clinical and molecular analysis of additional family members may be useful in some cases. A second problem relies on the presence of homoallelism, *i.e.*, homozygosity for two normal alleles with exactly the same size, which occurs in about 10% of all test results [31]. When such a result shows up the following doubt may be raised: "Is this result correct or due to technical issues the expanded allele was not detected?". The study of intragenic polymorphisms, which allow the distinction between the two normal chromosomes in the presumed homoallelic individual, and/or the application of additional techniques (*e.g.*, Southern blot analysis) may help solving this problem [31]. Furthermore, the existence of somatic mosaicism in MJD [81] (or in other SCAs, *e.g.*, [82, 83]), which originates differences in (CAG)n length among subpopulations of lymphocytes as well as between lymphocytes (where length is usually determined) and central nervous system (CNS) cells, imposes limitations in sizing precision of the CAG repeats. However, for molecular diagnosis purposes, an error of ±1 CAG repeat is acceptable [31].

GENE THERAPY STRATEGIES

Studies on conditional transgenic mouse models of "polyglutamine" SCAs (*e.g.*, of MJD [84] and of SCA1 [85]) have demonstrated that shutting off expression of the mutant transgene dramatically slows disease progression or even reverses the disease pathology, highlighting the potential of gene silencing as a therapeutic strategy. Recent advances have been made in this field, and several promising and powerful technologies are emerging to suppress the expression of mutant genes at the mRNA level *in vivo*, by means of short single- or double-stranded RNA or DNA molecules, such as small interfering RNAs (siRNAs) and administration of antisense oligonucleotides (ASOs). Nearly all patients with "polyglutamine" SCAs are heterozygous, having one wild-type and one mutant allele in the affected gene, and it is still not clear whether the loss of the wild-type allele product can produce a deleterious effect. Therefore, discrimination between wild-type and mutant transcripts should be taken into consideration when developing gene therapies, in order to preserve native protein expression and function. Strategies based on the presence of a SNP have been proposed to ensure allele discrimination [86]. In the case of MJD, the report that the "C" variant of a SNP, located immediately downstream of the CAG repeat tract, is present in more than 70% of the expanded MJD alleles [87, 88], raised good perspectives for the discrimination of *ATXN3* alleles. Targeting that SNP with a siRNA assay produced promising results in a rat model of MJD, in which good therapeutic efficacy and selectivity were observed [89]. Transposing this to MJD patients, it would only be efficient in heterozygous subjects with the "C" variant in *cis* with the expanded *ATXN3* allele. A couple of years later, the same research group [90], using the same rat model, tried a non-allele-specific *ATXN3* silencing strategy, suggesting it could also result safe and effective. Given the fact that mouse [91] and *Caenorhabditis elegans* [92] knockout models for ataxin-3 are viable and display no overt phenotype at basal condition, might support the idea that non-allele-specific silencing could be effectively applied. However, it has been shown that lack of *ATXN3* leads to increased cell death, in both human and mouse cell lines [93], not supporting the hypothesis of ataxin-3 as a non-essential protein. Another strategy for allele-specific silencing of the mutant *ATXN3* mRNA, via ASOs that discriminates between the wild-type and the expanded alleles on the basis of the CAG repeat length in cell lines, has also been successfully applied [94]. Notwithstanding, the search for *ATXN3* mRNA variation is still important for the development of targeted approaches. The recent identification of a high number of *ATXN3* alternative splicing variants [27] may also raise new possibilities. The use of gene silencing strategies in humans remains hampered by the unavailability of safe, precise, and robust methods of delivery to the CNS, and also by the uncertainty over long-term safety. Concerns related to non-specific off-target effects (*e.g.*, the siRNA affecting genes other than the diseased target) as well as to the safety of gene therapy itself (*e.g.*, increased risk of cancer due to transgene integration into and inactivation of tumor suppressor genes) [95]. Despite the theoretical complications and practical issues facing these therapeutic strategies for SCAs, and other CNS diseases, that need to be surpassed before an effective treatment of patients, it is now abundantly clear that such approaches hold tremendous promises.

CONCLUSION

Despite the fact that SCAs are well defined genetic entities, a differential diagnosis based on clinical data is considered very difficult or unfeasible. In many subtypes the causative mutation is already known, enabling molecular diagnosis or even pre-symptomatic test by direct detection of the mutation. Regardless of multiple efforts employed in understanding major genotype-phenotype correlations, namely on what concerns the study of intragenic variation and modifier genes, there is still insufficient information to allow for precise predictions of disease onset, but the knowledge of genetic variation on the basis of the clinical heterogeneity of these disorders is continuously growing. Furthermore, gene therapy approaches represent a tremendous promise for a near future. In this chapter, we have addressed several roles and aspects of genetics with respect to MJD that may be useful for other SCAs as well as for a vaster group of neurodegenerative disorders.

ACKNOWLEDGMENTS

C.B. is a postdoctoral fellow of "Fundação para a Ciência e a Tecnologia" – FCT [SFRH/BPD/63121/2009].

REFERENCES

[1] Schoenberg, B. S. (1978) Epidemiology of the inherited ataxias. *Adv. Neurol.* 21, 15-32.

[2]   Tallaksen, C. M. (2008) [Hereditary ataxias]. *Tidsskr. Nor. Laegeforen.* 128, 1977-1980.

[3]   Espinos, C. and Palau, F. (2009) Genetics and pathogenesis of inherited ataxias and spastic paraplegias. *Adv. Exp. Med. Biol.* 652, 263-296.

[4]   Soong, B. W. and Paulson, H. L. (2007) Spinocerebellar ataxias: an update. *Curr. Opin. Neurol.* 20, 438-446.

[5]   Tsuji, S., Onodera, O., Goto, J. and Nishizawa, M. (2008) Sporadic ataxias in Japan - a population-based epidemiological study. *Cerebellum.* 7, 189-197.

[6]   Carlson, K. M., Andresen, J. M. and Orr, H. T. (2009) Emerging pathogenic pathways in the spinocerebellar ataxias. *Curr. Opin. Genet. Dev.* 19, 247-253.

[7]   Schols, L., Bauer, P., Schmidt, T., Schulte, T. and Riess, O. (2004) Autosomal dominant cerebellar ataxias: clinical features, genetics, and pathogenesis. *Lancet Neurol.* 3, 291-304.

[8]   Durr, A. (2010) Autosomal dominant cerebellar ataxias: polyglutamine expansions and beyond. *Lancet Neurol.* 9, 885-894.

[9]   Silveira, I., Coutinho, P., Maciel, P., Gaspar, C., Hayes, S., Dias, A., Guimaraes, J., Loureiro, L., Sequeiros, J. and Rouleau, G. A. (1998) Analysis of SCA1, DRPLA, MJD, SCA2, and SCA6 CAG repeats in 48 Portuguese ataxia families. *Am. J. Med. Genet.* 81, 134-138.

[10]   Vale, J., Bugalho, P., Silveira, I., Sequeiros, J., Guimaraes, J. and Coutinho, P. (2009) Autosomal dominant cerebellar ataxia: frequency analysis and clinical characterization of 45 families from Portugal. *Eur. J. Neurol.* 17, 124-128.

[11]   Jardim, L. B., Silveira, I., Pereira, M. L., Ferro, A., Alonso, I., do Ceu Moreira, M., Mendonca, P., Ferreirinha, F., Sequeiros, J. and Giugliani, R. (2001) A survey of spinocerebellar ataxia in South Brazil - 66 new cases with Machado-Joseph disease, SCA7, SCA8, or unidentified disease-causing mutations. *J. Neurol.* 248, 870-876.

[12]   Teive, H. A., Munhoz, R. P., Raskin, S. and Werneck, L. C. (2008) Spinocerebellar ataxia type 6 in Brazil. *Arq Neuropsiquiatr.* 66, 691-694.

[13]   Lima, M., Mayer, F., Coutinho, P. and Abade, A. (1997) Prevalence, geographic distribution, and genealogical investigation of Machado-Joseph disease in the Azores (Portugal). *Hum. Biol.* 69, 383-391.

[14]   Bettencourt, C., Santos, C., Kay, T., Vasconcelos, J. and Lima, M. (2008) Analysis of segregation patterns in Machado-Joseph disease pedigrees. *J. Hum. Genet.* 53, 920-923.

[15]   Lima, L. and Coutinho, P. (1980) Clinical criteria for diagnosis of Machado-Joseph disease: report of a non-Azorena Portuguese family. *Neurology.* 30, 319-322.

[16]   Carvalho, D. R., La Rocque-Ferreira, A., Rizzo, I. M., Imamura, E. U. and Speck-Martins, C. E. (2008) Homozygosity enhances severity in spinocerebellar ataxia type 3. *Pediatr. Neurol.* 38, 296-299.

[17]   Coutinho, P. (1992) Doença de Machado-Joseph: Tentativa de definição. PhD Dissertation, *Instituto de Ciências Biomédicas Abel Salazar*, Porto.

[18]   Kieling, C., Prestes, P. R., Saraiva-Pereira, M. L. and Jardim, L. B. (2007) Survival estimates for patients with Machado-Joseph disease (SCA3). *Clin. Genet.* 72, 543-545.

[19]   Coutinho, P. and Andrade, C. (1978) Autosomal dominant system degeneration in Portuguese families of the Azores Islands. A new genetic disorder involving cerebellar, pyramidal, extrapyramidal and spinal cord motor functions. *Neurology.* 28, 703-709.

[20] Suite, N. D., Sequeiros, J. and McKhann, G. M. (1986) Machado-Joseph disease in a Sicilian-American family. *J. Neurogenet.* 3, 177-182.

[21] Sakai, T. and Kawakami, H. (1996) Machado-Joseph disease: A proposal of spastic paraplegic subtype. *Neurology.* 46, 846-847.

[22] Sequeiros, J. (1989) Análise genética da variação fenotípica na doença de Machado-Joseph. PhD Dissertation, *Instituto de Ciências Biomédicas de Abel Salazar*, Universidade do Porto.

[23] Almaguer Mederos, L. E., Proenza, C. L., Almira, Y. R., Batallan, K. E., Falcon, N. S., Gongora, E. M., Almarales, D. C., Perez, L. V. and Herrera, M. P. (2008) Age-dependent risks in genetic counseling for spinocerebellar ataxia type 2. *Clin. Genet.* 74, 571-573.

[24] Takiyama, Y., Nishizawa, M., Tanaka, H., Kawashima, S., Sakamoto, H., Karube, Y., Shimazaki, H., Soutome, M., Endo, K., Ohta, S. and et al. (1993) The gene for Machado-Joseph disease maps to human chromosome 14q. *Nat. Genet.* 4, 300-304.

[25] Kawaguchi, Y., Okamoto, T., Taniwaki, M., Aizawa, M., Inoue, M., Katayama, S., Kawakami, H., Nakamura, S., Nishimura, M., Akiguchi, I. and et al. (1994) CAG expansions in a novel gene for Machado-Joseph disease at chromosome 14q32.1. *Nat. Genet.* 8, 221-228.

[26] Ichikawa, Y., Goto, J., Hattori, M., Toyoda, A., Ishii, K., Jeong, S. Y., Hashida, H., Masuda, N., Ogata, K., Kasai, F., Hirai, M., Maciel, P., Rouleau, G. A., Sakaki, Y. and Kanazawa, I. (2001) The genomic structure and expression of MJD, the Machado-Joseph disease gene. *J. Hum. Genet.* 46, 413-422.

[27] Bettencourt, C., Santos, C., Montiel, R., Costa Mdo, C., Cruz-Morales, P., Santos, L. R., Simoes, N., Kay, T., Vasconcelos, J., Maciel, P. and Lima, M. (2010) Increased transcript diversity: novel splicing variants of Machado-Joseph disease gene (ATXN3). *Neurogenetics.* 11, 193-202.

[28] Paulson, H. L., Das, S. S., Crino, P. B., Perez, M. K., Patel, S. C., Gotsdiner, D., Fischbeck, K. H. and Pittman, R. N. (1997) Machado-Joseph disease gene product is a cytoplasmic protein widely expressed in brain. *Ann. Neurol.* 41, 453-462.

[29] Mauri, P. L., Riva, M., Ambu, D., De Palma, A., Secundo, F., Benazzi, L., Valtorta, M., Tortora, P. and Fusi, P. (2006) Ataxin-3 is subject to autolytic cleavage. *FEBS J.* 273, 4277-4286.

[30] Bettencourt, C., Silva-Fernandes, A., Montiel, R., Santos, C., Maciel, P. and Lima, M. (2007) Triplet Repeats: Features, Dynamics and Evolutionary Mechanisms. In Recent Advances in Molecular Biology and Evolution: *Applications to Biological Anthropology* (Santos, C. and Lima, M., eds.). pp. 83-114, Research Signpost, Kerala.

[31] Maciel, P., Costa, M. C., Ferro, A., Rousseau, M., Santos, C. S., Gaspar, C., Barros, J., Rouleau, G. A., Coutinho, P. and Sequeiros, J. (2001) Improvement in the molecular diagnosis of Machado-Joseph disease. *Arch. Neurol.* 58, 1821-1827.

[32] Gu, W., Ma, H., Wang, K., Jin, M., Zhou, Y., Liu, X., Wang, G. and Shen, Y. (2004) The shortest expanded allele of the MJD1 gene in a Chinese MJD kindred with autonomic dysfunction. *Eur. Neurol.* 52, 107-111.

[33] Padiath, Q. S., Srivastava, A. K., Roy, S., Jain, S. and Brahmachari, S. K. (2005) Identification of a novel 45 repeat unstable allele associated with a disease phenotype at the MJD1/SCA3 locus. *Am. J. Med. Genet. B Neuropsychiatr. Genet.* 133B, 124-126.

[34] Quan, F., Egan, R., DB, J. and Popovich, B. (1997) An unusually small 55 repeat MJD1 CAG allele in a patient with Machado-Joseph disease [abstract]. *Am. J. Hum. Genet.* 61, A318.

[35] Takiyama, Y., Sakoe, K., Nakano, I. and Nishizawa, M. (1997) Machado-Joseph disease: cerebellar ataxia and autonomic dysfunction in a patient with the shortest known expanded allele (56 CAG repeat units) of the MJD1 gene. *Neurology.* 49, 604-606.

[36] van Alfen, N., Sinke, R. J., Zwarts, M. J., Gabreels-Festen, A., Praamstra, P., Kremer, B. P. and Horstink, M. W. (2001) Intermediate CAG repeat lengths (53,54) for MJD/SCA3 are associated with an abnormal phenotype. *Ann. Neurol.* 49, 805-807.

[37] van Schaik, I. N., Jobsis, G. J., Vermeulen, M., Keizers, H., Bolhuis, P. A. and de Visser, M. (1997) Machado-Joseph disease presenting as severe asymmetric proximal neuropathy. *J. Neurol. Neurosurg. Psychiatry.* 63, 534-536.

[38] Oda, M., Maruyama, H., Komure, O., Morino, H., Terasawa, H., Izumi, Y., Imamura, T., Yasuda, M., Ichikawa, K., Ogawa, M., Matsumoto, M. and Kawakami, H. (2004) Possible reduced penetrance of expansion of 44 to 47 CAG/CAA repeats in the TATA-binding protein gene in spinocerebellar ataxia type 17. *Arch. Neurol.* 61, 209-212.

[39] Zuhlke, C., Dalski, A., Schwinger, E. and Finckh, U. (2005) Spinocerebellar ataxia type 17: report of a family with reduced penetrance of an unstable Gln49 TBP allele, haplotype analysis supporting a founder effect for unstable alleles and comparative analysis of SCA17 genotypes. *BMC Med. Genet.* 6, 27.

[40] Matsuura, T., Fang, P., Pearson, C. E., Jayakar, P., Ashizawa, T., Roa, B. B. and Nelson, D. L. (2006) Interruptions in the expanded ATTCT repeat of spinocerebellar ataxia type 10: repeat purity as a disease modifier? *Am. J. Hum. Genet.* 78, 125-129.

[41] Raskin, S., Ashizawa, T., Teive, H. A., Arruda, W. O., Fang, P., Gao, R., White, M. C., Werneck, L. C. and Roa, B. (2007) Reduced penetrance in a Brazilian family with spinocerebellar ataxia type 10. *Arch. Neurol.* 64, 591-594.

[42] Stevanin, G., Giunti, P., Belal, G. D., Durr, A., Ruberg, M., Wood, N. and Brice, A. (1998) De novo expansion of intermediate alleles in spinocerebellar ataxia 7. *Hum. Mol. Genet.* 7, 1809-1813.

[43] Lima, M., Costa, M. C., Montiel, R., Ferro, A., Santos, C., Silva, C., Bettencourt, C., Sousa, A., Sequeiros, J., Coutinho, P. and Maciel, P. (2005) Population genetics of wild-type CAG repeats in the Machado-Joseph disease gene in Portugal. *Hum. Hered.* 60, 156-163.

[44] Tsuji, S. (1997) Molecular genetics of triplet repeats: unstable expansion of triplet repeats as a new mechanism for neurodegenerative diseases. *Intern. Med.* 36, 3-8.

[45] Giunti, P., Sabbadini, G., Sweeney, M. G., Davis, M. B., Veneziano, L., Mantuano, E., Federico, A., Plasmati, R., Frontali, M. and Wood, N. W. (1998) The role of the SCA2 trinucleotide repeat expansion in 89 autosomal dominant cerebellar ataxia families. Frequency, clinical and genetic correlates. *Brain.* 121 (Pt 3), 459-467.

[46] Stevanin, G., Durr, A. and Brice, A. (2000) Clinical and molecular advances in autosomal dominant cerebellar ataxias: from genotype to phenotype and physiopathology. *Eur. J. Hum. Genet.* 8, 4-18.

[47] Maschke, M., Oehlert, G., Xie, T. D., Perlman, S., Subramony, S. H., Kumar, N., Ptacek, L. J. and Gomez, C. M. (2005) Clinical feature profile of spinocerebellar ataxia type 1-8 predicts genetically defined subtypes. *Mov. Disord.* 20, 1405-1412.

[48] van de Warrenburg, B. P., Hendriks, H., Durr, A., van Zuijlen, M. C., Stevanin, G., Camuzat, A., Sinke, R. J., Brice, A. and Kremer, B. P. (2005) Age at onset variance analysis in spinocerebellar ataxias: a study in a Dutch-French cohort. *Ann. Neurol.* 57, 505-512.

[49] Globas, C., du Montcel, S. T., Baliko, L., Boesch, S., Depondt, C., DiDonato, S., Durr, A., Filla, A., Klockgether, T., Mariotti, C., Melegh, B., Rakowicz, M., Ribai, P., Rola, R., Schmitz-Hubsch, T., Szymanski, S., Timmann, D., Van de Warrenburg, B. P., Bauer, P. and Schols, L. (2008) Early symptoms in spinocerebellar ataxia type 1, 2, 3, and 6. *Mov. Disord.* 23, 2232-2238.

[50] Maciel, P., Gaspar, C., DeStefano, A. L., Silveira, I., Coutinho, P., Radvany, J., Dawson, D. M., Sudarsky, L., Guimaraes, J., Loureiro, J. E. and et al. (1995) Correlation between CAG repeat length and clinical features in Machado-Joseph disease. *Am. J. Hum. Genet.* 57, 54-61.

[51] Maruyama, H., Nakamura, S., Matsuyama, Z., Sakai, T., Doyu, M., Sobue, G., Seto, M., Tsujihata, M., Oh-i, T., Nishio, T. and et al. (1995) Molecular features of the CAG repeats and clinical manifestation of Machado-Joseph disease. *Hum. Mol. Genet.* 4, 807-812.

[52] Bettencourt, C., Santos, C., Montiel, R., Kay, T., Vasconcelos, J., Maciel, P. and Lima, M. (2010) The (CAG)n tract of Machado-Joseph Disease gene (ATXN3): a comparison between DNA and mRNA in patients and controls. *Eur. J. Hum. Genet.* 18, 621-623.

[53] Takiyama, Y., Igarashi, S., Rogaeva, E. A., Endo, K., Rogaev, E. I., Tanaka, H., Sherrington, R., Sanpei, K., Liang, Y., Saito, M. and et al. (1995) Evidence for inter-generational instability in the CAG repeat in the MJD1 gene and for conserved haplotypes at flanking markers amongst Japanese and Caucasian subjects with Machado-Joseph disease. *Hum. Mol. Genet.* 4, 1137-1146.

[54] Kubis, N., Durr, A., Gugenheim, M., Chneiweiss, H., Mazzetti, P., Brice, A. and Bouche, P. (1999) Polyneuropathy in autosomal dominant cerebellar ataxias: phenotype-genotype correlation. *Muscle. Nerve.* 22, 712-717.

[55] Cancel, G., Durr, A., Didierjean, O., Imbert, G., Burk, K., Lezin, A., Belal, S., Benomar, A., Abada-Bendib, M., Vial, C., Guimaraes, J., Chneiweiss, H., Stevanin, G., Yvert, G., Abbas, N., Saudou, F., Lebre, A. S., Yahyaoui, M., Hentati, F., Vernant, J. C., Klockgether, T., Mandel, J. L., Agid, Y. and Brice, A. (1997) Molecular and clinical correlations in spinocerebellar ataxia 2: a study of 32 families. *Hum. Mol. Genet.* 6, 709-715.

[56] David, G., Durr, A., Stevanin, G., Cancel, G., Abbas, N., Benomar, A., Belal, S., Lebre, A. S., Abada-Bendib, M., Grid, D., Holmberg, M., Yahyaoui, M., Hentati, F., Chkili, T., Agid, Y. and Brice, A. (1998) Molecular and clinical correlations in autosomal dominant cerebellar ataxia with progressive macular dystrophy (SCA7). *Hum. Mol. Genet.* 7, 165-170.

[57] Lerer, I., Merims, D., Abeliovich, D., Zlotogora, J. and Gadoth, N. (1996) Machado-Joseph disease: correlation between the clinical features, the CAG repeat length and homozygosity for the mutation. *Eur. J. Hum. Genet.* 4, 3-7.

[58] Sobue, G., Doyu, M., Nakao, N., Shimada, N., Mitsuma, T., Maruyama, H., Kawakami, S. and Nakamura, S. (1996) Homozygosity for Machado-Joseph disease gene enhances phenotypic severity. *J. Neurol. Neurosurg. Psychiatry.* 60, 354-356.

[59] Hubener, J. and Riess, O. (2010) Polyglutamine-induced neurodegeneration in SCA3 is not mitigated by non-expanded ataxin-3: conclusions from double-transgenic mouse models. *Neurobiol. Dis.* 38, 116-124.

[60] Sato, K., Kashihara, K., Okada, S., Ikeuchi, T., Tsuji, S., Shomori, T., Morimoto, K. and Hayabara, T. (1995) Does homozygosity advance the onset of dentatorubral-pallidoluysian atrophy? *Neurology.* 45, 1934-1936.

[61] Ikeuchi, T., Takano, H., Koide, R., Horikawa, Y., Honma, Y., Onishi, Y., Igarashi, S., Tanaka, H., Nakao, N., Sahashi, K., Tsukagoshi, H., Inoue, K., Takahashi, H. and Tsuji, S. (1997) Spinocerebellar ataxia type 6: CAG repeat expansion in alpha1A voltage-dependent calcium channel gene and clinical variations in Japanese population. *Ann. Neurol.* 42, 879-884.

[62] Ragothaman, M. and Muthane, U. (2008) Homozygous SCA 2 mutations changes phenotype and hastens progression. *Mov. Disord.* 23, 770-771.

[63] Hire, R., Katrak, S., Vaidya, S., Radhakrishnan, K. and Seshadri, M. (2011) Spinocerebellar ataxia type 17 in Indian patients: two rare cases of homozygous expansions. *Clin. Genet.* 80, 472–477.

[64] Bettencourt, C., Fialho, R. N., Santos, C., Montiel, R., Bruges-Armas, J., Maciel, P. and Lima, M. (2008) Segregation distortion of wild-type alleles at the Machado-Joseph disease locus: a study in normal families from the Azores islands (Portugal). *J. Hum. Genet.* 53, 333-339.

[65] Igarashi, S., Takiyama, Y., Cancel, G., Rogaeva, E. A., Sasaki, H., Wakisaka, A., Zhou, Y. X., Takano, H., Endo, K., Sanpei, K., Oyake, M., Tanaka, H., Stevanin, G., Abbas, N., Durr, A., Rogaev, E. I., Sherrington, R., Tsuda, T., Ikeda, M., Cassa, E., Nishizawa, M., Benomar, A., Julien, J., Weissenbach, J., Wang, G. X., Agid, Y., St George-Hyslop, P. H., Brice, A. and Tsuji, S. (1996) Intergenerational instability of the CAG repeat of the gene for Machado-Joseph disease (MJD1) is affected by the genotype of the normal chromosome: implications for the molecular mechanisms of the instability of the CAG repeat. *Hum. Mol. Genet.* 5, 923-932.

[66] Durr, A., Stevanin, G., Cancel, G., Duyckaerts, C., Abbas, N., Didierjean, O., Chneiweiss, H., Benomar, A., Lyon-Caen, O., Julien, J., Serdaru, M., Penet, C., Agid, Y. and Brice, A. (1996) Spinocerebellar ataxia 3 and Machado-Joseph disease: clinical, molecular, and neuropathological features. *Ann. Neurol.* 39, 490-499.

[67] França Jr MC, D'Abreu A, Maurer-Morelli CV, Bonadia LC, Silveira MS, Nucci A, Marques Jr W, Emmel VE, Jardim LB, Pereira MLS and I., L.-C. (2009) Significant effect of normal CAG repeat in the MJD1 gene in age at onset in patients with Machado-Joseph disease [Abstract]. In V International Workshop on MJD. pp. 81, S. Miguel - Azores (Portugal).

[68] DeStefano, A. L., Cupples, L. A., Maciel, P., Gaspar, C., Radvany, J., Dawson, D. M., Sudarsky, L., Corwin, L., Coutinho, P., MacLeod, P. and et al. (1996) A familial factor independent of CAG repeat length influences age at onset of Machado-Joseph disease. *Am. J. Hum. Genet.* 59, 119-127.

[69] Bettencourt, C., Santos, C., Kay, T., Silva, C., Vasconcelos, J., Santos, J., Maciel, P. and Lima, M. (2005) Clinical presentation and size of the CAG tract in Machado-Joseph disease patients from the Azores Islands (Portugal). Açoreana 10, 311-318.

[70] Emmel, V. E., Alonso, I., Jardim, L. B., Saraiva-Pereira, M. L. and Sequeiros, J. (2011) Does DNA methylation in the promoter region of the ATXN3 gene modify age at onset in MJD (SCA3) patients? *Clin. Genet.* 79, 100-102.

[71] Jardim, L., Silveira, I., Pereira, M. L., do Ceu Moreira, M., Mendonca, P., Sequeiros, J. and Giugliani, R. (2003) Searching for modulating effects of SCA2, SCA6 and DRPLA CAG tracts on the Machado-Joseph disease (SCA3) phenotype. *Acta. Neurol. Scand.* 107, 211-214.

[72] Pulst, S. M., Santos, N., Wang, D., Yang, H., Huynh, D., Velazquez, L. and Figueroa, K. P. (2005) Spinocerebellar ataxia type 2: polyQ repeat variation in the CACNA1A calcium channel modifies age of onset. *Brain.* 128, 2297-2303.

[73] Nishimura, M., Kawakami, H., Maruyama, H., Izumi, Y., Kuno, S., Kaji, R. and Nakamura, S. (2001) Influence of interleukin-1beta gene polymorphism on age-at-onset of spinocerebellar ataxia 6 (SCA6) in Japanese patients. *Neurosci. Lett.* 307, 128-130.

[74] Bettencourt, C., Raposo, M., Kazachkova, N., Cymbron, T., Santos, C., Kay, T., Vasconcelos, J., Maciel, P., Donis, K. C., Saraiva-Pereira, M. L., Jardim, L. B., Sequeiros, J. and Lima, M. (2011) The APOE ε2 allele increases the risk of earlier age at onset in Machado-Joseph Disease. *Arch. Neurol.* 68, 1580-1583.

[75] Lopes-Cendes, I., Silveira, I., Maciel, P., Gaspar, C., Radvany, J., Chitayat, D., Babul, R., Stewart, J., Dolliver, M., Robitaille, Y., Rouleau, G. A. and Sequeiros, J. (1996) Limits of clinical assessment in the accurate diagnosis of Machado-Joseph disease. *Arch. Neurol.* 53, 1168-1174.

[76] Sequeiros, J., Maciel, P., Taborda, F., Ledo, S., Rocha, J. C., Lopes, A., Reto, F., Fortuna, A. M., Rousseau, M., Fleming, M., Coutinho, P., Rouleau, G. A. and Jorge, C. S. (1998) Prenatal diagnosis of Machado-Joseph disease by direct mutation analysis. *Prenat. Diagn.* 18, 611-617.

[77] Drusedau, M., Dreesen, J. C., De Die-Smulders, C., Hardy, K., Bras, M., Dumoulin, J. C., Evers, J. L., Smeets, H. J., Geraedts, J. P. and Herbergs, J. (2004) Preimplantation genetic diagnosis of spinocerebellar ataxia 3 by (CAG)(n) repeat detection. *Mol. Hum. Reprod.* 10, 71-75.

[78] Lima, M., Kay, T., Vasconcelos, J., Mota-Vieira, L., Gonzalez, C., Peixoto, A., Abade, A., MacLeod, P., Graca, R. and Santos, J. (2001) Disease knowledge and attitudes toward predictive testing and prenatal diagnosis in families with Machado-Joseph disease from the Azores Islands (Portugal). *Community Genet.* 4, 36-42.

[79] Gonzalez, C., Lima, M., Kay, T., Silva, C., Santos, C. and Santos, J. (2004) Short-term psychological impact of predictive testing for Machado-Joseph disease: depression and anxiety levels in individuals at risk from the Azores (Portugal). *Community Genet.* 7, 196-201.

[80] Paneque, M., Lemos, C., Escalona, K., Prieto, L., Reynaldo, R., Velazquez, M., Quevedo, J., Santos, N., Almaguer, L. E., Velazquez, L., Sousa, A., Fleming, M. and Sequeiros, J. (2007) Psychological follow-up of presymptomatic genetic testing for spinocerebellar ataxia type 2 (SCA2) in Cuba. *J. Genet. Couns.* 16, 469-479.

[81] Cancel, G., Gourfinkel-An, I., Stevanin, G., Didierjean, O., Abbas, N., Hirsch, E., Agid, Y. and Brice, A. (1998) Somatic mosaicism of the CAG repeat expansion in spinocerebellar ataxia type 3/Machado-Joseph disease. *Hum. Mutat.* 11, 23-27.

[82] Ito, Y., Tanaka, F., Yamamoto, M., Doyu, M., Nagamatsu, M., Riku, S., Mitsuma, T. and Sobue, G. (1998) Somatic mosaicism of the expanded CAG trinucleotide repeat in

mRNAs for the responsible gene of Machado-Joseph disease (MJD), dentatorubral-pallidoluysian atrophy (DRPLA), and spinal and bulbar muscular atrophy (SBMA). *Neurochem. Res.* 23, 25-32.

[83] Matsuura, T., Sasaki, H., Yabe, I., Hamada, K., Hamada, T., Shitara, M. and Tashiro, K. (1999) Mosaicism of unstable CAG repeats in the brain of spinocerebellar ataxia type 2. *J. Neurol.* 246, 835-839.

[84] Boy, J., Schmidt, T., Wolburg, H., Mack, A., Nuber, S., Bottcher, M., Schmitt, I., Holzmann, C., Zimmermann, F., Servadio, A. and Riess, O. (2009) Reversibility of symptoms in a conditional mouse model of spinocerebellar ataxia type 3. *Hum. Mol. Genet.* 18, 4282-4295.

[85] Bonini, N. M. and La Spada, A. R. (2005) Silencing polyglutamine degeneration with RNAi. *Neuron.* 48, 715-718.

[86] Miller, V. M., Xia, H., Marrs, G. L., Gouvion, C. M., Lee, G., Davidson, B. L. and Paulson, H. L. (2003) Allele-specific silencing of dominant disease genes. *Proc. Natl. Acad. Sci. USA* 100, 7195-7200.

[87] Gaspar, C., Lopes-Cendes, I., Hayes, S., Goto, J., Arvidsson, K., Dias, A., Silveira, I., Maciel, P., Coutinho, P., Lima, M., Zhou, Y. X., Soong, B. W., Watanabe, M., Giunti, P., Stevanin, G., Riess, O., Sasaki, H., Hsieh, M., Nicholson, G. A., Brunt, E., Higgins, J. J., Lauritzen, M., Tranebjaerg, L., Volpini, V., Wood, N., Ranum, L., Tsuji, S., Brice, A., Sequeiros, J. and Rouleau, G. A. (2001) Ancestral origins of the Machado-Joseph disease mutation: a worldwide haplotype study. *Am. J. Hum. Genet.* 68, 523-528.

[88] Martins, S., Calafell, F., Gaspar, C., Wong, V. C., Silveira, I., Nicholson, G. A., Brunt, E. R., Tranebjaerg, L., Stevanin, G., Hsieh, M., Soong, B. W., Loureiro, L., Durr, A., Tsuji, S., Watanabe, M., Jardim, L. B., Giunti, P., Riess, O., Ranum, L. P., Brice, A., Rouleau, G. A., Coutinho, P., Amorim, A. and Sequeiros, J. (2007) Asian origin for the worldwide-spread mutational event in Machado-Joseph disease. *Arch. Neurol.* 64, 1502-1508.

[89] Alves, S., Nascimento-Ferreira, I., Auregan, G., Hassig, R., Dufour, N., Brouillet, E., Pedroso de Lima, M. C., Hantraye, P., Pereira de Almeida, L. and Deglon, N. (2008) Allele-specific RNA silencing of mutant ataxin-3 mediates neuroprotection in a rat model of Machado-Joseph disease. *PLoS One.* 3, e3341.

[90] Alves, S., Nascimento-Ferreira, I., Dufour, N., Hassig, R., Auregan, G., Nobrega, C., Brouillet, E., Hantraye, P., Pedroso de Lima, M. C., Deglon, N. and de Almeida, L. P. (2010) Silencing ataxin-3 mitigates degeneration in a rat model of Machado-Joseph disease: no role for wild-type ataxin-3? *Hum. Mol. Genet.* 19, 2380-2394.

[91] Schmitt, I., Linden, M., Khazneh, H., Evert, B. O., Breuer, P., Klockgether, T. and Wuellner, U. (2007) Inactivation of the mouse Atxn3 (ataxin-3) gene increases protein ubiquitination. *Biochem. Biophys. Res. Commun.* 362, 734-739.

[92] Rodrigues, A. J., Coppola, G., Santos, C., Costa Mdo, C., Ailion, M., Sequeiros, J., Geschwind, D. H. and Maciel, P. (2007) Functional genomics and biochemical characterization of the C. elegans orthologue of the Machado-Joseph disease protein ataxin-3. *FASEB J.* 21, 1126-1136.

[93] Rodrigues, A. J., do Carmo Costa, M., Silva, T. L., Ferreira, D., Bajanca, F., Logarinho, E. and Maciel, P. (2010) Absence of ataxin-3 leads to cytoskeletal disorganization and increased cell death. *Biochim. Biophys. Acta.* 1803, 1154-1163.

[94] Hu, J., Matsui, M., Gagnon, K. T., Schwartz, J. C., Gabillet, S., Arar, K., Wu, J., Bezprozvanny, I. and Corey, D. R. (2009) Allele-specific silencing of mutant huntingtin and ataxin-3 genes by targeting expanded CAG repeats in mRNAs. *Nat. Biotechnol.* 27, 478-484.

[95] Underwood, B. R. and Rubinsztein, D. C. (2008) Spinocerebellar ataxias caused by polyglutamine expansions: a review of therapeutic strategies. *Cerebellum.* 7, 215-221.

In: Ataxia: Causes, Symptoms and Treatment
Editor: Sung Hoi Hong

ISBN: 978-1-61942-867-6
© 2012 Nova Science Publishers, Inc.

Chapter 8

NEUROIMAGING IN SPINOCEREBELLAR ATAXIA TYPE 3: CLINICAL AND ANATOMICAL CORRELATES

Anelyssa D'Abreu, Fernando Cendes
and Iscia Lopes-Cendes
Faculty of Medical Sciences, University of Campinas-UNICAMP,
Campinas, SP, Brazil

ABSTRACT

Spinocerebellar ataxia 3 (SCA3) is a clinically heterogeneous neurodegenerative disorder characterized by ataxia, ophthalmoplegia, peripheral neuropathy, pyramidal dysfunction and movement disorders. It has an autosomal dominant inheritance and it results from a CAG repeat expansion mutation in the protein coding region of the *ATXN3* gene located at chromosome 14q32. Early neuropathological and neuroimaging studies mostly concentrated on the cerebellum, brainstem, spinal cord and basal ganglia; however, recent observations have demonstrated a more widespread cerebral involvement in SCA3. Visual analysis usually displays atrophy of the pons, cerebellar peduncles, frontal and temporal lobes, globus pallidus, as well as decreased anteroposterior and transverse diameters of the midbrain and decrease anteroposterior diameter of the medulla oblongata. Brain SPECT showed perfusion abnormalities in the parietal lobes, inferior portion of the frontal lobes, mesial and lateral portions of the temporal lobes, basal ganglia, and cerebellar hemispheres and vermis, while 18F-Dopa uptake (PET) was significantly decreased in the cerebellum, brainstem and nigro-striatal dopaminergic system, cerebral cortex and the striatum. Magnetic resonance spectroscopy (MRS) of the deep white matter demonstrated changes suggestive of axonal dysfunction in normal appearing white matter. Voxel-based morphometry (VBM) studies have conflicting results probably reflecting differences in sample sizes and characteristics. Different studies using texture analysis, manual volumetry and VBM demonstrated thalamic involvement in SCA3. The objective of this review is to discuss neuroimaging findings in SCA3 and how they contribute to a better understanding of the disease pathophysiology and future research directions.

INTRODUCTION

Machado-Joseph disease or spinocerebellar ataxia type 3 (MJD/SCA3) is an autosomal dominant disorder resulting from a trinucleotide repeat expansion (CAG) located in the 10th exon of the *ATXN3* gene. The causative gene, *ATXN3*, is mapped to chromosome 14q32.1 [1] and encodes the protein named ataxin-3. In MJD/SCA3, the normal CAG alleles range between 12 and 44 repeats; intermediate alleles from 45 to 51 repeats present reduced penetrance, while CAG expansions over approximately 52 CAG repeats present penetrance of 100%, which is age dependant[2]. Increased expanded repeat length in successive generations clinically translates into the phenomenon of anticipation, which is characterized by a tendency for earlier disease onset and more severe phenotype (figure 1)[3]. The clinical onset is usually in the 3rd or 4th decades with cerebellar ataxia [4]. Oculomotor abnormalities are frequent and the most common complaint is diplopia [4]. ''Bulging eyes appearance'' (a combination of lid retraction and poor blinking), gaze-evoked nystagmus, abnormal saccades, decrease smooth pursuit gain, impaired vestibulo-ocular reflex and supranuclear vertical gaze palsy are observed in the neurological examination [4, 5]. We also observe pyramidal dysfunction [6],dystonia and parkinsonism[6, 7]. Peripheral nerve involvement occurs in approximately 60% of patients [8] and is mostly determined by duration of disease[9]. Non-motor symptoms have also been reported in MJD/SCA3, such as autonomic dysfunction[10], excessive daytime sleepiness[11], restless legs syndrome [12], REM sleep behavior disorder[11], insomnia [13] cognitive and behavioral abnormalities [14, 15], depressive symptoms[16], chronic pain[17], cramps[18] and fatigue[19]. The most comprehensive neuropathological study in MJD/SCA3 used unconventional thick serial tissue sections in addition to conventional techniques. They demonstrated gray matter degeneration in multiple areas involved in the cerebellothalamocortical motor loop; the basal ganglia-thalamocortical motor loop; the visual, auditory, somatosensory, oculomotor and vestibular system; the ingestion-related and precerebellar brainstem system; the pontine noradrenergic system and the dopaminergic and cholinergic midbrain system.

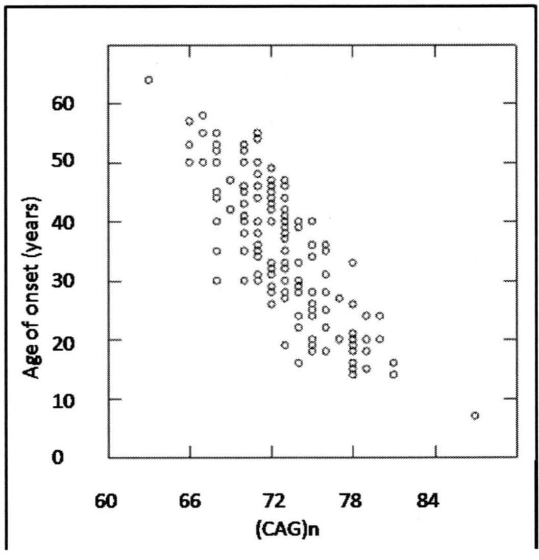

Figure 1. Inverse correlation between age of onset and CAG repeat length.

White matter degeneration was only observed in the cerebellum, spinal cord and brainstem. No neocortical alterations were noticed [20]. Imaging studies have much contributed to a better understanding of disease pathology, and the purpose of this chapter is to review neuroimaging findings in MJD/SCA3 and discuss possible future research steps in this area.

IMAGING STUDIES IN MJD/SCA3:

1. Visual Analysis

Magnetic resonance imaging (MRI) of minimally symptomatic patients or patients with new-onset symptoms may be normal. However patients with longer or more severe disease may present cerebellar atrophy; atrophy of the dorsal pons and of the medulla; enlargement of the forth ventricule, atrophy of the cerebellar peduncle, mild enlargement of the brain sulci and frontal atrophy (figure 2) [21].

Atrophy of the pontine tegmentum can be more evident than of the pontine base [22]. Nonspecific hyperintense lesions in the deep white matter have also been observed in middle-aged patients. [21].

A linear high intensity signal was observed at the media margin of the globus pallidus (internal segment), which was consistent with the degeneration of the lenticular fasciculus (LF), observed in the autopsy [23]. This finding however has been observed in Parkinson`s disease and normal controls [24]; suggesting the hyperintensity is frequent but not specific for MJD/SCA3 [25].

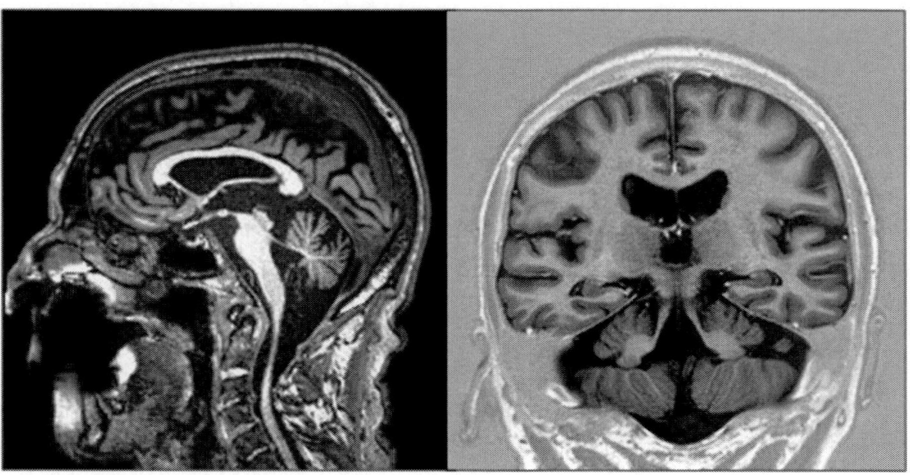

Figure 2. MJD/SCA3 patient with marked cerebellar and brainstem atrophy.

2. Manual Volumetry

Thirty-one MJD/SCA3 patients were compared to 20 patients with sporadic olivopontocerebellar atrophy, and 26 control subjects. Measurements included the anteroposterior and transverse diameters of the pons, midbrain, medulla oblongata, fourth ventricle, the width of the middle and superior cerebellar peduncle; the diameter of the dentate nucleus, red nucleus, and globus pallidus. Authors blindly used a graded semi-quantitatively approach from 0 to 3 (none- severe) to evaluate the degree of atrophy in the frontal, temporal, parietal, and occipital lobes[26]. Main findings were severe atrophy of the brainstem, mostly at pontine tegmentum and moderate atrophy of the cerebellum, followed by moderate to severe atrophy in the frontal and temporal lobes, and significant atrophy in the superior and middle cerebellar peduncles and globus pallidus. Decreased anteroposterior and transverse diameters of the midbrain and decrease anteroposterior diameter of the medulla oblongata were also described. Most importantly however, was the clinical-anatomical correlation described: pontine and midbrain atrophy were age-dependent while the decrease in the anteroposterior and transverse diameters of the globus pallidus and the degree of temporal or occipital lobe atrophy correlated with duration of illness. A high signal intensity in the transverse pontine fibers was observed in 14 (45.2%) of 31 patients with MJD/SCA3 [26].

Expanded CAG repeat length also plays an important role in disease progression. Thirty MJD/SCA3 individuals had the ratio of their anteroposterior diameter of the pontine tegmentum and the midbrain to the distance between the nasion and the inion subtracted from the grand mean of the same ratio in the control group. This value was called the degree of atrophy.

The ratio of the area of the pontine base and the vermis to the area of the posterior fossa was also subtracted from the grand mean of the same ratio in all controls. The quotient of the degree of atrophy divided by age at the time of examination was correlated with the expanded CAG length. There were significant correlations between the expanded CAG length and the degree of atrophy adjusted for age in the pontine tegmentum, pontine base, midbrain and vermis. Duration-adjusted degree of atrophy did not correlate with expanded CAG length in any structure [27].

Another study suggests that age was also a major determinant of cerebral involvement, along with expanded CAG repeat length [27, 28]. The sagital area of the pontine base and tegmentum, midbrain and vermis of 21 MJD/SCA3 patients independently correlated with the natural logarithm of the age at scanning. Multiple regression analysis demonstrated that the expanded CAG inversely correlated with the midsagittal area of the pontine tegmentum and of the vermis.

The progression of atrophy does not seem to be uniform in various brain regions. A longitudinal study of 7 patients showed that while the atrophy of the pontine base and the cerebellum significantly correlated with age, atrophy of the midbrain and pontine tegmentum did not seem to show progression [29]. Another study demonstrated that the pontine tegmentum atrophy in MJD/SCA3 was present early in the course of the disease, while the area of the pontine base remained in the control range after symptoms onset for a long period. The area of the pontinetegmentumnever superimposed with the measured area of the pontine tegmentum in controls [30]. Thought the ratio of atrophy of the tegmentum divided by age correlated with expanded CAG length, the pontine base ratio, correlated negatively with disease duration.

Clear clinical-anatomical correlation studies are few. One study involving manual segmentation of the thalamus demonstrated decreased thalamic volumes in MJD/SCA3, which correlated with the presence of dystonia [31].

3. Voxel-Based Morphometry (VBM)

There are four studies that used VBM in MJD/SCA3 [32-35]. Three of those compare MJD/SCA3 with other spinocerebellar ataxias (SCAs)- SCA1 [33, 35], SCA2 [33] and SCA6 [34, 35]- in an attempt to establish disease biomarkers and to differentiate patterns of atrophy within them. While in one study atrophy was restricted to brainstem and vermis [34], other found loss of grey matter volume in the cerebellum (hemispheres and vermis), but nearly no atrophy in the pons, basal ganglia and neocortex [35]. Goel et al. described not only involvement of the cerebellar hemispheres and vermis, but also bilateral superior temporal gyrus, bilateral inferior temporal gyrus and cingulate gyrus atrophy [33].

White matter loss was either restricted to the brainstem, cerebellar peduncles and cerebellar hemispheres (34, 35) or absent [33]. Compared to other SCAs, SCA1 and SCA6 lead to a more pronounced atrophy in the cerebellar hemispheres [35, 36] than SCA3. Grey matter loss in the cerebellum is also more important in SCA6 [34, 35]. SCA2 had a similar pattern of atrophy to SCA1 [33].

A more comprehensive study was carried out in 45 MJD/SCA3 patients and 51 controls, in which authors observed significant grey matter atrophy at frontal, parietal, temporal and occipital lobes, limbic cortex, subcortical grey matter, cerebellum and brainstem (figure 3). White matter atrophy was restricted to the cerebellum [32].

Age, expanded CAG length and disease duration were significant factors in the prediction of grey matter density, yet, age and expanded CAG length were the most important ones. White matter abnormalities were observed in the deep cerebellum. Longitudinal evaluation approximately 1 year after the first MRI did not reveal significant progression, probably due to ceiling effect.

Differences in findings among studies probably result from sample size (9 [34], 10 [33], 24 [35] and 45 patients [32]); variable clinical markers, such as age, age of symptom onset, disease duration and clinical phenotype.

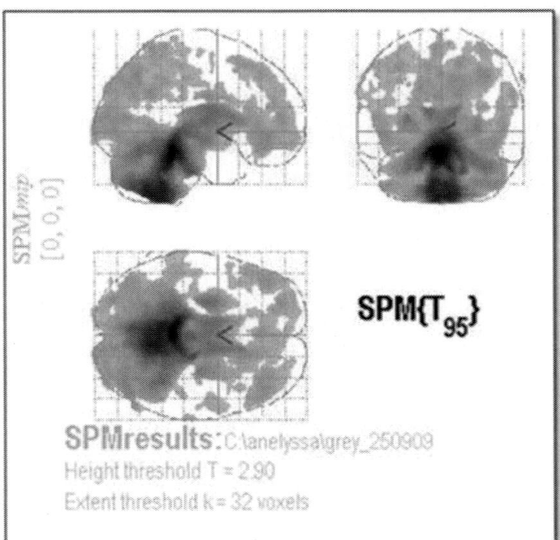

Figure 3. Output from statistical parametric mapping (SPM). Grey areas represent grey matter atrophy.

4. Spectroscopy

There are few studies using spectroscopy in MJD/SCA3. In a large sample of forty MJD/SCA3 patients, researches acquired single voxel 1H-MRS using point resolved spectroscopy (PRESS) at the superior-posterior region of the left hemisphere at the level of the corpus callosum [21]. The main finding was decreased levels of NAA/Cr in the deep white mater of patients with MJD/SCA3, which did not correlate with expanded CAG repeat length or clinical characteristics. This finding suggests neuronal dysfunction in a normal appearing area of the brain and indicates a widespread brain damage. Yabe et al. obtained 31P-MRS in the calf muscle of 8 male patients with MJD/SCA3 and 11 healthy men before, during, and after a 4 minute plantar flexion exercise [37]. They calculated the ratio of phosphocreatine to phosphocreatine plus inorganic phosphate {PCr/(Pi + PCr)}, the ratio Pi/PCr, and the maximum rate (Vmax) of mitochondrial ATP production. There was a significant difference between MJD/SCA3 and controls in PCr/(Pi + PCr) ratio at rest and Vmax. Interestingly, Vmax was inversely correlated with the scale for the assessment and rating of ataxia scores (SARA). MJD/SCA3 showed a reduction in Vmax over the course of 2 years. These data suggest that 31P-MRS may be potentially used as a surrogate marker for MJD/SCA3.

5. PET/SPECT

Brain SPECT demonstrated perfusion abnormalities in the parietal lobes, inferior portion of the frontal lobes, mesial and lateral portions of the temporal lobes, basal ganglia, and cerebellar hemispheres and vermis [38]. A statistically significant relationship was observed between the perfusion of the left parietal lobe and extrapyramidal syndrome and between the length of the expanded CAG repeat and the perfusion of the lateral portion of the right temporal lobe.

18F-Dopa uptake in MJD/SCA3 was significantly diminished in the cerebellum, brainstem and nigrostriatal dopaminergic system, the cerebral cortex and the striatum [39]. PET with fluorine-18-fluorodeoxyglucose (FDG) in 12 symptomatic patients with MJD/SCA3 showed reduced brain glucose metabolism at the bilateral anterior lobe and right posterior lobe of the cerebellum, the bilateral parahippocampal gyrus and the right lentiform nucleus [40]. PET-FDG study in seven asymptomatic MJD/SCA3 patients showed subclinical changes of FDG consumption decreased in the cerebellar hemispheres, brainstem, and occipital, parietal and temporal cortices of asymptomatic MJD/SCA3 gene carriers compared to controls, suggesting preclinical disease activity [41]. Regional FDG uptake ratios between asymptomatic gene carriers and MJD/SCA3 showed also significant differences in the neocortex and the cerebellum. Discriminant function analysis between the asymptomatic mutation carriers, controls and symptomatic MJD/SCA3 found that the best discriminant between controls and symptomatic subjects was the cerebellar FDG uptake ratios (sensitivity and specificity of 100%). In asymptomatic carriers and symptomatic patients, cerebellar FDG uptake ratios were consistent with clinical status in 14 out of 15 subjects (sensitivity of 100% and specificity of 85.7%). A similar study used 99mTc- TRODAT-1 brain SPECTto assess uptake values in bilateral striatal areas in 5 asymptomatic MJD/SCA3 gene carriers, 10 age-matched MJD/SCA3 patients, and 10 age-matched healthy control subjects [42]. Uptake values of the asymptomatic gene carriers and symptomatic individual exhibited a significant reduction compared to the control group. As expected the reduction was more severe in the patient group. Authors concluded that impairment of presynaptic dopamine function occurs at an early stage, prior to symptom onset.

6.   Texture Analysis

There is only one study using texture analysis in MJD/SCA3 [43].Texture analysis is a computerized method used to quantify texture properties of a digital image (coarseness, rugosity, smoothness etc). This work used a statistical approach based on the gray-level cooccurrence (GLC) matrix, which extracted texture information established on the gray-level distribution of pairs of pixels. Differences between patients and controls were observed in the bilateral caudate nuclei, thalami and putamen, while no differences were found for the corpus callosum, confirming previous reports.

CONCLUSION

Prior to neuroimaging studies the general agreement about the pathology of MJD/SAC3 was that the involvement was mostly restricted to the cerebellum, brainstem and basal ganglia. Conversely, different neuroimaging techniques demonstrated further involvement of the thalamus and the neocortex, suggesting a much more widespread pathology then previously acknowledged.

Nonetheless, few studies have addressed the asymptomatic MJD/SCA3 mutation carrier or performed longitudinal evaluation. Even fewer address the correlation between clinical scales and neuroimaging findings. It is still unclear how the disease progresses in the brain, and if different phenotypes represent different affected brain areas. The search for a possible biomarker is still ongoing, which would be extremely helpful in future clinical trials.

REFERENCES

[1]   Kawaguchi Y, Okamoto T, Taniwaki M, Aizawa M, Inoue M, Katayama S, et al. Cag Expansions in a Novel Gene for Machado-Joseph Disease at Chromosome 14q32.1. *Nat. Genet.* 1994 Nov;8(3):221-8.

[2]   Todd PK, Paulson HL. RNA-Mediated Neurodegeneration in Repeat Expansion Disorders. *Ann. Neurol.* 2010 Mar;67(3):291-300.

[3]   Maruyama H, Nakamura S, Matsuyama Z, Sakai T, Doyu M, Sobue G, et al. Molecular features of the CAG repeats and clinical manifestation of Machado-Joseph disease. *Human Molecular Genetics.* 1995;4(5):807-12.

[4]   D'Abreu A, Franca MC, Paulson HL, Lopes-Cendes I. Caring for Machado-Joseph disease: Current understanding and how to help patients. *Parkinsonism and Related Disorders.* 2010;16(1):2-7.

[5]   Gordon CR, Joffe V, Vainstein G, Gadoth N. Vestibulo-ocular arreflexia in families with spinocerebellar ataxia type 3 (Machado-Joseph disease). *Journal of Neurology Neurosurgery and Psychiatry.* 2003;74(10):1403-6.

[6]   Jardim LB, Pereira ML, Silveira I, Ferro A, Sequeiros J, Giugliani R. Neurologic findings in Machado-Joseph disease - Relation with disease duration, subtypes, and (CAG)(n). *Archives of Neurology.* 2001;58(6):899-904.

[7]   Rosenberg RN. Machado-Joseph disease: an autosomal dominant motor system degeneration. *Mov. Disord.* 1992;7(3):193-203.

[8]   Klockgether T, Schols L, Abele M, Burk K, Topka H, Andres F, et al. Age related axonal neuropathy in spinocerebellar ataxia type 3/Machado-Joseph disease (SCA3/MJD). *J. Neurol. Neurosurg. Psychiatry.* 1999 Feb;66(2):222-4.

[9]   Schmitz-Hubsch T, Coudert M, Bauer P, Giunti P, Globas C, Baliko L, et al. Spinocerebellar ataxia types 1, 2, 3, and 6: disease severity and nonataxia symptoms. *Neurology.* 2008 Sep 23;71(13):982-9.

[10]   Yeh TH, Lu CS, Chou YH, Chong CC, Wu T, Han NH, et al. Autonomic dysfunction in Machado-Joseph disease. *Arch. Neurol.* 2005 Apr;62(4):630-6.

[11]   Friedman JH, Fernandez HH, Sudarsky LR. REM behavior disorder and excessive daytime somnolence in Machado-Joseph disease (SCA-3). *Mov. Disord.* 2003 Dec;18(12):1520-2.

[12]   Schols L, Haan J, Riess O, Amoiridis G, Przuntek H. Sleep disturbance in spinocerebellar ataxias: is the SCA3 mutation a cause of restless legs syndrome? *Neurology.* 1998 Dec;51(6):1603-7.

[13]   D'Abreu A, Franca M, Conz L, Friedman JH, Nucci AM, Cendes F, et al. Sleep symptoms and their clinical correlates in Machado-Joseph disease. *Acta Neurologica Scandinavica.* 2009;119(4):277-80.

[14]   Zawacki TM, Grace J, Friedman JH, Sudarsky L. Executive and emotional dysfunction in Machado-Joseph disease. *Mov. Disord.* 2002 Sep;17(5):1004-10.

[15]   Kawai Y, Takeda A, Abe Y, Washimi Y, Tanaka F, Sobue G. Cognitive impairments in Machado-Joseph disease. *Arch. Neurol.* 2004 Nov;61(11):1757-60.

[16]   Schmitz-Hubsch T, Coudert M, Tezenas du Montcel S, Giunti P, Labrum R, Durr A, et al. Depression comorbidity in spinocerebellar ataxia. *Mov. Disord.* 2011 Apr;26(5):870-6.

[17]   Franca MC, D'Abreu A, Friedman JH, Nucci A, Lopes-Cendes I. Chronic pain in Machado-Joseph disease. *Archives of Neurology.* 2007;64(12):1767-70.

[18]   Franca MC, Dabreu A, Nucci A, Lopes-Cendes I. Muscle excitability abnormalities in Machado-Joseph disease. *Archives of Neurology.* 2008;65(4):525-9.

[19]   Friedman JH, Amick MM. Fatigue and daytime somnolence in Machado Joseph disease(Spinocerebellar ataxia type 3). *Movement Disorders.* 2008;23(9):1323-4.

[20]   Rub U, Brunt ER, Deller T. New insights into the pathoanatomy of spinocerebellar ataxia type 3 (Machado-Joseph disease). *Current Opinion in Neurology.* 2008;21(2):111-6.

[21]   D'Abreu A, Franca M, Appenzeller S, Lopes-Cendes I, Cendes F. Axonal Dysfunction in the Deep White Matter in Machado-Joseph Disease. *Journal of Neuroimaging.* 2009;19(1):9-12.

[22]   Tokumaru AM, Kamakura K, Maki T, Murayama S, Sakata I, Kaji T, et al. Magnetic resonance imaging findings of Machado-Joseph disease: Histopathologic correlation. *Journal of Computer Assisted Tomography.* 2003;27(2):241-8.

[23] Yamada S, Nishimiya J, Nakajima T, Taketazu F. Linear high intensity area along the medial margin of the internal segment of the globus pallidus in Machado-Joseph disease patients. *Journal of Neurology Neurosurgery and Psychiatry.* 2005;76(4):573-5.

[24] Shirai W, Ito S, Hattori T. Linear T2 hyperintensity along the medial margin of the globus pallidus in patients with Machado-Joseph disease and Parkinson disease, and in healthy subjects. *American Journal of Neuroradiology.* 2007;28:1993-5.

[25] Ito S, Shirai W, Hattori T. Linear T2 hyperintensity along the medial margin of the globus pallidus is highly sensitive but not specific for Machado-Joseph disease. *Movement Disorders.* 2006;21:P1082.

[26] Murata Y, Yamaguchi S, Kawakami H, Imon Y, Maruyama H, Sakai T, et al. Characteristic magnetic resonance imaging findings in Machado-Joseph disease. *Archives of Neurology.* 1998;55(1):33-7.

[27] Abe Y, Tanaka F, Matsumoto M, Doyu M, Hirayama M, Kachi T, et al. CAG repeat number correlates with the rate of brainstem and cerebellar atrophy in Machado-Joseph disease. *Neurology.* 1998;51(3):882-4.

[28] Onodera O, Idezuka J, Igarashi S, Takiyama Y, Endo K, Takano H, et al. Progressive atrophy of cerebellum and brainstem as a function of age and the size of the expanded CAG repeats in the MJD1 gene in Machado-Joseph disease. *Ann. Neurol.* 1998;43(3):288-96.

[29] Horimoto Y, Matsumoto M, Yuasa H, Kojima A, Nokura K, Katada E, et al. Brainstem in Machado-Joseph disease: atrophy or small size? *European Journal of Neurology.* 2008;15(1):102-5.

[30] Yoshizawa T, Watanabe M, Frusho K, Shoji S. Magnetic resonance imaging demonstrates differential atrophy of pontine base and tegmentum in Machado-Joseph disease. *Journal of the neurological sciences.* 2003;215(1-2):45-50.

[31] D'Abreu A, Franca MC, Yasuda CL, Souza MSA, Lopes-Cendes I, Cendes F. Thalamic Volume and Dystonia in Machado-Joseph Disease. *Journal of Neuroimaging.* 2011;21(2):e91-e3.

[32] D'Abreu A, França Jr. MC, Yasuda CL, Campos BAG, Lopes-Cendes I, Cendes F. Neocortical atrophy in Machado-Joseph Disease: a longitudinal neuroimaging study. *Journal of Neuroimaging* (2011) DOI: 101111/j1552-6569201100614x. 2011.

[33] Goel G, Pal PK, Ravishankar S, Venkatasubramanian G, Jayakumar PN, Krishna N, et al. Gray matter volume deficits in spinocerebellar ataxia: An optimized voxel based morphometric study. *Parkinsonism and Related Disorders* (2011), doi:101016/jparkreldis201104008. 2011.

[34] Lukas C, Schols L, Bellenberg B, Rub U, Przuntek H, Schmid G, et al. Dissociation of grey and white matter reduction in spinocerebellar ataxia type 3 and 6: A voxel-based morphometry study. *Neuroscience Letters.* 2006;408(3):230-5.

[35] Schulz JB, Borkert J, Wolf S, Schmitz-Hubsch T, Rakowicz M, Mariotti C, et al. Visualization, quantification and correlation of brain atrophy with clinical symptoms in spinocerebellar ataxia types 1, 3 and 6. *Neuroimage.* 2010;49(1):158-68.

[36] Lukas C, Hahn HK, Bellenberg B, Hellwig K, Globas C, Schimrigk SK, et al. Spinal cord atrophy in spinocerebellar ataxia type 3 and 6 - Impact on clinical disability. *Journal of Neurology.* 2008;255(8):1244-9.

[37] Yabe I, Tha KK, Yokota T, Sato K, Soma H, Takei A, et al. Estimation of Skeletal Muscle Energy Metabolism in Machado-Joseph Disease Using P-31-MR Spectroscopy. *Movement Disorders.* 2011;26(1):165-8.

[38] Etchebehere EC CF, Lopes-Cendes I, Pereira JA, Lima MC, Sansana CR, Silva CA, Camargo MF, Santos AO, Ramos CD, Camargo EE. Brain single-photon emission computed tomography and magnetic resonance imaging in Machado-Joseph disease. *Archives of Neurology.* 2001;58(8):1257-63.

[39] Taniwaki T ST, Kobayashi T, Kuwabara Y, Otsuka M, Ichiya Y, Masuda K, Goto I. Positron emission tomography (PET) in Machado-Joseph disease. *Journal of the neurological sciences.* 1997;145(1):63-7.

[40] Wang PS, Liu RS, Yang BH, Soong BW. Regional patterns of cerebral glucose metabolism in spinocerebellar ataxia type 2, 3 and 6 - A voxel-based FDG-positron emission tomography analysis. *Journal of Neurology.* 2007;254(7):838-45.

[41] Soong BW LR. Positron emission tomography in asymptomatic gene carriers of Machado–Joseph disease. *J Neurol Neurosurg Psychiatry.* 1998;64:499-504.

[42] Yen TC, Tzen KY, Chen MC, Chou YHW, Chen RS, Chen CJ, et al. Dopamine transporter concentration is reduced in asymptomatic Machado-Joseph disease gene carriers. *Journal of Nuclear Medicine.* 2002;43(2):153-9.

[43] De Oliveira MS DAA, França Jr MC, Lopes-Cendes I, Cendes F, Castellano G. MRI-Texture Analysis of Corpus Callosum, Thalamus, Putamen, and Caudate in Machado-Joseph Disease. *J. Neuroimaging.* 2010 Dec 1 doi: 101111/j1552-6569201000553x 2010.

In: Ataxia: Causes, Symptoms and Treatment
Editor: Sung Hoi Hong

ISBN: 978-1-61942-867-6
© 2012 Nova Science Publishers, Inc.

Chapter 9

COMPUTATIONAL ANALYSIS OF ATAXIN PROTEINS: NEW INSIGHT INTO THEIR FUNCTIONAL PERFORMANCE AND ATAXIA DEVELOPMENT

E. Pirogova[1], V. Vojisavljevic[1], J. L. Hernández Cáceres[2] and I. Cosic[1]*
[1]School of Electrical and Computer Engineering, RMIT University,
Melbourne, Victoria, Australia
[2]Centre for Cybernetics Applications to Medicine CECAM-ISCMH, Havana Cuba

ABSTRACT

People affected by ataxia, a genetic neurological disorder, have problems with coordination. Ataxia is the principal symptom of a group of neurological disorders known as cerebellar ataxias. Most of them are progressive. In ataxia, a neurodegenerative process leads to changes in a motor cortex responsible for balance and coordination. Recently several genes that cause autosomal dominant ataxia development were identified. These abnormal genes share a common ability to produce abnormal ataxin protein sequences that affect nerve cells in the cerebellum and spinal cord. Here, using signal processing methods we analysed ataxin proteins and identified the characteristic features corresponding to their biological activities. The Resonant Recognition Model (RRM) is a physico-mathematical approach developed for analysis of protein interactions. By incorporating Smoothed Pseudo Wigner - Ville distribution (SPWV) in the RRM, we can predict locations of active/binding sites along the protein molecule. The findings of this study showed that our computational predictions correspond closely with the experimentally identified locations of the active regions for the selected ataxin-1 and ataxin-3 protein groups. We also present and discuss the results of possible interactions between the ataxin-1 and growth factor independent transcriptional regulator-1 (Gfi-1) proteins known to be responsible for the selective Purkinje cell degeneration in ataxia disorder. In addition, we demonstrate that by using our recently developed protein classification methodology, we can distinguish between different ataxin protein functional groups that correspond to different neurological disorders. By employing

---

* ph. 61 3 9925-3015, fax 61 3 9925-2007

Hierarchical classification methodology and using the Euclidian distance as a measure of the distance between vectors representing the distribution of amino acid residues along the ataxin proteins, it is possible to extract ataxin proteins' specific features into an adjoin 10-dimensional vector that represents the distribution of electron ion potentials along a proteins' backbone, and thus classify ataxin proteins by their different functionalities. The developed classification system is tested here on known ataxin proteins. The results obtained provide a valuable insight into the functional performance of ataxin proteins. The presented novel computational approach can be used to predict unknown protein-protein interactions of ataxin with other proteins that can potentially influence its function and thus, contribute to ataxia disorder development.

Keywords: signal processing, protein function, characteristic frequency, ataxia, Gfi-1

1. INTRODUCTION

Ataxia defines a symptom of incoordination, which can be associated with infections, injuries or diseases. Ataxia also denotes a group of specific degenerative diseases of the nervous system called the hereditary and sporadic ataxias. Spinocerebellar ataxias (SCAs) are a class of neurodegenerative disorders, characterized by the loss of balance, progressive motor dysfunction and degeneration of the cerebellar purkinje cells (PC) [1]. Excessive repeats of particular amino acids in the primary structures of ataxin proteins have been found to be responsible for ataxia disorder development. However, what causes mutations to occur in these proteins is still unknown. Over the last decade, a growing number of inherited neurodegenerative diseases, including Huntington's disease and several forms of SCAs, have been shown to be related to a polymorphic CAG-triplet repeat motif inside the coding region of particular genes [1, 2]. Abnormal expansion beyond a threshold number of 35–40 triplets translates into lengthening of the otherwise harmless polyglutamine tract. Although the proteins associated with ataxia disorders are mutually unrelated, it was shown that these diseases share several common features and appear to progress via a similar pathogenic mechanism [1-6].

Functional activities of majority of ataxin proteins are quite diverse due to a large variety of possible roles they perform. For instance, it was established that ataxin-6 (ATX6) is a subunit of a P/Q type calcium channel, and mutated versions of the channel are more permeable to calcium [7]. Ataxin-1 (ATX1) has been implicated as having a significant role in protein ubiquitination pathways [8]; RNA metabolism [9]; regulation of growth factor independent transcription factor Gfi-1, a protein essential for cerebellar Purkinje cell survival [10], protein folding [11] and hormonal receptor regulation [12]. It was suggested that ATX1 is phosphorylated via a calcium-dependent mechanism [13]. A role in RNA (or DNA) metabolism has been proposed for ATX1 [12, 13], ATX2 [14], ATX3 [15-17] and ATX7 [19], whereas participation in ubiquitin proteasome pathways has been suggested for ATX1 [8] and ATX3 [15-18]. With such diversity of putative mechanisms for a single protein's function, it is difficult to grasp a plausible hypothesis for the pathophysiology associated with the presence of long glutamine repeats. On the other hand, available evidence shows that we cannot rule out the possibility of common bioactivity being shared by different ataxin proteins. Thus, understanding the complexity and unclear nature of ataxia disorder development at the molecular level remains an unresolved objective [20]. One of the issues arising from the latest advances in genome research is that the genetic bases of a disorder are now known even though the function of the codified protein(s) or pathophysiologic mechanisms triggered by the corresponding mutated proteins, have not been determined. A pathological hallmark of most polyglutamine diseases is the presence of nuclear and cytoplasmic inclusions which contain the mutated polyglutamine protein. However, for some patients with ataxia disorder, the molecular analysis of their mutant proteins revealed no cytoplasmic inclusions in the ataxin primary sequences. This fact underpins the complicated and unclear nature of ataxia disorder [20].

Experimental findings have shown the presence of pathological effects in mice models where loss of Gfi-1 mimics spinocerebellar ataxia type 1 (SCA1) phenotypes in Purkinje cells and leads to Purkinje cell degeneration. This indicates that the ATX1/Gfi-1 interaction might contribute to the selective Purkinje cell degeneration in SCA1. Moreover, it has been proposed that the AXH domain of ATX1 mediates neurodegeneration through its interaction with Gfi-1/Senseless proteins [10]. Published research has shown that different types of ataxia disorder may influence different parts of the nervous system. However, it is still not clear which parts of the nervous system are most affected by ataxia progression [1, 3].

In this chapter we present and discuss the results of our computational study of different ataxin proteins. The Resonant Recognition Model (RRM) [21] was used to determine ataxin proteins' characteristic frequencies and predict the locations of protein active/binding site(s) within their primary structures.

The RRM is based on Fourier transforms [21, 22]. The main disadvantage of a Fourier Transform is that the information about frequency characteristic along the series is hidden, and we can obtain only averaged time and frequency content of the analysed signal. In the last 20 years, time-frequency distribution methods have become powerful alternative tools for signal analysis.

A time-frequency transform presents energy distribution of a signal over the time and frequency domains [23]. In our study, we applied the time-frequency signal processing technique to selected proteins, aiming to demonstrate how a signal's energy is distributed over the time-frequency space. By incorporating Smoothed Pseudo Wigner–Ville distribution (SPWV) in the standard RRM approach, we overcome the problem of non-localised events currently present in the model and improve the RRM predictive capabilities and accuracy for investigation of the physical characteristics of proteins [24].

Using the computational approach we identified the characteristic frequencies of ataxin proteins, as a whole functional group, which correspond to their common biological activity. We selected and analysed different ataxin subgroups, associated with different neurological disorder types. While doing so, we anticipated that we would be able to distinguish between disorder types by determining their specific characteristic features/frequencies. We also analysed possible interactions between ataxin and Gfi-1 gene proteins that leads to spinocerebellar ataxia type 1 (SCA1) phenotypes in Purkinje cells and thus, to Purkinje cell degeneration. In our study we also employed a new Hierarchical classification methodology for analysis of the functional behaviour of the selected ataxin proteins. The findings of this computational study may shed new light on the functional behaviour of ataxin proteins, and open up new possibilities for ataxia treatment.

2. MATERIALS AND METHODS

2.1. Resonant Recognition Model

Proteins, the building blocks of any living organism, show great diversity and versatility due to the properties of their constitutive elements, amino acids. The crucial problem of understanding how a protein function is 'encrypted' in the protein's primary structure has not been entirely resolved as yet. Even though experimental methods such as X-ray crystallography and nuclear magnetic resonance (NMR) have been successful in the determination of the 3D structures of proteins, these techniques are expensive and highly time consuming. Thus, there is an urgent need for theoretical approaches suitable for the computational analysis of the structural and functional performances of different protein families. The RRM is a physico-mathematical approach that interprets protein sequences as linear information using digital signal processing methods [21, 22, 25-31]. The RRM postulates that protein (DNA) interactions entail a mechanism of resonant energy transfer between the interacting molecules at the frequency specific for each observed function/interaction. In this model, the protein primary structure is represented by a numerical series by assigning to each amino acid in the sequence a physical parameter value relevant to the protein's biological activity. Through using the RRM, it has been hypothesised that there is a significant correlation between spectra of the numerical presentation of amino acids and their biological activity [21, 25]. It has been found that proteins with the same biological function have a common frequency component in their numerical spectra. This frequency is considered to be a characteristic feature of a protein's biological function or interaction [26-32]. The RRM procedure involves two stages of calculations. First, the original amino acid sequence is transformed into a numerical sequence by assigning to each amino acid a particular value of the physical parameter relevant to a protein's biological function. Here, the energy of delocalised electrons (calculated as the electron–ion interaction pseudopotential, EIIP [33] of each amino acid residue is used. The EIIP parameter describes the average energy states of all valence electrons in a particular amino acid. The EIIP values for each amino acid were calculated from the general model of pseudopotentials [33]:

$$\langle k+q|w|k \rangle = 0.25 \frac{Z \sin(1.04 * \pi Z)}{2\pi}$$

where q is a change of momentum k of the delocalised electron in the interaction with potential w, and

$$Z = \frac{\sum_i Z}{N}$$

where Z_i is the number of valence electrons of the ith atom of each amino acid and N is the total number of atoms in the amino acid. Thus, the resulting numerical series represents the distribution of the free electron energies along the protein. The numerical sequences obtained are analysed using Fourier Transforms (FT) to extract information pertinent to the biological function. As the average distance between amino acid residues in a protein sequence is about 3.8 Å, it can be assumed that the points in the derived numerical sequence are equidistant. For further numerical analysis, the distance between points in these numerical sequences is set at an arbitrary value, d = 1. Peak frequencies in the amplitude cross-spectral function define common frequency components of the two sequences analysed. In order to determine the common frequency components for a group of protein sequences, we have calculated the values of multiple cross-spectral function coefficients, M_n which are defined as follows [22, 25]:

$$|M_n|=|X1_n|.|X2_n|...|XM_n| \quad n=1,2,...,N/2$$

where l_n is the number of cross correlated proteins, Mn represents the nth spectral component in the cross-spectral function and Xk,n is the nth spectral component of the kth protein. Peak frequencies in such a multiple cross-spectral function denote common frequency components for all the sequences analysed. The multiple cross-spectral function for a large group of sequences with the same biological function has been named 'consensus spectrum'. The presence of a distinct peak frequency in a consensus spectrum implies that all of the analysed sequences within the group have one frequency component in common. This frequency is related to the biological function provided the following criteria are met:

(1) One peak only exists for a group of protein sequences sharing the same biological function.
(2) No significant peak exists for biologically unrelated protein sequences.
(3) Peak frequencies are different for different biological functions.

In our previous research [26-32] the above criteria have been implemented, and the following fundamental conclusion was drawn: each specific biological function of a given protein or DNA is characterised by a single frequency. Our previous research showed that proteins with the same biological function have a common frequency in their numerical spectra, and each specific biological function of a protein or regulatory DNA sequence(s) is characterised by a single frequency [25]. The results of our previous studies with a number of different protein families revealed that proteins and their interacting targets (receptors, binding proteins and inhibitors) display the same characteristic frequency in their interactions. However, it is obvious that one protein can participate in more than one biological process, i.e. revealing more than one biological function. Therefore, it has been postulated that the RRM frequency characterises a particular biological process of interaction between selected bio-molecules. Further research in this direction led to the conclusion that interacting molecules have the same characteristic frequency but opposite phases at that frequency [21, 25]. Thus, the RRM characteristic frequencies represent a protein's general functions as well as the mutual recognition between a particular protein and its target (receptor, ligand, etc.). As this recognition arises from the matching of periodicities within the distribution of energies of free electrons along the interacting proteins, it can be regarded as the resonant recognition. Once the characteristic frequency for the particular biological function or interaction is determined, it becomes possible to identify the individual 'hot spot' amino acids that contributed most to this specific characteristic frequency and thus, possibly to the observed biological behaviour of the protein. These "key" amino acids are found to be clustered in and around a protein's active sites. By knowing a protein's specific characteristic frequency we can also identify the protein's active sites (functional epitopes) and design bioactive peptide analogues [21, 26, 28, 31).

2.2. Time–Frequency Analysis

The Wigner quasi-distribution was initially introduced to replace the classical phase-space distribution in statistical physics with corresponding quantum analogue [34]. Von Neumann [24] established a method where two nonsimultaneously measurable quantum mechanical quantities, such as coordinates and momentum, can be measured simultaneously with limited precision. He also showed that all measurements, with limited accuracy, can be replaced by the absolutely accurate measurements of other quantities, which are related to their non-simultaneously measurable quantities. Although due to the uncertainty principle, the concept of phase space in quantum mechanics is somewhat problematic, various functions which bear some resemblance to true phase–space distribution functions of the non-quantum world were introduced. They proved to be useful not only as calculation tools, but also provided insights into the relations between classical and quantum mechanics. The first of such functions was introduced by Wigner [34] to study quantum corrections in classical statistical mechanics. It is now known as the Wigner function. It may be shown [24, 34] that the phase–space distribution, which is produced in simultaneous measurements of position and momentum, can be represented as a convolution of the Wigner function of the considered quantum state and the Wigner function of the filter state, which represents a measuring apparatus. In general, Wigner–Ville distribution (WVD) describes the frequency content changes as a function of time. The distribution is the actual energy intensity of various frequency components of the signal at a given position along the protein assuming that the average distance between amino acids in the protein molecule is set at an arbitrary value d = 1. In practical calculations, convolution of the signal generates the cross term that represents interference of the signals, and consequently, significantly decreases the resolution of the signal. A number of methods have been developed to reduce the cross-term [34]. In this study we replaced the WVD by the Smoothed Pseudo Wigner-Ville distribution (SPWVD) [24], where some window functions are convolved with the WVD to restrain and decrease the effect of the interference terms. Here we analysed the 1D signal EIIP [i], where the i term stands for the EIIP numerical value of the ith amino acid along the protein molecule. The time unit is substituted by the space unit which represents the distance between two consecutive amino acids in the protein. The distance between neighbouring amino acids is considered as a constant value.

Supposing EIIP[i], i = 1, 2, …,N is the numerical sequence of the electron–ion interaction potentials of amino acids along a polypeptide chain; then the SPWVD is given by S(t, f) [24]:

$$S(t,f) = \int_{-\infty}^{\infty} h(\tau) \int_{-\infty}^{\infty} g(s-t) z(s+\tau/2) z(s+\tau/2)^* ds\, e^{-j2\pi\nu\tau} d\tau$$

where z is an analytical (complex) signal obtained from the numerical signal EIIP[i], which represents a sequence of electron ion potentials of an amino acid of the particular protein. The 's' is a time lag or a shift in the space domain (positions of amino acids). In the discrete form, the SPWVD can be calculated as follows:

$$W(n,m) = \frac{1}{2} N \sum_{k=-N+1}^{N+1} |h(k)|^2 \sum_{p=-M+1}^{M-1} g(p) z(n+p+k) z^*(n+p-k) e^{-\frac{2i\pi km}{M}}$$

where z is a complex signal generated from the numerical sequence EIIP[i] by using a Hilbert transform and z* is a complex conjugated from the signal and $h(k)$ and $g(p)$ represent independent frequency and time (space) smoothing, respectively. In this study, as the smoothing functions, we used the Gauss filters, which are defined as:

$$h(k) = e^{(-k^2/2\sigma)/(\sigma\sqrt{2\pi})} \quad \text{and} \quad g(p) = e^{(-p^2/2\sigma)/(\sigma\sqrt{2\pi})}$$

where σ is the standard deviation and k and p are the average values in the frequency and distance sets. These selected parameters of the filters should satisfy the following criteria:

- The length of the windows of space domain filter $g(p)$ has to be longer than the length of the functionally important part of a protein.
- Long windows (compared to the whole signal's length) can decrease time and frequency resolution and thus, suppress a non-stationary character of the signal.

We found that a standard deviation of 20 for time (space) and 10 for frequency would satisfy both criteria. The resulting SPWVD could be shown in a t–f plane as a contour plot according to the values of S(t, f) (Figures 1b, 2b), which represents the distribution of the signal energy in the space domain. By choosing the standard deviation of the Gaussian functions h and g, we are practically adjusting between the resolution in frequency and space domain interferences.

2.3. Hierarchical Classification Methodology

To classify feature vectors, representing different ataxin proteins, we employed a proximity matrix which uses the Euclidian distances between ataxin proteins as follows [35]:

$$\|a-b\| = \sqrt{\sum_{17} (a_i - b_i)^2}$$

where a is the feature vector corresponding to the ataxin protein A, b is the feature vector corresponding to the protein B, and a_i and b_i are the ith components of the vectors a and b. On the basis of the computed feature vectors it is possible then to generate a cluster using a hierarchical clustering with complete linkage.

RESULTS AND DISCUSSION

It was reported that excessive repeats of particular amino acids in the primary structures of ataxin proteins lead to ataxia disorder development [1-6]. In this study, we applied the RRM to structure-function analysis of ataxin proteins aiming to understand the changes in their functionality caused by polyglutamine repeats and thus, understand the reasons for ataxia disorder developments.

The computational analysis of twenty seven ataxin proteins (animal sequences, all of different origins) was carried out. The primary structures of the ataxins were collected from the NCBI Entrez Protein Database. A multiple cross-spectral analysis was performed for all the selected ataxin proteins as well as for their subgroups (ATA-1, ATA-2, ATA-3, ATA-7 and ATA-10) using the EIIP values (Figures 1a, 2a, 3).

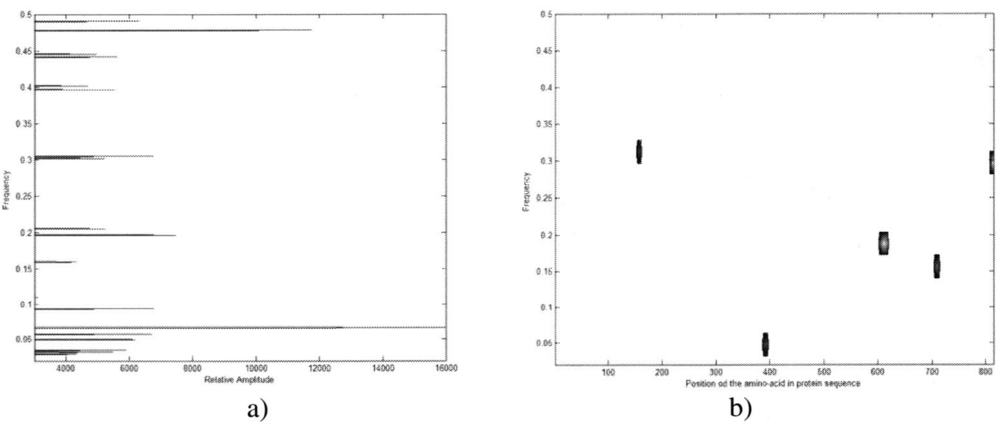

a)   b)

Figure 1. a) Multiple cross-spectral function of ataxin-1 proteins; b) SPWVD spectral density of Ataxin-1 human protein.

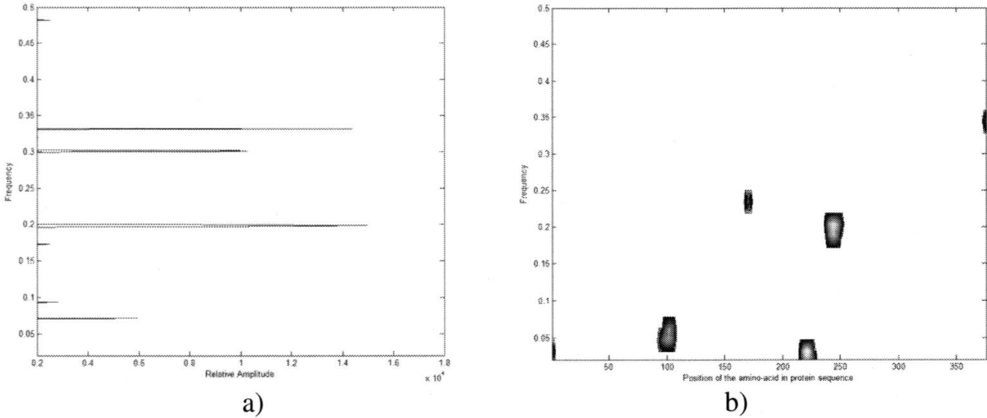

a)   b)

Figure 2. a) Multiple cross-spectral function of ataxin-3 proteins; b) SPWVD spectral density of Ataxin-3 human protein.

Table 1. RRM characteristic frequencies identified for Ataxin-1, Ataxin-3 subgroups and for the combined group of Ataxin proteins (ATA-1, ATA-, ATA-3, ATA-7 and ATA-10)

	ATA-1 s	ATA-3	Ataxin proteins
f_1	0.067	0.070	0.069
f_2	0.197	0.197	0.197
f_3	0.305	0.331	0.331

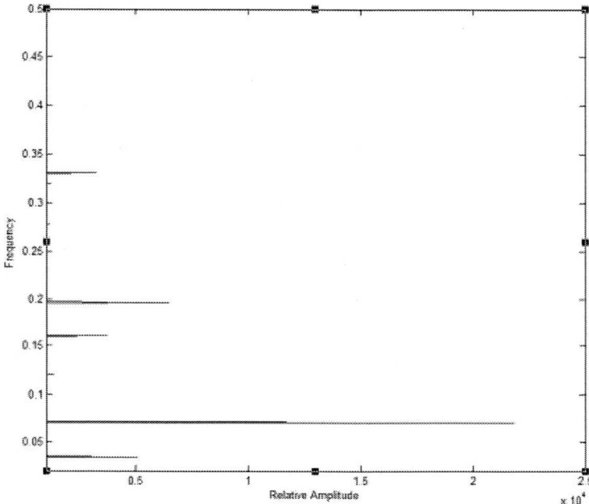

Figure 3. Multiple cross-spectral function of twenty seven ataxin proteins (ATA1, ATA2, ATA3, ATA7 and ATA10).

Characteristic frequencies of twenty seven ataxin proteins and their subgroups were obtained and are shown in Table 1. The characteristic frequencies having the highest power density in the spectrum of twenty seven ataxin proteins were identified at f_1 = 0.069, f_2 = 0.197 and f_3 = 0.331 (Table 1). According to the RRM criteria, peak frequencies are different for different biological functions.

These three peaks determined by the multiple cross-spectral function which correspond to different biological activities, are the characteristic features of ataxin subgroups, included in the whole functional group of twenty seven ataxin proteins. It is of interest to note that these peaks (f_1 = 0.069, f_2 = 0.197 and f_3 = 0.331) identified as the characteristics frequencies of ataxin-1 and ataxin-3 subgroups can be observed in Figures 1a, 2a and 3, respectively, but these frequencies have different values of spectral density. For analysis of the selected protein sequences, e.g. ataxin-1 human and ataxin-3 human, we used the SPWVD in frequency–space/time domain. By applying this procedure for the structure–function analysis of a single protein, we can determine the positions of amino acids along the protein sequence with the highest time density distribution power S(t, f) (Figures 1b, 2b). This can be achieved by using the contour plot in a frequency - space plane that can show an area within the protein sequence which has the most significant effect on a particular frequency component (shown as the brightest region in Figures 1b and 2b).

Table 2. Experimentally defined domains and binding/active sites of Ataxin-1 and Ataxin-3 human protein sequences

Ataxin 1 human		Ataxin 3 human	
Amino acid position	Domain or active/binding site description	Amino acid position	Domain or active/binding site description
562-693	Active site	1-180	Josephin domain
494-604	Self association	224-243	Catalytic activity
538-815	Interaction with USP7	244-263	--‖--
540-766	RNA binding	342-360	--‖--

Our computational predications have been compared with experimental findings. The analysis of ataxin-1 human (Table 2; Figure 1b) showed that for the frequency $f_2 = 0.197$ the predicted location of the active site is at 610–630 amino acids. An analysis of ataxin-3 human revealed that for the same frequency $f_2 = 0.197$, the determined regions of catalytic activity are at 230–260 and the Josephin domain is at 90–110 amino acids. These computational predictions are in accordance with the experimental findings (Table 2).

In the case of ataxia disorders, mutations in the genes can also increase the toxic effects of the proteins they produce [1, 2]. Although the analysed ataxin proteins are discernable by the diversity of their functions and no homologous sequences were selected for analysis, the RRM approach was successfully applied for the determination of ataxin characteristic frequencies corresponding to their multifunctional activity. We have also determined the characteristic frequencies of different ataxin functional subgroups. As mentioned earlier on the basis of the determined RRM characteristic frequency for a particular biological function or interaction, it becomes possible to identify the individual "hot spot" amino acids or domains that contribute most to the characteristic frequency and thus, to the protein's biological function. We achieved this by analysing ataxin-1 human and ataxin-3 human sequences using the SPWV distribution, when the functionally important regions in these proteins were identified. Previously we used the RRM, based on Fourier Transformation, for structure–function analysis of different proteins. However, due to limitations of the classical non-localised spectral transformations, in this study we applied the SPWV distribution instead of the 1D FT. This new tool has been tested here with the ataxin proteins chosen as the example protein group. The results revealed that application of the SPWV distribution to studied proteins improved both the accuracy and efficiency of the RRM predictive capabilities for protein active/binding sites allocation. Thus, we conclude that by using SPWV distribution for computational analysis of ataxin proteins, we not only can predict the functionally important amino acids (as done in the standard RRM using the Inverse Fourier Transform), but also can define the active regions along the protein molecule. Another advantage of the SPWV is that we can also reduce the number of analysed proteins required for accurate predictions. In particular, we can calculate the RRM frequency by using a limited number of protein sequences (from one to three proteins sequences). In addition, it was also shown that our computational predictions correspond closely with experimentally identified locations of the active or binding sites for the selected protein examples.

Recent studies suggest that the polyglutamine string in the ataxin-1 protein induces binding to and reduces the level of the Gfi-1 protein that is essential for survival of Purkinje cells by amplifying ataxin-1's effects on Gfi-1. Previous research has shown that an excess of the normal ataxin-1 protein could cause the same kind of neuron degeneration as the mutated protein, indicating that another part of the ataxin-1 protein might be the primary cause of cell death in SCA1, such as the AXH domain region [10]. Ataxin-1's effects on Gfi-1 are seemingly one of the main causes of neurodegeneration in SCA1. These findings complement several other recent studies indicating that normal proteins can cause neurodegenerative disease if they are present in excessive amounts and that some gene mutations cause disease by enhancing the protein's normal activity [10, 36]. A similar disease mechanism, for example, has been found in Parkinson's disease, where an extra copy of the normal alpha-synuclein gene can cause a development of the disease [37].

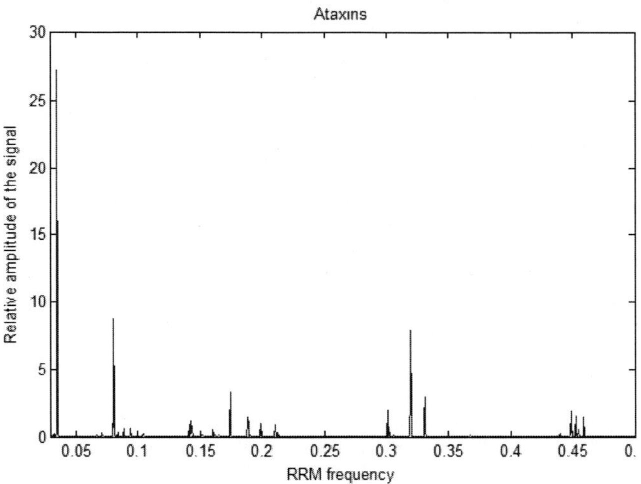

Figure 4. Multiple cross-spectral function of six ataxin-1 protein sequences.

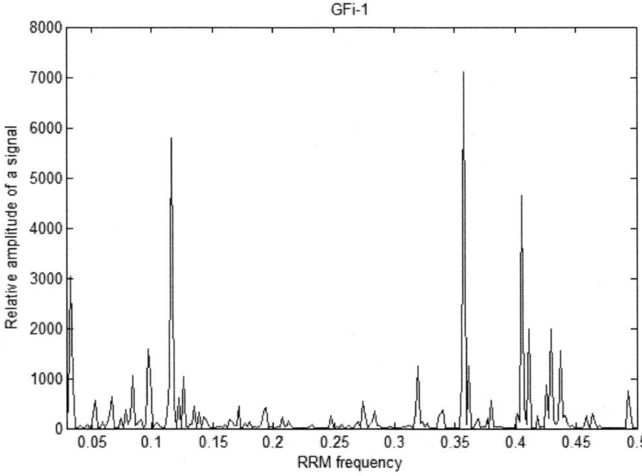

Figure 5. Multiple cross-spectral function of six GFi-1 protein sequences.

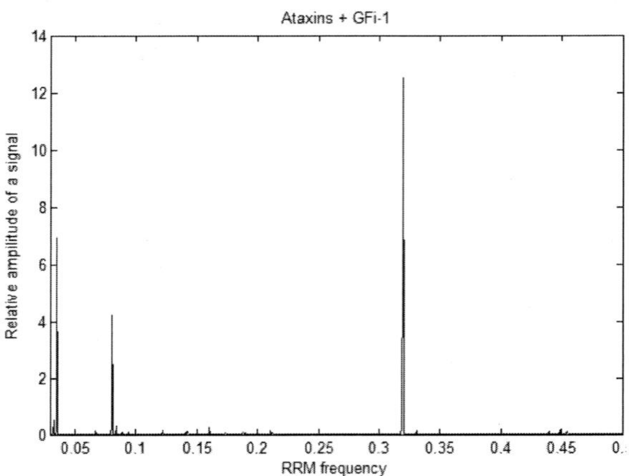

Figure 6. Multiple cross-spectral function of the ataxin and Gfi-1 protein sequences (12 sequences).

Also, an extra copy of the APP gene (due to an extra copy of chromosome 21) in patients with Down syndrome can trigger Alzheimer's disease [38]. Mutations in ataxin, alpha-synuclein and APP genes also increase the toxic effects of the proteins they produce [7].

These findings suggest that research that investigates normal functions of mutated proteins may help to give better understanding of the causes and progression of ataxia disorder [1-4]. In the case of hereditary ataxia, a potential target for new drug therapy is examination of proteins that can interact with ataxin-1 and thus, contribute to SCA1 development. Gfi-1 governs such diverse cell processes as self-renewal of hematopoietic stem cells, proliferation, apoptosis, differentiation, and cell fate specification. However, the molecular basis of its transcriptional functions has remained elusive [10]. Here we applied the RRM approach to investigate the structure-function relationship of six ataxin-1 and six Gfi-1 protein sequences (all from different origins). A multiple cross-spectral analysis was performed for each selected protein group as well as for their mutual combination using the EIIP values (Figure 4-Figure 6). Prominent characteristics frequencies for ataxin-1 were identified at $f_1 = 0.069$, $f_2 = 0.197$ and $f_3 = 0.331$ (Table 1). For the selected six ataxin-1 sequences the eaks were identified at $f_1=0.015$, $f_2=0.070$ and $f_3=0.3298$ (Figure 4).

From Figure 5 we can observe that these peaks present in the multiple cross-spectral function of six Gfi-1 proteins but with different values of spectral density. According to the RRM concept, this fact implies that the selected ataxin-1 and Gfi-1 proteins can recognise each other at the distance and interact on the basis of the common frequencies. Multiple cross-spectral analysis performed for the combined groups of twelve ataxin-1 and Gfi-1 proteins identified the characteristic frequencies to be at $f_1=0.015$, $f_2=0.070$ and $f_3=0.3298$ (shown in Figure 6). The analysis of the RRM cross-spectral functions for the group of twenty two selected ataxin proteins revealed the difference in primary structures amongst several sub-group of ataxins. To investigate further the ontogenic connections amongst different ataxins, firstly we encoded biological sequences of twenty two ataxins into the feature vectors. Secondly, we classified the vectors using a well- known hierarchical classifying methodology [35]. However, the appropriate design of the suitable feature vector for the selected proteins is not an easy task. In this study we employed a novel encoding method based on our earlier experience with the RRM approach, where the EIIP is used as an amino acid physico-chemical parameter. The newly developed classification methodology consists of several steps:

(1) Translation of protein primary sequences into numerical sequences by assigning the EIIP values to each amino acid in a given protein sequence.
(2) Use of binary "coif" wavelet as a filter applied to the numerical sequence of the EIIP in order to calculate spectral energies corresponding to different bands in a frequency domain.
(3) Calculate Square Energy Operator (SEO) which represents the rate of change of the spectral energy in a particular frequency band.
(4) On the basis of calculated SEO parameters it becomes possible to construct a specific feature vector, which can represent a particular protein sequence.
(5) By using the constructed specific feature vectors, we can classify the selected group of ataxin proteins using the Hierarchical classification method.

In summary, the proposed approach enables us to reveal hidden information about the relationship between structural motifs within ataxin primary sequence and their corresponding functional behaviour. The ataxin protein sequences used for computational analysis are given below:

>1 ATX1 human ataxin 1815 aa
>2 ATX1 mouse ataxin 1792 aa
>3 ATX1 rat ataxin 1789 aa
>4 ATX1 gibbon ataxin 156 aa
>5 ATX1 lemur catta ataxin 146 aa
>6 ATX1 tamarin ataxin 151 aa
>7 ATX1 macaca thibetana ataxin 153 aa
>8 ATX1 orangutan ataxin 166 aa
>9 ATX2 human ataxin 1312 aa
>10 ATX2 mouse ataxin 1285 aa
>11 ATX2 horse ataxin 46 aa
>12 ATX2 caenorhabditis elegans ataxin 959 aa
>13 ATX3 chicken ataxin 363 aa
>14 ATX3 human ataxin 376 aa
>15 ATX3 mouse ataxin 355 aa
>16 ATX3 rat ataxin 355 aa
>17 ATX3 xenopus tropicalis ataxin 356 aa
>18 ATX3 zebrafish ataxin 306 aa
>19 ATX7 human ataxin 892 aa
>20 ATX7 mouse ataxin 867 aa
>21 ATX10 human ataxin 475 aa
>22 ATX10 mouse ataxin 475 aa
>23 ATX10 rat ataxin 475 aa

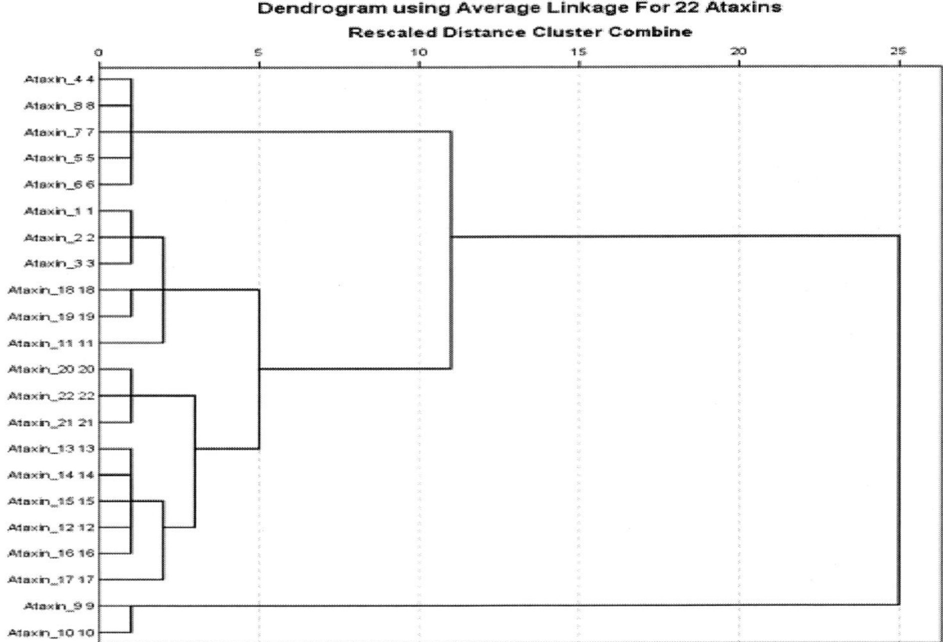

Figure 7. Dendogram using average linkage for the selected twenty two ataxin proteins.

The results of clustering of twenty two selected ataxin proteins are shown in Figure 7. By applying cluster analysis and proposing to group the ataxin proteins into 3 major clusters, we obtained a high similarity, in terms of the feature vector space, between the following proteins: (i) ataxin 4, 5, 6, 7, and 8 (these ataxin proteins are from monkey origin and short in length; (ii) ataxin 1, 2, 3, and11 (these ataxin proteins are from human origin); (iii) ataxin 12, 13, 14, 15,16, 17, 18, and 19 (all ATA3 proteins); and (iv) a very distant group which consist of ataxins 9, 10 (human and mouse ATA2). The findings obtained clearly show that the employed classification methodology, based on spectral energy bands distribution along proteins and EIIP parameter, is an efficient tool for distinguishing between functionally different ataxin proteins corresponding to different types of ataxia disorder.

CONCLUSION

Although the analysed ataxin proteins are discernable by the diversity of their functions and no homologous sequences were selected for analysis, the RRM approach was successfully applied for the determination of ataxin characteristic frequencies corresponding to their multifunctional activity. We have also determined the characteristic frequencies of different ataxin functional sub-groups. Once the RRM characteristic frequency for a particular biological function or interaction has been determined, it is possible to identify the individual amino acids, the so-called "hot spots", or domains that most contribute to the characteristic frequency and thus to the protein's biological function. We achieved this by analysing Ataxin-1 human and ataxin-3 human sequences using the SPWV distribution.

It was shown previously that the RRM approach, based on Fast Fourier Transform (FFT), can be successfully applied to structure-function analysis of different proteins. However, due to limitations of the classical non-localised spectral transformations, in this study we applied the SPWV distribution instead of the one-dimensional FFT. This new tool has been tested for structure-function analysis of the selected ataxin proteins and their different functional subgroups. The results revealed that application of the SPWV distribution to studied proteins improved both the accuracy and efficiency of the RRM predictive capabilities for protein active/binding sites allocation. Thus, we conclude that by using SPWV distribution for computational analysis of ataxin proteins, we can not only predict the functionally important amino acids (as done in the standard RRM using the Inverse Fast Fourier Transform (IFFT), but also define the active regions along the protein molecule. Another advantage of the SPWV is that we can also reduce the number of analysed proteins required for accurate predictions. In particular, we can calculate the RRM frequency by using a limited number of protein sequences (from one to three proteins sequences). In addition, it was also shown that our computational predictions correspond closely with the experimentally identified locations of the active/binding sites for the selected protein examples.

We have determined the characteristic frequencies of different functional sub-groups of ataxin proteins (ATA1, ATA3) as well as the characteristic frequency of the entire functional protein group. The dominant characteristic frequency was identified at f=0.069 that corresponds to the common bioactivity of ataxin proteins, the ability to affect nerve cell functions leading to the development of ataxia disorders. In addition, the possible interactions between ataxin-1 and Gfi-1 proteins have been studied. The common frequencies of ataxin-1 and Gfi-1 proteins were identified implying that ataxin-1 can be involved in interactive biological process with Gfi-1. These computational findings are in accordance with experimental findings published by other researchers. This chapter has also presented and discussed a newly developed protein classification methodology. The results obtained revealed that it is suitable for classification of the selected proteins based on their distinct functional performance. The classification presents a valuable tool for researchers aiming at distinguishing between proteins with defined primary structures but unknown functions.

REFERENCES

[1] Lunkes A, Mandel J.L (1997) Polyglutamines, nuclear inclusions and neurodegeneration. *Nat. Med.* 3:1201-1202.

[2] Lin X, Antalffy B, Kang D, Orr HT, Zoghbi, HY (2000) Polyglutamine expansion downregulates specific neuronal genes before pathologic changes in SCA1. *Nature Neurosci.* 3, 157-163.

[3] Bird T D (2005) MD Hereditary Ataxia Overview. GeneReviews.

[4] Schols L., Bauer P, Schmidt T et al (2004) Autosomal dominant cerebellar ataxias: clinical features, genetics, and pathogenesis. *Lancet Neurol.* 3:291-304.

[5] Giunti P, Sabbadini G, Sweeney MG et al. (2003) Expansion of the poly Q repeat in ataxin-2 alters its Golgi localization, disrupts the Golgi complex and causes cell death. *Human Molecular Genetics*, 12(13):1485-1496.

[6]   Huynh DP, Yang H T, Vakharia H (2003) Expansion of the polyQ repeat in ataxin-2 alters its Golgi localization, disrupts the Golgi complex and causes cell death. *Hum. Mol. Genet.* 12:1485–1496.

[7]   Piedras-Rentería ES, Watase K, Harata N et al (2001) Increased Expression of α1A Ca2+ Channel Currents Arising from Expanded Trinucleotide Repeats in Spinocerebellar Ataxia Type 6. *The Journal of Neuroscience* 21(23):9185–9193.

[8]   Davidson JD, Riley B, Burright EN et al (2000) Identification and characterization of an ataxin-1-interacting protein: A1Up, an ubiquitin like nuclear protein. *Human Molecular Genetics* 9(15): 2305-2312.

[9]   Irwin S, Vandelft M, Pinchev D et al (2005) RNA association and nucleocytoplasmic shuttling by ataxin-1. *Journal of Cell Science* 118:233-242.

[10]   Tsuda H, Jafar-Nejad H, Patel AJ et al (2005). The AXH domain of Ataxin-1 mediates neurodegeneration through its interaction with Gfi-1/Senseless proteins. *Cell* 122 (4): 633–44.

[11]   Cummings CJ, Mancini MA, Antalffy B et al (1998) Chaperone suppression of aggregation and altered subcellular proteasome localization imply protein misfolding in SCA1. *Nature Genet.* 19:148–154.

[12]   Tsai C.-C, Kao H Y, Mitzutani A et al (2004) Ataxin 1, a SCA1 neurodegenerative disorder protein, is functionally linked to the silencing mediator of retinoid and thyroid hormone receptors. *PNAS* 101(12):4047-4052.

[13]   Kaytor MD, Byam CE, Tousey SK et al (2005) A cell-based screen for modulators of ataxin-1 phosphorylation. *Human Molecular Genetics* 14(8):1095-1105.

[14]   Shibata H, Huynh DP, Pulst, S M (2000) A novel protein with RNA-binding motifs interacts with ataxin-2. Hum. Mol. Genet. 9:1303-1313

[15]   Li F, Macfarlan T, Pittman RN et al (2002) Ataxin-3 Is a Histone binding Protein with Two Independent Transcriptional Corepressor Activities. *Biol. Chem.* 277(47):45004-45012.

[16]   Burnett B, Li F, Pittman RN (2003) The polyglutamine neurodegenerative protein ataxin-3 binds polyubiquitylated proteins and has ubiquitin protease activity. *Hum. Mol. Genet.* 12(23):3195-3205.

[17]   Mao Y, Senic-Matuglia F, Di Fiore PP et al (2005) Deubiquitinating function of ataxin-3: Insights from the solution structure of the Josephin domain. *PNAS*, 36:12700-12705.

[18]   Chai Y, Koppenhafer S L, Shoesmith S J et al (1999) Evidence for proteasome involvement in polyglutamine disease: localization to nuclear inclusions in SCA3/MJD and suppression of polyglutamine aggregation in vitro. *Hum. Mol. Genet.* 8:673-682.

[19]   Helmlinger D, Hardy S., Sasorith S et al (2004) Ataxin-7 is a subunit of GCN5 histone acetyltran-sferase-containing complexes. *Hum. Mol. Genet.* 3(12):1257-1265.

[20]   Koyano S, Iwabuchi K, Yagishita et al (2002) Paradoxical absence of nuclear inclusion in cerebellar Purkinje cells of hereditary ataxias linked to CAG expansion. *J. Neurol. Neurosurg. Psychiatry.* 73:450-452.

[21]   Cosic I (1994) Macromolecular Bioactivity: Is it Resonant Interaction between Macromolecules? - Theory and Applications, IEEE Trans. on *Biomedical Engineering* 41:1101-1114.

[22]   Cosic I (1995) Virtual Spectroscopy for Fun and Profit. *Biotechnology* 13:236-238.

[23] Boashash B (2005) *Time-Frequency Signal Analysis and Processing Prentice Hall PTR.*

[24] Lalovic D, Davidovic DM, Bijedic N (2003) Quantum mechanics in terms of non negative smoothed Wigner functions, Phys. Rev. A 46:1206–1212.

[25] Cosic I (1997) *The resonant recognition model of macromolecular activity*, Birkhauser, Basel.

[26] Cosic I, Drummond AE, Underwood JR et al (1994) A New Approach to Growth Factor Analogue Design: Modelling of FGF Analogues, *Molecular and Cellular Biochemistry* 130:1-9.

[27] Ciblis P, Cosic I (1997) The Possibility of Soliton/Exciton Transfer in Proteins, *Journal of Theoretical Biology* 184:331-338.

[28] De Trad CH, Fang Q, Cosic I (2000) The Resonant Recognition Model (RRM) Predicts Amino Acid Residues in Highly Conservative Regions of the Hormone Prolactin (PRL). *Biophysical Chemistry* 84(2):149-157.

[29] Cosic I (2001) The Resonant Recognition Model of Bio-molecular Interactions: possibility of electromagnetic resonance. *Polish Journal of Medical Physics and Engineering* 7(1):73-87.

[30] De Trad CH, Fang Q, Cosic I (2002) Protein sequences comparison based on the wavelet transform approach. *Protein Engineering* 15(3):193-203.

[31] Pirogova E, Fang Q, Akay M et al (2002) Investigation of the structure and function relationships of Oncogene proteins. *Proceeding of the IEEE* 90(12):1859-1867.

[32] Pirogova E, Simon GP, Cosic I (2003) Investigation of the applicability of Dielectric Relaxation properties of amino acid solutions within the Resonant Recognition Model, *IEEE Transactions on Nanobioscience* 2(2):63-69.

[33] Veljkovic V, Slavic M (1972) General Model of Pseudopotentials, *Physical Review Let.* 29, 105.

[34] Wigner E P (1932) *On the Quantum Correction for Thermodynamic Equilibrium Phys. Rev.* 40: 749.

[35] Hastie T., Tibshirani R., Friedman J. The Elements of Statistical Learning: Data Mining, Inference, and Prediction. Springer, New York, 2001. xvi + 533 pp. ISBN 0-387-95284-5.

[36] Gatchel J R, Zoghbi HY (2005) Diseases of unstable repeat expansion: mechanisms and common principles. *Nat. Rev. Genet.*. 6(10):743-755.

[37] Klegeris A, Giasson, B I, Zhang H et al (2006). Alpha-synuclein and its disease-causing mutants induce ICAM-1 and IL-6 in human astrocytes and astrocytoma cells. *FASEB J.* 20(12):2000-2008.

[38] Theuns J, Brouwers N, Engelborghs S, Sleegers K, Bogaerts V, Corsmit E, de Pooter T, van Duijn CM, de Deyn PP, van Broeckhoven C (2006) Promoter mutations that increase amyloid precursor-protein expression are associated with Alzheimer disease. *Am. J. Hum. Genet.* 78(6): 936-946.

In: Ataxia: Causes, Symptoms and Treatment
Editor: Sung Hoi Hong

ISBN: 978-1-61942-867-6
© 2012 Nova Science Publishers, Inc.

Chapter 10

THE *PCD* HAMSTER: A NEW MODEL OF SPINOCEREBELLAR ATAXIA WITH POTENTIAL APPLICATION FOR DRUG EVALUATION

Kenji Akita and Hitomi Ohta
Biomedical Institute, Research Center,
Hayashibara Biochemical Laboratories, Inc.
Okayama, Japan

ABSTRACT

The hamster Purkinje Cell Degeneration (*hm*PCD) is a line of spontaneous ataxic mutation in the Syrian hamster. *Nna1* gene expression in the *hm*PCD brain is suppressed similar to that in the authentic *pcd* mutant mice. The influence of the causal allele in the *hm*PCD is considerably milder than the previously described alleles of the *pcd* mouse strains. The homozygous mutants of *hm*PCD develop a progressive but moderate ataxia that becomes apparent within the first two months of life. The major pathology in the mutant hamster is substantial corticocerebellar atrophy, which is attributable to primary loss of Purkinje neurons. The characteristic discordant movement can be quantitatively assessed by several behavioral tests; thus, the *hm*PCD would be applicable to study the effectiveness of pharmacological agents for ataxia. Recently, we demonstrated that daily administrations of NK-4, a neurotrophic cyanine dye compound, considerably delayed the onset of ataxia in the *hm*PCD. The behavioral outcomes were well supported by the histological findings of the cerebellum. NK-4 significantly suppressed degenerative loss of Purkinje neurons, which resulted in reduced cerebellar atrophy. Our results suggest that the *hm*PCD is a unique animal model for validating the efficacy of drugs targeting spinocerebellar ataxia and identify NK-4 as a promising candidate.

INTRODUCTION

Cerebellar ataxias are characterized by loss of balance and motor coordination due to dysfunction of the cerebellum and its afferent and efferent connections. Although no effective treatment is currently available for most ataxic syndromes or related neurodegenerative disorders [1], increased understanding of the pathogenic mechanisms of ataxias may lead to the discovery of novel therapeutic drugs in the near future.

Animal models allow one to identify pathways that affect disease onset and progression, to test and screen for pharmacological agents that affect pathogenic processes, and to validate potential targets using genetic and pharmacological approaches [2]. Of several mutant strains of ataxic mice that have been identified to date, only some of them are genetically and pathologically well characterized [3]. Of these, the Purkinje cell degeneration (*pcd*) mutant mouse [4, reviewed in 5] has been used to demonstrate the therapeutic potential of cerebellar cell-grafting [6-8] and insulin-like growth factor-1 (IGF-1) treatment [9,10] in the restoration of behavioral function. A recent, open label clinical trial of subcutaneous IGF-1 injection for the treatment of spinocerebellar ataxia (SCA) 3 and SCA7 suggested significant improvement of ataxic rating scores in patients with SCA3, and the stabilization of disease progression in both SCA3 and SCA7 [11].

In this chapter, a new line of ataxic mutant in the Syrian hamster (*Mesocricetus auratus*) is introduced that is characterized by substantial corticocerebellar atrophy with progressive loss of the cerebellar Purkinje cell population. Importantly, expression of *Nna1* (**n**ervous system **n**uclear protein induced by **a**xotomy **1**), the causative gene of the *pcd* phenotypes reported in mice [12,13], was dramatically reduced in the brain of mutant hamsters [14,15]. We, therefore, referred to the ataxic mutant line as *hm*PCD (hamster PCD) and describe its general properties and potential utility.

ATAXIC MUTANT HAMSTERS (HMPCD)*

Pcd Mutation on Mice

Mullen *et al.* reported that ataxia associated with the spontaneous *pcd* mutation in mice is an autosomal recessive trait [4]. Homozygotes of the original *pcd*[1J] mice (hereafter, *pcd* mice unless otherwise specified**) have a normal appearance but are smaller in size than their unaffected littermates [4]. These animals exhibit an abrupt and almost complete loss of cerebellar Purkinje cells and a progressive degeneration of granule cells, probably as a secondary consequence of Purkinje cell degeneration [16]. The cerebellum of mutant mice is essentially normal until the second postnatal week, after which most Purkinje cells rapidly degenerate. In parallel with the abrupt loss of Purkinje cells, locomotive discordance becomes obvious during the third to fourth postnatal week (Figure 1B).

In addition to the distinct degeneration of the cerebellar Purkinje and granule cells, the *pcd* mice also display progressive, partial degeneration profiles in other brain regions including thalamus [17], inferior olivary complex, deep cerebellar nuclei [18], retinal photoreceptor cells [4, 19] and mitral neurons in olfactory bulbs [4,20]. In non-neural systems, defective spermatogenesis is one of the major features of *pcd* mice. Male *pcd* mice are sterile due to the reduced number, reduced motility, and structural abnormalities of the sperm [4, 21]. The *Nna1* was originally identified as an inducible gene in a sciatic nerve transection paradigm [12]. *Nna1* is also known as ATP/GTP binding protein 1 (*Agtpbp-1*) [13] or cytosolic carboxypeptidase 1 (*CCP1*) [22]. In adult wild-type mice, a 4-kb *Nna1* transcript is expressed mainly in the brain, testis, and heart. In the *pcd* mice, expression of *Nna1* RNA was significantly reduced in the brain, which results in undetectable levels of Nna1 protein [5]. It is now accepted that the *pcd* phenotypes are the result of Nna1 protein loss-of-function because Purkinje cell-specific expression of a *Nna1* transgene successfully rescued the neuronal cell loss and ataxia in the *pcd*^{3J} mice [23].

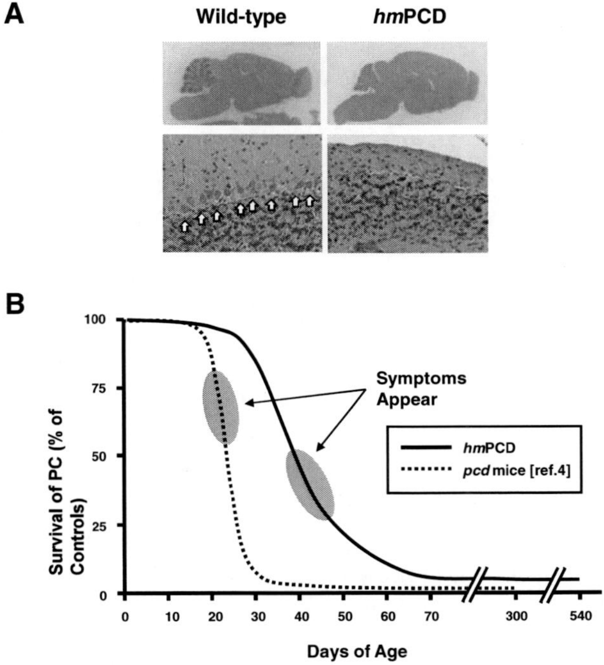

Figure 1. Cerebellar histological properties in hmPCDs. (A) Histological findings of the cerebella of a wild-type (left) and an ataxic mutant (hmPCD; right) in the Syrian hamster at 18 months of age. Arrows indicate Purkinje cells. Mid-sagittal sections (5 µm) were stained with hematoxylin and eosin. Bars indicate 600 µm for the upper panels and 30 µm for the lower panels, respectively. Adapted from Ohta H et al, PLoS ONE 6(2):e17137 [28]. (B) Illustrational comparison of Purkinje cell survival rates between the hmPCD (solid line) and the pcd mice (broken line). The curve of the pcd mice was adapted with permission from Mullen et al, Proc Natl Acad Sci USA 73:208-12 [4].

Although the molecular basis of Purkinje cell death in *pcd* has not been resolved, recent studies suggest that elevated autophagy responses including mitochondrial autophagy (also known as "mitophagy") are involved [24,25]. Because Nna1 protein functions as a peptidase [26] and is localized to mitochondria, the loss of function may lead to decreases in cellular levels of amino acids and altered bioenergetics, resulting in mitochondria dysfunction [25, 26].

General Properties of the hmPCD

In 2001, two male ataxic hamsters were found within a closed-colony for breeding. The mode of genetic transmission of the ataxic phenotype was autosomal recessive. By repeated mating of homozygous and/or heterozygous mutants, the mutant line *hm*PCD was established two years later. The body size of the *hm*PCD is about 20% smaller at ten weeks of age compared with the parental line but displays an otherwise normal appearance under conventional breeding conditions. Both homozygous males and females are fertile and live a normal lifespan of ~two years. The major clinical sign of the mutant hamster is a moderate ataxia of gait, including unsteady walking and stumbling as well as a slight trembling of the head. The hindlimb locomotor defects are marked compared with forelimbs while postural reflex movements are normal. Mutant males tend to develop ataxia a little earlier than females with symptoms becoming apparent around seven weeks of age and then progressing slowly. With increasing age, the gait becomes broad-based and frequently off-balanced with lateral deviations and uneven strides. Other than these ataxia-related symptoms, no behavioral abnormalities have been confirmed in the *hm*PCD. Although some spinocerebellar ataxias are often discussed in relation to neurochemical deficiencies [27], a detailed neurochemical analysis of the *hm*PCD has not been conducted.

Histology and Genetics

The histological abnormality of the *hm*PCD is limited to the cerebellum. There are no morphological malformations nor are gross abnormalities observed in the skeletal system, muscular system, reproductive organs or other splanchnic organs. The adult *hm*PCDs exhibited significant atrophy in the cerebellum compared with wild-type hamsters (Figure 1A). There was a remarkable reduction in the cerebellar cortical region, apparent as a reduction in the thickness of both molecular and granule cell layers while the area of the deep cerebellar nuclei was not changed significantly. The average cerebellar mass of the *hm*PCD at 10 weeks of age is reduced by ~25-30% compared with age- and sex-matched wild-type control hamsters. With the exception of the cerebellum, the central nervous system of both young and older *hm*PCDs appeared normal.

In the *hm*PCD, the Purkinje cell number decreases starting from the third postnatal week and continues over the next several weeks. The most critical period of neuronal degeneration is around five weeks of age. By the time that ataxic hamsters reached 18 months of age, more than 90% of the Purkinje cells had disappeared in all lobules of the cerebellum. In contrast to the considerable early degenerative loss of Purkinje neurons, a moderate reduction of cerebellar granule cells was also observed. The granule cell density of the *hm*PCDs was reduced by approximately 20% at 9 weeks of age. A mild degeneration of granule cells is likely to occur in *hm*PCDs probably due to the lack of support from Purkinje cells.

Molecular analysis revealed that expression of the *Nna1* gene was significantly reduced in the brain of *hm*PCDs. This strongly suggests that suppressed *Nna1* gene expression is implicated in the degenerative loss of Purkinje cells in *hm*PCDs, similar to the *pcd* mice. Determination of the genetic defect responsible for the ataxic phenotype requires more detailed examination; however, it is probable that the *pcd*-type mutation is at least involved in the pathogenesis of ataxia in the *hm*PCDs.

In wild-type adult male hamster, a 4-kb *Nna1* transcript was abundantly expressed in the testis and whole brain, with low levels detected in skeletal muscle, and negligible expression detected in the heart, liver, stomach, kidney, lung, small intestine, spleen, thymus, and adrenal gland. A testis specific 1-kb transcript that appears to be an alternatively spliced form of the *Nna1* gene was also detected, but the functional significance of this RNA was unclear.

Phenotypic Comparison to the *Pcd* Mice

The ataxic symptom in the *pcd* mice is moderate, beginning in the third to fourth postnatal week. In contrast, the *hm*PCD develops ataxia at the seventh postnatal week, much later than the *pcd* mice. Therefore, the timing of the onset of ataxia is substantially different. Figure 1B shows time courses of Purkinje neuronal loss in these two animal models, and it provides reasonable support for this notion. Purkinje cell death begins in *pcd* mice at 18 days of age, and by 29 days of age > 90% of the Purkinje cells have been lost [4]. In the *hm*PCD, however, there was no significant sign of Purkinje cell death at 18 days of age; approximately 80% of Purkinje cells were alive at 32 days of age; and more than 30% were still alive at 46 days of age. A recent study revealed that ~10% of Purkinje cells still survived in 18-month-old mutants [28]. Thus, degeneration of Purkinje cells progresses considerably slower in the *hm*PCDs compared with the *pcd* mice, which likely delays ataxia development in the *hm*PCD. Both mutant animals lose most Purkinje neurons in their early adulthood; however, late-onset degeneration profiles are dissimilar. The reduction of granule cell density in the *hm*PCDs seems moderate compared with that in the *pcd* mice, in which approximately 95% of granule cells degenerated by 20 months of age [29]. Other than reduction of granule cell density, the *pcd* mutant mice also exhibit late-onset degeneration of deep cerebellar nuclei, inferior olivary complex, thalamic neurons, retinal photoreceptor cells, and mitral neurons in olfactory bulb [4,16-21]. The degenerative profile in these regions of *hm*PCDs > 1 year old was still subtle. Testicular expression of *Nna1* should correlate with normal spermatogenesis, because *hm*PCDs with strong *Nna1* expression in the testis are fertile and an exceptional non-sterile strain of *pcd* mouse (*pcd*^{2J}) expresses stable amounts of testicular *Nna1* [12].

* The *hm*PCD has not been commercially supplied or deposited to any other research institutes.

**Twelve distinct *pcd* alleles have been reported according to the latest version (May 18, 2011) of a web catalogue released from The Jackson Laboratory (http://www.informatics.jax.org/searches/allele_report.cgi?_ Marker_key=79447).

APPLICATION TO DRUG EVALUATION

In this section, we describe our recent study, the first to demonstrate the use of the ataxic *hm*PCD to validate the efficacy of pharmacological agents [28].

A Neurotrophic Dye Compound NK-4

NK-4, a photosensitizing cyanine dye (Fig. 2) has been used as an active ingredient of over the counter (OTC) medicine in Japan for treating allergy, and for promoting wound healing since the 1950s [30]. Recently, we screened more than 250 cyanine dyes for their neurotrophin-like activity and found that NK-4 and some other related compounds exhibited remarkable neurotrophic potency [28, 31, 32].

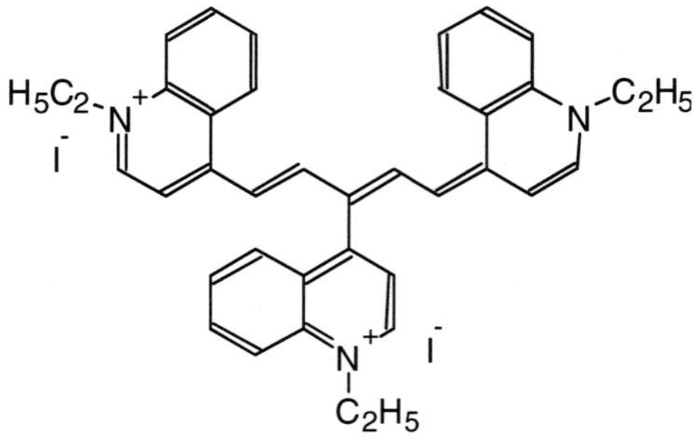

Figure 2. Chemical structure of NK-4. NK-4 is a divalent cationic pentamethine trinuclear cyanine dye that contains three quinolinium rings, N-alkyl side chains and two iodine anions. Formal nomenclature of NK-4 is as follows: 4,4'-[3-{2-(1-ethyl-4(1H)-quinolylidene)ethylidene}propenylene]bis(1-ethylquinolinium iodide).

NK-4 promoted cell growth and NGF-primed neurite-outgrowth in PC12 cells via activation of the PI3K-Akt signaling pathway at nanomolar concentrations. It also showed free radical scavenging, anti-amyloid β (Aβ) fibril formation and acetylcholinesterase inhibitory activities *in vitro*. In addition, NK-4 attenuated ischemia-induced brain injury in rats [31], ameliorated cognitive impairments in both an amyloid precursor protein (APP) transgenic mouse model and an intracerebroventricular Aβ injection-induced model of Alzheimer's disease [32].

Effect of NK-4 on Ataxia in the *hmPCD*

The *hm*PCDs were treated with 20 or 100 μg/kg of NK-4 (i.p.) once a day for seven weeks, starting from three weeks of age [28]. Motor coordination was assessed by the rota-rod test and inclined plane task. As shown in Figure 3, a low dose of NK-4 elicited a moderate, but significant effect in the attenuation of motor function deterioration. Animals given a high dose of NK-4 exhibited more remarkable effects. Although NK-4 could not reverse the symptom completely, the deterioration of rota-rod performance was considerably delayed. Judging from the time courses in the rota-rod test (Figure 3, upper panel), the delay period in disease progression was more than 4 weeks for the NK-4 high dosing group. Assuming that life spans of human and hamsters are 75 and 2 years, respectively, the month-long delay for hamsters would be equivalent to 3 years for human. Therefore, the effect of NK-4 in the delay of ataxia progression would be significant. Inclined plane task also revealed improved ability in the NK-4-treated animals to hold their posture on an inclined floor (Figure 3, lower panel). The tolerable inclinations stayed constant throughout the test period in saline-treated *hm*PCDs. On the other hand, wild-type hamsters and NK-4-treated *hm*PCDs showed gradual increases in their tolerable inclination during the test period. The degrees of tolerable inclination in NK-4-treated *hm*PCDs were significantly larger than those of saline-treated *hm*PCDs at 5 weeks of age or later.

The *hm*PCDs treated with NK-4 (both high and low doses) had significantly larger cerebellar volumes compared with those from saline-treated controls at 10 weeks of age (Figure 4A). The mitigative effect on the cerebellar atrophy suggests that NK-4 has neuroprotective activity in this model. Treatment with NK-4 significantly attenuated the loss of calbindin-positive Purkinje cells compared with saline-treated controls (Figure 4B).

The dendrites of Purkinje cells from NK-4-treated *hm*PCDs were significantly thicker and longer and displayed a higher density than those from saline-treated *hm*PCD controls. In addition, NK-4 treatment also prevented the reduction of granule cell density in the cerebellum of the *hm*PCD (Figure 4C) in a dose-dependent fashion.

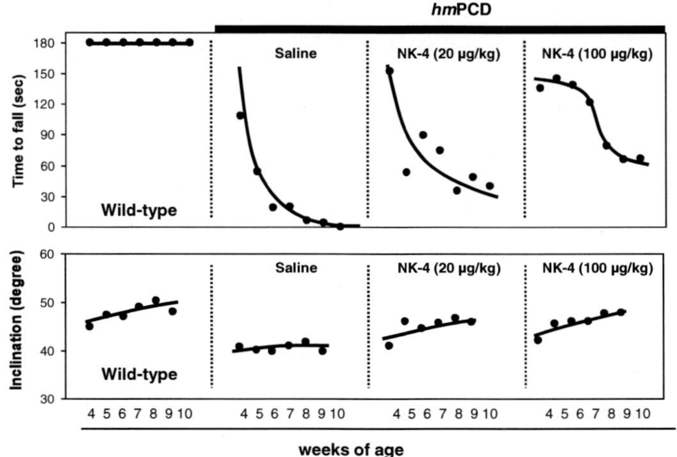

Figure 3. Ameliorative effects of NK-4 on motor discoordination in hmPCDs. Rota-rod performance (upper) and maximum inclinations on inclined plan task (lower) of hmPCDs were shown. In rota-rod test, each hamster was placed on a rotating rod (diameter; 60 mm) at a constant speed of 6 rpm, and the time spent on the rod was recorded with an upper cutoff limit of 180 sec. One session consisted of six consecutive trials, and the sixth record was used for evaluation. In inclined plane task, each hamster was placed on a flat board covered with rubber (300 × 300 mm). The board was gradually inclined until the animal was unable to maintain a head up position for 5 sec, and the maximum inclination from three consecutive trials was recorded. All the hamsters were pre-trained at 3 weeks of age prior to the trials in both tests (n = 5 or 6 in each group).

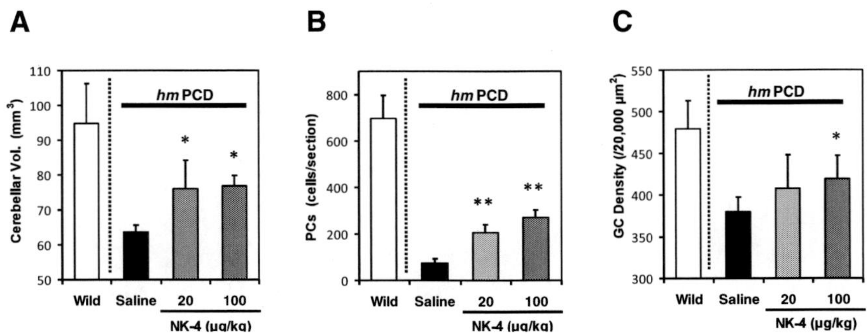

Figure 4. Neuroprotective effects of NK-4 in hmPCDs. Measurement of cerebellar volumes (A), Purkinje cell counts (B) and granule cell densities (C) in the hmPCDs at 10 weeks of age. Cerebellar volumes were calculated based on a following equation: $V = 0.5 \times (\text{minor axis})^2 \times (\text{major axis})$. Purkinje cells were counted in all lobules of the cerebellar mid-sagittal sections. The granule cell densities were calculated by counting the number of granule cells within the middle part of granule cell layer. Values are means ± SD (n = 5 or 6 in each group). * P < 0.05 and ** P < 0.01 vs. saline-treated hmPCD group. Adapted from Ohta H et al, PLoS ONE 6(2):e17137 [28].

These lines of evidence clearly indicate that NK-4 has a beneficial effect to maintain synaptic connections between Purkinje cells and other types of neurons in the cerebellum and/or medulla in *hm*PCDs.

CONCLUSION

To date, numerous laboratory animals with neurological mutations have been described. These animal models are characterized by selective neuronal loss and/or dysfunctions resulting from discrete, genetically induced lesions, and they have served as valuable experimental models for the analysis of the developmental, differentiational, and degenerative mechanisms relevant to neuronal systems.

The *hm*PCD is a new animal model for the study of ataxia and characterization of this mutant line suggests that it may be analogous to the *pcd* mutant mice. The advantage of the *hm*PCD over existing *pcd* mouse strains is the slower and milder degeneration of cerebellar Purkinje neurons, which recapitulates one of the key aspects of human disease. Thus, the *hm*PCD model could provide a more preferable *in vivo* system to validate pharmacological agents that ameliorate late-onset progressive cerebellar ataxia. Administration of the neurotrophic cyanine dye compound, NK-4 to the *hm*PCD significantly delayed the onset of ataxia and decreased levels of neurodegeneration and atrophy in the cerebellum.

Taken together, these observations suggest that the cyanine dye compound is a promising candidate for the treatment of ataxia and that the *hm*PCD line could be used to quantitatively assess the efficacy of existing therapeutic candidates or to screen for novel pharmacological agents. Further work is necessary to characterize the genetic, pathological, and biochemical properties of the *hm*PCD, and will lead to additional insights into the biology of chronic neurodegenerative disorders.

ACKNOWLEDGMENTS

The authors thank Dr. T. Ohta (Hayashibara Biochemical Laboratories Inc.) for critical reading of the manuscript. The authors also thank Dr. R. J. Mullen, Dr. E. M. Eicher and Dr. R. L. Sidman for their kind support.

REFERENCES

[1] Evidente VGH, Gwinn-Hardy KA, Caviness JN et al (2000) Hereditary ataxias. *Mayo Clin. Proc.* 75:475–90.

[2] Marsh JL, Lukacsovoch T, Thompson LM (2009) Animal model of polyglutamine disease and therapeutic approaches. *J. Biol. Chem.* 284:7431-5.

[3] Lalonde R, Strazielle C (2007) Spontaneous and induced mouse mutations with cerebellar dysfunctions: behavior and neurochemistry. *Brain Res.* 1140:51–74.

[4] Mullen RJ, Eicher EM, Sidman RL (1976) Purkinje cell degeneration, a new neurological mutation in the mouse. *Proc. Natl. Acad. Sci. USA* 73:208–12.

[5]   Wang T, Morgan JI (2007) The Purkinje cell degeneration (*pcd*) mouse: An unexpected molecular link between neuronal degeneration and regeneration. *Brain Res.* 1140:26–40.

[6]   Triarhou LC, Zhang W, Lee WH (1995) Graft-induced restoration of function in hereditary cerebellar ataxia. *Neuroreport* 6:1827-32.

[7]   Zhang W, Lee WH, Triarhou LC (1996) Grafted cerebellar cells in a mouse model of hereditary ataxia express IGF-I system genes and partially restore behavioral function. *Nat. Med.* 2:65-71.

[8]   Triarhou LC, Zhang W, Lee WH (1996) Amelioration of the behavioral phenotype in genetically ataxic mice through bilateral intracerebellar grafting of fetal Purkinje cells. *Cell Transplant.* 5:269-77.

[9]   Carrascosa C, Torres-Aleman I, Lopez-Lopez C et al (2004) Microspheres containing insulin-like growth factor I for treatment of chronic neurodegeneration. *Biomaterials* 25:707-14.

[10] Fernandez AM, Carro EM, Lopez-Lopez C, Torres-Aleman I (2005) Insulin-like growth factor I treatment for cerebellar ataxia: Addressing a common pathway in the pathological cascade? *Brain Res. Rev.* 50:134-141.

[11] Arpa J, Sanz-Gallego I, Medina-Báez, J et al (2011) Subcutaneous insulin-like growth factor-1 treatment in spinocerebellar ataxias: an open label clinical trial *Movement Disorder* 26:358-9.

[12] Fernandez-Gonzalez A, La Spada AR, Treadaway J et al (2002) Purkinje cell degeneration (*pcd*) phenotypes caused by mutations in the axotomy-induced gene, *Nna1. Science* 295:1904–6.

[13] Harris A, Morgan JI, Pecot M et al (2000) Regenerating motor neurons express *Nna1*, a novel ATP/GTP-binding protein related to zinc carboxypeptidase. *Mol. Cell Neurosci.* 16:578–96.

[14] Akita K, Arai S, Ohta T et al (2007) Suppressed *Nna1* gene expression in the brain of ataxic Syrian hamsters. *J. Neurogenet.* 21:19–29.

[15] Akita K, Arai S (2009) The ataxic Syrian hamster: An animal model homologous to the *pcd* mutant mouse? *Cerebellum* 8:202–10.

[16] Triarhou LC, Norton J, Alyea CJ et al (1985) A quantitative study of the granule cells in Purkinje cell degeneration (*pcd*) mutant. *Ann Neurol* 18:146.

[17] O'Gorman S, Sidman RL (1985) Degeneration of thalamic neurons in "Purkinje cell degeneration" mutant mice. I. Distribution of neuron loss. *J. Comp. Neurol.* 234:277–97.

[18] Ghetti B, Norton J, Triarhou LC (1987) Nerve cell atrophy and loss in the inferior olivary complex of "Purkinje cell degeneration" mutant mice. *J. Comp. Neurol.* 260:409–22.

[19] La Vail MM, Blanks JC, Mullen RJ (1982) Retinal degeneration in the *pcd* cerebellar mutant mouse. I. Light microscopic and autoradiographic analysis. *J. Comp. Neurol.* 212:217–30.

[20] Greer CA, Shepherd GM (1982). Mitral cell degeneration and sensory function in the neurological mutant mouse Purkinje cell degeneration (*PCD*). *Brain Res.* 235:156–61.

[21] Handel MA, Dawson M (1981) Effects on spermiogenesis in the mouse of a male sterile neurological mutation, Purkinje cell degeneration. *Gamete Res.* 4:185–92.

[22] Kalinina E, Biswas R, Berezniuk I et al (2007) A novel subfamily of mouse cytosolic carboxypeptidases. *FASEB J.* 21:836-50.

[23] Wang T, Parris J, Li L et al (2006) The carboxypeptidase-like substrate-binding site in *Nna1* is essential for the rescue of the Purkinje cell degeneration (*pcd*) phenotype. *Mol. Cell Neurosci.* 33:200–13.

[24] Rodriguez de la Vega M, Sevilla RG, Hermoso A (2007) Nna1-like proteins are active metallocarboxypeptidases of a new and diverse M14 subfamily. *FASEB J.* 20:851–65.

[25] Chakrabarti L, Zahra R, Jackson SM et al (2010) Mitochondrial dysfunction in NnaD mutant flies and Purkinje cell degeneration mice reveals a role for Nna proteins in neural bioenergetics. *Neuron* 66:835-47.

[26] Berezniuk I, Sironi J, Callaway MB et al (2010) CCP1/Nna1 functions in protein turnover in mouse brain: Implication for cell death in Purkinje cell degeneration mice. *FASEB J.* 24:1813–23.

[27] Botez MI, Botez-Marquard T, Mayer P et al (1998) The treatment of spinocerebellar ataxias: facts and hypotheses. *Med. Hypotheses* 51:381-4.

[28] Ohta H, Arai S, Akita K et al (2011) Neurotrophic effects of a cyanine dye via the PI3K-Akt pathway: Attenuation of motor discoordination and neurodegeneration in an ataxic animal model. *PLoS ONE* 6:e17137.

[29] Triarhou LC (1998) Rate of neuronal fallout in a transsynaptic cerebellar model. *Brain Res. Bull.* 47:219–22.

[30] Suzue K (1969) Medical research for photosensitizing dyes. *Kankohshikiso* 71:22-42 (in Japanese).

[31] Koya-Miyata S, Ohta H, Akita K et al (2010) Cyanine dyes attenuate cerebral ischemia and reperfusion injury in rats. *Biol. Pharm. Bull.* 33:1872-7.

[32] Ohta H, Arai S, Akita K et al (2012) Effects of NK-4 in a transgenic mouse model of Alzheimer's disease. *PLoS ONE* DOI 10.1371/journal.pone.0030007 (in press).

In: Ataxia: Causes, Symptoms and Treatment
Editor: Sung Hoi Hong

ISBN: 978-1-61942-867-6
© 2012 Nova Science Publishers, Inc.

Chapter 11

STEM CELL REPLACEMENT THERAPY AS A POTENTIAL TREATMENT FOR SCA1 DISEASE

Sung Hoi Hong[1], and Seongman Kang[2]*
[1]Department of Biomedical Science, College of Health Science,
Korea University, Jeongneung-dong, Seongbuk-gu,
South Korea
[2]Graduate School of Biotechnology, Korea University, Anam-dong,
Seongbuk-gu, South Korea

ABSTRACT

Spinocerebellar ataxia type 1 (SCA1) is an autosomal dominant neurodegenerative disorder caused by expansion of CAG trinucleotide repeats in the ataxin-1 gene and is characterized by cerebellar ataxia and progressive motor deterioration. The ataxin-1 protein is involved in transcription and RNA processing. SCA1 pathogenesis appears to be related to a gain-of-function effect that is caused by toxic mutant ataxin-1-derived aggregates or cellular dysfunction through an abnormal interaction between mutated and normal proteins. Recent studies have clarified the molecular mechanisms of SCA1 pathogenesis, which provide direction for future treatments. Therapeutic hope has come from observations including the reduction of aggregates and alleviation of the pathogenic phenotype by the application of potent inhibitors and RNA interference. However, no treatment is currently available for SCA1 disease. In this chapter, we discuss the potential of stem cells as a therapeutic approach to SCA1.

Keywords: SCA1 disease, polyglutamine, aggregates, cell replacement therapy, stem cells

* Correspondence to: Sunghoi Hong Department of Biomedical Science, College of Health Science, Korea University, Jeongneung-dong, Seongbuk-gu, Seoul 136-703, South Korea, Tel: 82-2-940-2816, Fax: 82-2-917-2388, E-mail: shong21@korea.ac.kr

INTRODUCTION

Spinocerebellar ataxia type 1 (SCA1) is an inherited neurodegenerative disorder characterized by motor symptoms with some cognitive deficits [Burk et al., 2003; Orr, 2000; Zoghbi and Orr, 2000]. SCA1 disease is caused by the expansion of an unstable CAG trinucleotide repeat, which encodes the amino acid glutamine in the ataxin-1 protein [Banfi et al., 1994; Orr et al., 1993]. A typical feature of SCA1 pathogenesis is progressive degeneration of cerebellar Purkinje cells and brainstem neurons [Orr and Zoghbi, 2001; Zoghbi and Orr, 2000]. It has been established that the polyglutamine repeat plays a key role in the pathogenesis of polyglutamine diseases, although its effects are strongly modulated by the protein context within which it resides [Michalik and Van Broeckhoven, 2003].

The mutant ataxin-1-derived nuclear inclusion that was detected in Purkinje cells of an SCA1 transgenic model suggested that the aggregate formed by the expanded polyglutamine may be cytotoxic [Perutz, Johnson, Suzuki, and Finch, 1994; Thakur and Wetzel, 2002], although nuclear localization, modifications, and aberrant protein-protein interactions appear to be required to initiate SCA1 pathogenesis both *in vivo* and *in vitro* [Chen et al., 2003; Emamian et al., 2003; Hong, Kim, Ka, Choi, and Kang, 2002; Klement et al., 1998; Lee, Hong, Kim, and Kang, 2011; Lim et al., 2008; Matilla et al., 1997; Tsuda et al., 2005].

Nevertheless, no treatment is currently available for SCA1 disease, although pathological studies of SCA1 are ongoing. In this chapter, we summarize the current information on SCA1 disease and discuss the potential of cell replacement for SCA1 disease therapy.

Causes and Pathogenesis of SCA1 Disease

SCA1 is an inherited and incurable dominantly neurodegenerative disorder, characterized by progressive motor dysfunction and cognitive deficits [Burk et al., 2003; Orr, 2000; Zoghbi, 1995; Zoghbi and Orr, 2000]. Onset is typically in mid-life, and death usually occurs 10–30 years after symptom onset. At the pathological level, the most frequent and severe alterations observed in patients with SCA1 are the loss of Purkinje cells in the cerebellar cortex and the degeneration of neurons in the inferior olivary nuclei, cerebellar dentate nuclei, and red nuclei [Orr and Zoghbi, 2001; Zoghbi and Orr, 2000]. SCA1 is caused by an instability in a CAG trinucleotide-repeat tract [Orr and Zoghbi, 2007; Zoghbi and Orr, 2000, 2009]. The triplet repeat consists of a row of three nucleotide bases in the disease gene, which encode the ataxin-1 protein including the amino acid glutamine [Zoghbi and Orr, 2000].

The CAG triplet repeat varies 6–35 times in normal genes but is expanded well beyond normal length in mutant genes that encompass 40 to more than 100 triplets [Chung et al., 1993]. Interestingly, the longer the expansion, the more severe the disease, and the earlier the onset. This repeat is unstable and expands as it is passed from one generation to the next, particularly if the affected parent is male, explaining the phenomenon of anticipation [Zoghbi and Orr, 1995]. The expansion of triplet repeat tracts may be caused by errors in replication machinery [Kang, Jaworski, Ohshima, and Wells, 1995]. It has been established that the polyglutamine repeat by itself plays a key role in SCA1 pathogenesis, although its effects are strongly modulated by the protein context within which it resides [Michalik and Van Broeckhoven, 2003].

A pathological hallmark of SCA1 is the presence of small and large aggregates containing the mutant ataxin-1 protein [Skinner et al., 1997]. In the case of SCA1 transgenic mice and patients containing mutant ataxin-1 (82Q), the aggregates are positive for ubiquitin and the components of proteasome and the HDJ-2/HSDJ chaperone protein [Cummings et al., 1998] that are involved in quality control of protein surveillance machinery. Since the aggregates were first identified, they have been viewed as playing a key role in polyglutamine-mediated pathogenesis [Zoghbi and Orr, 2009]. However, the primary pathogenic role of the aggregates remains unclear.

Many ataxin-1- interacting proteins have been identified using various experimental tools to assess the biological and pathological functions of ataxin-1 in SCA1 disease, such as yeast two-hybrid systems.

In our previous study [Kang and Hong, 2009], many ataxin-1-interacting proteins that are regulated by the length of the polyglutamine tract were summarized, suggesting that the expanded polyglutamine could change the conformation of the ataxin-1 protein and trigger a series of aberrant interactions with cellular proteins. Among the known ataxin-1-interacting proteins, most are involved in the regulation of transcription [Cvetanovic et al., 2007; Goold et al., 2007; Lee, Hong, and Kang, 2008; Lee et al., 2011; Serra et al., 2006; Tsuda et al., 2005], RNA processing [Hong, Ka, Kim, Park, and Kang, 2003; Irwin et al., 2005; Lim et al., 2008; Okazawa et al., 2002], protein modifications [Al-Ramahi et al., 2006; Chen et al., 2003; Emamian et al., 2003; Hong, Lee, Cho, and Kang, 2008; Kang and Hong, 2010; Riley, Zoghbi, and Orr, 2005; Ueda et al., 2002], stabilization [Chen et al., 2003; Hong et al., 2002], and signal transduction [Gatchel et al., 2008; Goold et al., 2007; Serra et al., 2004].

However, the pathological mechanism of SCA1 disease that could be caused by the expanded polyglutamine tract in ataxin-1 proteins has not been studied clearly .

Potent Inhibitors of SCA1 Disease

Potential therapies for SCA1 have been intensively studied using animal models and cell culture systems. Increased levels of particular molecular chaperones such as heat shock protein 70 (HSP70) and HSP40 suppress both the aggregation and toxicity of mutant ataxin-1 in cell culture systems [Cummings et al., 1998] and in *Drosophila* and mouse models of Huntington's disease (HD) and SCA1 disease [Chan, Warrick, Gray-Board, Paulson, and Bonini, 2000; Fernandez-Funez et al., 2000; Muchowski et al., 2000]. Besides molecular chaperones, other polyglutamine mediated aggregation-suppressing agents, such as chemical chaperones [Yoshida, Yoshizawa, Shibasaki, Shoji, and Kanazawa, 2002], synthetic or recombinant peptides [Kazantsev et al., 2002; Ren, Nagai, Tucker, Strittmatter, and Burke, 2001; 2001; Vig et al., 2011], intracellular antibodies [Khoshnan, Ko, and Patterson, 2002; Lecerf et al., 2001], various disaccharides [Tanaka et al., 2004], and certain chemicals [Heiser et al., 2002; Sanchez, Mahlke, and Yuan, 2003] also attenuate polyglutamine toxicity. Alternatively, the histone deacetylase inhibitor suppresses polyglutamine toxicity in cells and in *Drosophila* models [McCampbell et al., 2001; Steffan et al., 2001].

Additionally, gene silencing of the mutant allele through RNA interference has proved to be a useful method to prevent target gene expression both *in vitro* (cell culture) and *in vivo* (brain) [Xia et al., 2004]. Introduction of recombinant adeno-associated viral vectors expressing short hairpin RNAs directed against the human mutant ataxin-1 gene improve the behavioral phenotype in SCA1 animal models [Xia et al., 2004]. However, in patients with SCA1, short hairpin RNAs would problematically target both the mutant and wild-type allele, although ataxin-1 knockout mice do not display the SCA1 phenotype.

An ideal treatment for polyglutamine diseases would be a combination of these and other therapeutic strategies. Compounds that inhibit the PI-3K/Akt pathway or small peptides that prevent 14-3-3/ataxin-1 interactions could play a role in SCA1 treatment [Paulson, 2003]. Furthermore, the androgen-blocking drug leuprorelin rescues the polyglutamine- dependent phenotype in a transgenic mouse model of spinal and bulbar muscular atrophy [Katsuno, Adachi, Inukai, and Sobue, 2003].

Lithium carbonate alleviates the severe motor dysfunction and cognitive impairment in $Sca1^{154Q/2Q}$ mice [Watase et al., 2007]. Lithium exerts its neuroprotective effects in neurological diseases such as Alzheimer's diseases (AD), HD, and bipolar disorder [Chuang et al., 2002; X. Li, Ketter, and Frye, 2002; Phiel, Wilson, Lee, and Klein, 2003]. The mechanism of action of lithium as a mood-stabilizer has not been clarified, but, in part, it inhibits glycogen synthase kinase 3 beta and inositol production [Carmichael, Sugars, Bao, and Rubinsztein, 2002; Pilcher, 2003].

To date, there is no effective treatment that can cure or substantially prolong the life span of individuals affected with SCA1 or other progressive neurological diseases.

Stem cell Treatment for SCA1 Disease

Stem cell treatment for patients with neurological diseases, such as AD, Parkinson's disease, HD, and spinal cord injury, is attracting increased attention for its potential to cure pathological symptoms by replacing lost neurons [Dunnett and Rosser, 2007; Lindvall and Kokaia, 2010; Mendez et al., 2008]. Restoration of functional neurons in the cerebellum of patients with SCA1 could be accomplished by replacing new cerebellar progenitors that are derived from stem cells. The transplanted progenitors would be recognized and integrated by the host central nervous system, and could differentiate into mature Purkinje cells and other cerebellar neurons, but the neuronal axons would have to extend to form neuronal junctions.

One possible therapeutic tool in the treatment of SCA1 is cell transplantation therapy using fetal neural stem cells (NSCs) isolated from fetal neuroectoderm as a primordial cerebellar tissue. These cells are self-renewing, multipotent cells that are usually committed to main nervous system phenotypes. Transplantation of fetal NSCs into various ataxia murine models has been extensively studied over the last few decades [Grimaldi, Carletti, and Rossi, 2005; Triarhou, 1996] and has focused on the developmental potential of fetal neural cells as well as the role of the specific regional brain environment to determine the fate of cerebellar progenitors. To re-establish the functional circuits of damaged Purkinje cells in the cerebellum, many different groups have transplanted wild-type mouse intracerebellar embryonic cells into mutant animals with degenerated Purkinje cells [Carletti, Grimaldi, Magrassi, and Rossi, 2002; Gardette, Alvarado-Mallart, Crepel, and Sotelo, 1988; Keep, Alvarado-Mallart, and Sotelo, 1992; Mullen, Eicher, and Sidman, 1976; Sotelo, Alvarado-Mallart, Gardette, and Crepel, 1990; Triarhou, 1996]. The transplanted cells were engrafted and migrated to the adult cerebellar cortex to produce the typical Purkinje cell phenotype but failed to reach deep host cerebellar nuclei [Armengol, Sotelo, Angaut, and Alvarado-Mallart, 1989; Carletti et al., 2002; Sotelo and Alvarado-Mallart, 1991]. Functional connections between the deep host cerebellar nuclei and grafted cells has been achieved by transplanting fetal cerebellar progenitors directly into deep nuclei [Keep et al., 1992; Triarhou, 1996; Triarhou, Low, and Ghetti, 1992], indicating that the fetal neural progenitors recover both motor and cognitive symptoms caused by Purkinje cell loss [Keep et al., 1992; Sotelo et al., 1990; Triarhou, Zhang, and Lee, 1995; Zhang, Lee, and Triarhou, 1996]. These studies, performed over decades, have accumulated important data regarding the cerebellar developmental events and implantation of grafted neural progenitors for the successful clinical application of neural transplantation.

Adult NSCs are usually restricted to two areas of the brain such as the subventricular zone lining the lateral ventricles and the subgranular zone in the dentate gyrus of the hippocampus and also have self-renewal and multipotency [Doetsch, Caille, Lim, Garcia-Verdugo, and Alvarez-Buylla, 1999]. Recently, transplantation of NPCs derived from the subventricular zone of adult mice into the cerebellar white matter of SCA1 transgenic animals has resulted in improved motor skills compared with those in sham-treated controls [Chintawar et al., 2009], indicating that transplanted adult NSCs could be useful for treating SCA1 disease. However, most adult and fetal NSCs have limited expansion ability and differentiation capacity.

Instead, embryonic stem cells (ESCs) are pluripotent and can be differentiated into any cell type in the body, including neurons, and could be unlimitedly proliferated *in vitro*. The ability of ESCs represents a promising source for basic developmental study and cell replacement therapy for neurodegenerative disorders [Erceg et al., 2010; Hedlund, Hefferan, Marsala, and Isacson, 2007; Hong et al., 2007; Hong, Kang, Isacson, and Kim, 2008; Keirstead et al., 2005], including SCA1 and other cerebellar ataxias. The successful use of ESCs for treating cerebellar disorders depends on efficient differentiation of ESCs into functional cerebellar progenitor cells and their delivery to specific cerebellar regions. Recent studies have reported that a combination method of inducing signals with fibroblast growth factor and WNT and the cytokines bone morphogenetic protein, sonic hedgehog, and brain-derived neurotrophic factor generates functional cells from mouse and human ESCs with cerebellar characteristics that express specific markers and engraft after cell transplantation [Erceg et al., 2010; Muguruma et al., 2010; Su et al., 2006].

As most cerebellar ataxias are related to Purkinje cell loss, further investigations should focus on developing new protocols for efficient differentiation of human ESCs to produce higher yields of Purkinje cells.

However, many factors that are involved in the full differentiation and survival of transplanted cerebellar progenitor cells in a host brain should be completely understood to clinically apply stem cell therapy in the future. But, ES cells have the serious disadvantage of allogeneicity, which requires immunosuppression during cell replacement therapy.

An alternative strategy is to create patient-specific pluripotent stem cells with ESC properties. Induced pluripotent stem cells (iPSCs) provide a new hope for creating personalized pluripotent cells that can differentiate into any cell in the human body [Takahashi et al., 2007]. After iPSCs were first successfully produced in 2006 from mouse fibroblasts [Takahashi and Yamanaka, 2006], Yamanaka's group revolutionized stem cell research by generating human iPSCs through the introduction of four transcription factors, such as Oct3/4, Sox2, Klf4, and c-Myc, into human fibroblasts. These cells are similar to hESCs in morphology, expression of stem cell genes and proteins, epigenetic modification, differentiation into three lineages, and teratoma formation in immune-deficient mice, but the full extent of their relationship to ESCs is still being assessed [Takahashi et al., 2007]. Although a number of groups have evaluated the neural differentiation potential and function of human iPSCs in animal models of neurodegenerative diseases [Hargus et al., 2010; Tsuji et al., 2010; Wernig et al., 2008], the neural precursors that were derived from iPSCs have not yet been applied to any cerebellar ataxia model, so the clinical application of iPSCs is a future endeavor. A serious problem in the clinical application of iPSCs is the use of retroviral vectors that include potent oncogenes, such as c-Myc and Klf4, in current reprogramming protocols, which may themselves cause cancer by integrating into the cellular genome. Various studies have offered an alternative of using nonintegrating genetic episomal vectors [Yu et al., 2009] and liposome-based transfection or direct delivery of reprogramming proteins [Kim et al., 2009; Okita, Ichisaka, and Yamanaka, 2007; Zhou et al., 2009] or small molecules [W. Li et al., 2009; Shi, Desponts et al., 2008; Shi, Do et al., 2008]. Additionally, feeder-free and xeno-free culture conditions must be established to differentiate iPSCs into neural subtypes. Therefore, a number of issues need to be addressed to apply iPSCs to cell replacement therapy for cerebellar disorders and other neurological disorders, such as the use of appropriate cell types and gene delivery systems for more efficient and safe reprogramming, establishing protocols for more efficient differentiation of iPSCs into specific neural subtypes, and improving safety requirements to exclude cancer risks after transplantation.

CONCLUSION

To establish a functional cerebellum in a patient affected by Purkinje cell loss, the transplanted neural progenitors derived from stem cells should be reconnected to the region-specific neurons in the host brain. Although which type of stem cells is most appropriate for regenerative therapy of cerebellar disorders has not been determined, accelerated research in the stem cell field provides hope that efficient cell replacement therapy for cerebellar ataxia diseases will become a reality in the future.

ACKNOWLEDGMENTS

This work was supported by grants from the National Research Foundation of Korea (NRF) (20100023160 and 20100020349) of the Korea government.

REFERENCES

Al-Ramahi, I., Lam, Y. C., Chen, H. K., de Gouyon, B., Zhang, M., Perez, A. M., et al. (2006). CHIP protects from the neurotoxicity of expanded and wild-type ataxin-1 and promotes their ubiquitination and degradation. *J. Biol. Chem., 281*(36), 26714-26724.

Armengol, J. A., Sotelo, C., Angaut, P., and Alvarado-Mallart, R. M. (1989). Organization of Host Afferents to Cerebellar Grafts Implanted into Kainate Lesioned Cerebellum in Adult Rats. *Eur. J. Neurosci., 1*(1), 75-93.

Banfi, S., Servadio, A., Chung, M. Y., Kwiatkowski, T. J., Jr., McCall, A. E., Duvick, L. A., et al. (1994). Identification and characterization of the gene causing type 1 spinocerebellar ataxia. *Nat. Genet., 7*(4), 513-520.

Burk, K., Globas, C., Bosch, S., Klockgether, T., Zuhlke, C., Daum, I., et al. (2003). Cognitive deficits in spinocerebellar ataxia type 1, 2, and 3. *J. Neurol., 250*(2), 207-211.

Carletti, B., Grimaldi, P., Magrassi, L., and Rossi, F. (2002). Specification of cerebellar progenitors after heterotopic-heterochronic transplantation to the embryonic CNS in vivo and in vitro. *J. Neurosci., 22*(16), 7132-7146.

Carmichael, J., Sugars, K. L., Bao, Y. P., and Rubinsztein, D. C. (2002). Glycogen synthase kinase-3beta inhibitors prevent cellular polyglutamine toxicity caused by the Huntington's disease mutation. *J. Biol. Chem., 277*(37), 33791-33798.

Chan, H. Y., Warrick, J. M., Gray-Board, G. L., Paulson, H. L., and Bonini, N. M. (2000). Mechanisms of chaperone suppression of polyglutamine disease: selectivity, synergy and modulation of protein solubility in Drosophila. *Hum. Mol. Genet., 9*(19), 2811-2820.

Chen, H. K., Fernandez-Funez, P., Acevedo, S. F., Lam, Y. C., Kaytor, M. D., Fernandez, M. H., et al. (2003). Interaction of Akt-phosphorylated ataxin-1 with 14-3-3 mediates neurodegeneration in spinocerebellar ataxia type 1. *Cell, 113*(4), 457-468.

Chintawar, S., Hourez, R., Ravella, A., Gall, D., Orduz, D., Rai, M., et al. (2009). Grafting neural precursor cells promotes functional recovery in an SCA1 mouse model. *J. Neurosci., 29*(42), 13126-13135.

Chuang, D. M., Chen, R. W., Chalecka-Franaszek, E., Ren, M., Hashimoto, R., Senatorov, V., et al. (2002). Neuroprotective effects of lithium in cultured cells and animal models of diseases. *Bipolar. Disord., 4*(2), 129-136.

Chung, M. Y., Ranum, L. P., Duvick, L. A., Servadio, A., Zoghbi, H. Y., and Orr, H. T. (1993). Evidence for a mechanism predisposing to intergenerational CAG repeat instability in spinocerebellar ataxia type I. *Nat. Genet., 5*(3), 254-258.

Cummings, C. J., Mancini, M. A., Antalffy, B., DeFranco, D. B., Orr, H. T., and Zoghbi, H. Y. (1998). Chaperone suppression of aggregation and altered subcellular proteasome localization imply protein misfolding in SCA1. *Nat. Genet., 19*(2), 148-154.

Cvetanovic, M., Rooney, R. J., Garcia, J. J., Toporovskaya, N., Zoghbi, H. Y., and Opal, P. (2007). The role of LANP and ataxin 1 in E4F-mediated transcriptional repression. *EMBO Rep., 8*(7), 671-677.

Doetsch, F., Caille, I., Lim, D. A., Garcia-Verdugo, J. M., and Alvarez-Buylla, A. (1999). Subventricular zone astrocytes are neural stem cells in the adult mammalian brain. *Cell, 97*(6), 703-716.

Dunnett, S. B., and Rosser, A. E. (2007). Stem cell transplantation for Huntington's disease. *Exp. Neurol., 203*(2), 279-292.

Emamian, E. S., Kaytor, M. D., Duvick, L. A., Zu, T., Tousey, S. K., Zoghbi, H. Y., et al. (2003). Serine 776 of ataxin-1 is critical for polyglutamine-induced disease in SCA1 transgenic mice. *Neuron, 38*(3), 375-387.

Erceg, S., Ronaghi, M., Zipancic, I., Lainez, S., Rosello, M. G., Xiong, C., et al. (2010). Efficient differentiation of human embryonic stem cells into functional cerebellar-like cells. *Stem. Cells Dev., 19*(11), 1745-1756.

Fernandez-Funez, P., Nino-Rosales, M. L., de Gouyon, B., She, W. C., Luchak, J. M., Martinez, P., et al. (2000). Identification of genes that modify ataxin-1-induced neurodegeneration. *Nature, 408*(6808), 101-106.

Gardette, R., Alvarado-Mallart, R. M., Crepel, F., and Sotelo, C. (1988). Electrophysiological demonstration of a synaptic integration of transplanted Purkinje cells into the cerebellum of the adult Purkinje cell degeneration mutant mouse. *Neuroscience, 24*(3), 777-789.

Gatchel, J. R., Watase, K., Thaller, C., Carson, J. P., Jafar-Nejad, P., Shaw, C., et al. (2008). The insulin-like growth factor pathway is altered in spinocerebellar ataxia type 1 and type 7. *Proc. Natl. Acad. Sci. USA, 105*(4), 1291-1296.

Goold, R., Hubank, M., Hunt, A., Holton, J., Menon, R. P., Revesz, T., et al. (2007). Down-regulation of the dopamine receptor D2 in mice lacking ataxin 1. *Hum. Mol. Genet., 16*(17), 2122-2134.

Grimaldi, P., Carletti, B., and Rossi, F. (2005). Neuronal replacement and integration in the rewiring of cerebellar circuits. *Brain Res. Brain Res. Rev., 49*(2), 330-342.

Hargus, G., Cooper, O., Deleidi, M., Levy, A., Lee, K., Marlow, E., et al. (2010). Differentiated Parkinson patient-derived induced pluripotent stem cells grow in the adult rodent brain and reduce motor asymmetry in Parkinsonian rats. *Proc. Natl. Acad. Sci. USA, 107*(36), 15921-15926.

Hedlund, E., Hefferan, M. P., Marsala, M., and Isacson, O. (2007). Cell therapy and stem cells in animal models of motor neuron disorders. *Eur. J. Neurosci., 26*(7), 1721-1737.

Heiser, V., Engemann, S., Brocker, W., Dunkel, I., Boeddrich, A., Waelter, S., et al. (2002). Identification of benzothiazoles as potential polyglutamine aggregation inhibitors of Huntington's disease by using an automated filter retardation assay. *Proc. Natl. Acad. Sci. USA, 99 Suppl 4*, 16400-16406.

Hong, S., Hwang, D. Y., Yoon, S., Isacson, O., Ramezani, A., Hawley, R. G., et al. (2007). Functional analysis of various promoters in lentiviral vectors at different stages of in vitro differentiation of mouse embryonic stem cells. *Mol. Ther, 15*(9), 1630-1639.

Hong, S., Ka, S., Kim, S., Park, Y., and Kang, S. (2003). p80 coilin, a coiled body-specific protein, interacts with ataxin-1, the SCA1 gene product. *Biochim. Biophys. Acta., 1638*(1), 35-42.

Hong, S., Kang, U. J., Isacson, O., and Kim, K. S. (2008). Neural precursors derived from human embryonic stem cells maintain long-term proliferation without losing the potential to differentiate into all three neural lineages, including dopaminergic neurons. *J. Neurochem., 104*(2), 316-324.

Hong, S., Kim, S. J., Ka, S., Choi, I., and Kang, S. (2002). USP7, a ubiquitin-specific protease, interacts with ataxin-1, the SCA1 gene product. *Mol. Cell Neurosci., 20*(2), 298-306.

Hong, S., Lee, S., Cho, S. G., and Kang, S. (2008). UbcH6 interacts with and ubiquitinates the SCA1 gene product ataxin-1. *Biochem. Biophys. Res. Commun, 371*(2), 256-260.

Irwin, S., Vandelft, M., Pinchev, D., Howell, J. L., Graczyk, J., Orr, H. T., et al. (2005). RNA association and nucleocytoplasmic shuttling by ataxin-1. *J. Cell Sci., 118*(Pt 1), 233-242.

Kang, S., and Hong, S. (2009). Molecular pathogenesis of spinocerebellar ataxia type 1 disease. *Mol. Cells, 27*(6), 621-627.

Kang, S., and Hong, S. (2010). SUMO-1 interacts with mutant ataxin-1 and colocalizes to its aggregates in Purkinje cells of SCA1 transgenic mice. *Arch. Ital. Biol., 148*(4), 351-363.

Kang, S., Jaworski, A., Ohshima, K., and Wells, R. D. (1995). Expansion and deletion of CTG repeats from human disease genes are determined by the direction of replication in E. coli. *Nat. Genet., 10*(2), 213-218.

Katsuno, M., Adachi, H., Inukai, A., and Sobue, G. (2003). Transgenic mouse models of spinal and bulbar muscular atrophy (SBMA). *Cytogenet. Genome. Res., 100*(1-4), 243-251.

Kazantsev, A., Walker, H. A., Slepko, N., Bear, J. E., Preisinger, E., Steffan, J. S., et al. (2002). A bivalent Huntingtin binding peptide suppresses polyglutamine aggregation and pathogenesis in Drosophila. *Nat. Genet., 30*(4), 367-376.

Keep, M., Alvarado-Mallart, R. M., and Sotelo, C. (1992). New insight on the factors orienting the axonal outgrowth of grafted Purkinje cells in the pcd cerebellum. *Dev. Neurosci., 14*(2), 153-165.

Keirstead, H. S., Nistor, G., Bernal, G., Totoiu, M., Cloutier, F., Sharp, K., et al. (2005). Human embryonic stem cell-derived oligodendrocyte progenitor cell transplants remyelinate and restore locomotion after spinal cord injury. *J. Neurosci., 25*(19), 4694-4705.

Khoshnan, A., Ko, J., and Patterson, P. H. (2002). Effects of intracellular expression of anti-huntingtin antibodies of various specificities on mutant huntingtin aggregation and toxicity. *Proc. Natl. Acad. Sci. USA, 99*(2), 1002-1007.

Kim, D., Kim, C. H., Moon, J. I., Chung, Y. G., Chang, M. Y., Han, B. S., et al. (2009). Generation of human induced pluripotent stem cells by direct delivery of reprogramming proteins. *Cell Stem. Cell, 4*(6), 472-476.

Klement, I. A., Skinner, P. J., Kaytor, M. D., Yi, H., Hersch, S. M., Clark, H. B., et al. (1998). Ataxin-1 nuclear localization and aggregation: role in polyglutamine-induced disease in SCA1 transgenic mice. *Cell, 95*(1), 41-53.

Lecerf, J. M., Shirley, T. L., Zhu, Q., Kazantsev, A., Amersdorfer, P., Housman, D. E., et al. (2001). Human single-chain Fv intrabodies counteract in situ huntingtin aggregation in cellular models of Huntington's disease. *Proc. Natl. Acad. Sci. USA, 98*(8), 4764-4769.

Lee, S., Hong, S., and Kang, S. (2008). The ubiquitin-conjugating enzyme UbcH6 regulates the transcriptional repression activity of the SCA1 gene product ataxin-1. *Biochem. Biophys. Res. Commun, 372*(4), 735-740.

Lee, S., Hong, S., Kim, S., and Kang, S. (2011). Ataxin-1 occupies the promoter region of E-cadherin in vivo and activates CtBP2-repressed promoter. *Biochim. Biophys. Acta., 1813*(5), 713-722.

Li, W., Wei, W., Zhu, S., Zhu, J., Shi, Y., Lin, T., et al. (2009). Generation of rat and human induced pluripotent stem cells by combining genetic reprogramming and chemical inhibitors. *Cell Stem. Cell, 4*(1), 16-19.

Li, X., Ketter, T. A., and Frye, M. A. (2002). Synaptic, intracellular, and neuroprotective mechanisms of anticonvulsants: are they relevant for the treatment and course of bipolar disorders? *J. Affect. Disord., 69*(1-3), 1-14.

Lim, J., Crespo-Barreto, J., Jafar-Nejad, P., Bowman, A. B., Richman, R., Hill, D. E., et al. (2008). Opposing effects of polyglutamine expansion on native protein complexes contribute to SCA1. *Nature, 452*(7188), 713-718.

Lindvall, O., and Kokaia, Z. (2010). Stem cells in human neurodegenerative disorders--time for clinical translation? *J. Clin. Invest., 120*(1), 29-40.

Matilla, A., Koshy, B. T., Cummings, C. J., Isobe, T., Orr, H. T., and Zoghbi, H. Y. (1997). The cerebellar leucine-rich acidic nuclear protein interacts with ataxin-1. *Nature, 389*(6654), 974-978.

McCampbell, A., Taye, A. A., Whitty, L., Penney, E., Steffan, J. S., and Fischbeck, K. H. (2001). Histone deacetylase inhibitors reduce polyglutamine toxicity. *Proc. Natl. Acad. Sci. USA, 98*(26), 15179-15184.

Mendez, I., Vinuela, A., Astradsson, A., Mukhida, K., Hallett, P., Robertson, H., et al. (2008). Dopamine neurons implanted into people with Parkinson's disease survive without pathology for 14 years. *Nat. Med., 14*(5), 507-509.

Michalik, A., and Van Broeckhoven, C. (2003). Pathogenesis of polyglutamine disorders: aggregation revisited. *Hum. Mol. Genet., 12 Spec No 2*, R173-186.

Muchowski, P. J., Schaffar, G., Sittler, A., Wanker, E. E., Hayer-Hartl, M. K., and Hartl, F. U. (2000). Hsp70 and hsp40 chaperones can inhibit self-assembly of polyglutamine proteins into amyloid-like fibrils. *Proc. Natl. Acad. Sci. USA, 97*(14), 7841-7846.

Muguruma, K., Nishiyama, A., Ono, Y., Miyawaki, H., Mizuhara, E., Hori, S., et al. (2010). Ontogeny-recapitulating generation and tissue integration of ES cell-derived Purkinje cells. *Nat Neurosci, 13*(10), 1171-1180.

Mullen, R. J., Eicher, E. M., and Sidman, R. L. (1976). Purkinje cell degeneration, a new neurological mutation in the mouse. *Proc. Natl. Acad. Sci. USA, 73*(1), 208-212.

Okazawa, H., Rich, T., Chang, A., Lin, X., Waragai, M., Kajikawa, M., et al. (2002). Interaction between mutant ataxin-1 and PQBP-1 affects transcription and cell death. *Neuron, 34*(5), 701-713.

Okita, K., Ichisaka, T., and Yamanaka, S. (2007). Generation of germline-competent induced pluripotent stem cells. *Nature, 448*(7151), 313-317.

Orr, H. T. (2000). The ins and outs of a polyglutamine neurodegenerative disease: spinocerebellar ataxia type 1 (SCA1). *Neurobiol. Dis., 7*(3), 129-134.

Orr, H. T., Chung, M. Y., Banfi, S., Kwiatkowski, T. J., Jr., Servadio, A., Beaudet, A. L., et al. (1993). Expansion of an unstable trinucleotide CAG repeat in spinocerebellar ataxia type 1. *Nat. Genet., 4*(3), 221-226.

Orr, H. T., and Zoghbi, H. Y. (2001). SCA1 molecular genetics: a history of a 13 year collaboration against glutamines. *Hum. Mol. Genet., 10*(20), 2307-2311.

Orr, H. T., and Zoghbi, H. Y. (2007). Trinucleotide repeat disorders. *Annu. Rev. Neurosci., 30*, 575-621.

Paulson, H. (2003). Polyglutamine neurodegeneration: minding your Ps and Qs. *Nat. Med., 9*(7), 825-826.

Perutz, M. F., Johnson, T., Suzuki, M., and Finch, J. T. (1994). Glutamine repeats as polar zippers: their possible role in inherited neurodegenerative diseases. *Proc. Natl. Acad. Sci. USA, 91*(12), 5355-5358.

Phiel, C. J., Wilson, C. A., Lee, V. M., and Klein, P. S. (2003). GSK-3alpha regulates production of Alzheimer's disease amyloid-beta peptides. *Nature, 423*(6938), 435-439.

Pilcher, H. R. (2003). Drug research: the ups and downs of lithium. *Nature, 425*(6954), 118-120.

Ren, H., Nagai, Y., Tucker, T., Strittmatter, W. J., and Burke, J. R. (2001). Amino acid sequence requirements of peptides that inhibit polyglutamine-protein aggregation and cell death. *Biochem. Biophys. Res. Commun., 288*(3), 703-710.

Riley, B. E., Zoghbi, H. Y., and Orr, H. T. (2005). SUMOylation of the polyglutamine repeat protein, ataxin-1, is dependent on a functional nuclear localization signal. *J. Biol. Chem., 280*(23), 21942-21948.

Sanchez, I., Mahlke, C., and Yuan, J. (2003). Pivotal role of oligomerization in expanded polyglutamine neurodegenerative disorders. *Nature, 421*(6921), 373-379.

Serra, H. G., Byam, C. E., Lande, J. D., Tousey, S. K., Zoghbi, H. Y., and Orr, H. T. (2004). Gene profiling links SCA1 pathophysiology to glutamate signaling in Purkinje cells of transgenic mice. *Hum. Mol. Genet., 13*(20), 2535-2543.

Serra, H. G., Duvick, L., Zu, T., Carlson, K., Stevens, S., Jorgensen, N., et al. (2006). RORalpha-mediated Purkinje cell development determines disease severity in adult SCA1 mice. *Cell, 127*(4), 697-708.

Shi, Y., Desponts, C., Do, J. T., Hahm, H. S., Scholer, H. R., and Ding, S. (2008). Induction of pluripotent stem cells from mouse embryonic fibroblasts by Oct4 and Klf4 with small-molecule compounds. *Cell Stem. Cell, 3*(5), 568-574.

Shi, Y., Do, J. T., Desponts, C., Hahm, H. S., Scholer, H. R., and Ding, S. (2008). A combined chemical and genetic approach for the generation of induced pluripotent stem cells. *Cell Stem. Cell, 2*(6), 525-528.

Skinner, P. J., Koshy, B. T., Cummings, C. J., Klement, I. A., Helin, K., Servadio, A., et al. (1997). Ataxin-1 with an expanded glutamine tract alters nuclear matrix-associated structures. *Nature, 389*(6654), 971-974.

Sotelo, C., and Alvarado-Mallart, R. M. (1991). The reconstruction of cerebellar circuits. *Trends Neurosci., 14*(8), 350-355.

Sotelo, C., Alvarado-Mallart, R. M., Gardette, R., and Crepel, F. (1990). Fate of grafted embryonic Purkinje cells in the cerebellum of the adult "Purkinje cell degeneration" mutant mouse. I. Development of reciprocal graft-host interactions. *J. Comp. Neurol., 295*(2), 165-187.

Steffan, J. S., Bodai, L., Pallos, J., Poelman, M., McCampbell, A., Apostol, B. L., et al. (2001). Histone deacetylase inhibitors arrest polyglutamine-dependent neurodegeneration in Drosophila. *Nature, 413*(6857), 739-743.

Su, H. L., Muguruma, K., Matsuo-Takasaki, M., Kengaku, M., Watanabe, K., and Sasai, Y. (2006). Generation of cerebellar neuron precursors from embryonic stem cells. *Dev. Biol., 290*(2), 287-296.

Takahashi, K., Tanabe, K., Ohnuki, M., Narita, M., Ichisaka, T., Tomoda, K., et al. (2007). Induction of pluripotent stem cells from adult human fibroblasts by defined factors. *Cell, 131*(5), 861-872.

Takahashi, K., and Yamanaka, S. (2006). Induction of pluripotent stem cells from mouse embryonic and adult fibroblast cultures by defined factors. *Cell, 126*(4), 663-676.

Tanaka, M., Machida, Y., Niu, S., Ikeda, T., Jana, N. R., Doi, H., et al. (2004). Trehalose alleviates polyglutamine-mediated pathology in a mouse model of Huntington disease. *Nat. Med., 10*(2), 148-154.

Thakur, A. K., and Wetzel, R. (2002). Mutational analysis of the structural organization of polyglutamine aggregates. *Proc. Natl. Acad. Sci. USA, 99*(26), 17014-17019.

Triarhou, L. C. (1996). The cerebellar model of neural grafting: structural integration and functional recovery. *Brain Res. Bull., 39*(3), 127-138.

Triarhou, L. C., Low, W. C., and Ghetti, B. (1992). Intraparenchymal grafting of cerebellar cell suspensions to the deep cerebellar nuclei of pcd mutant mice, with particular emphasis on re-establishment of a Purkinje cell cortico-nuclear projection. *Anat. Embryol. (Berl), 185*(5), 409-420.

Triarhou, L. C., Zhang, W., and Lee, W. H. (1995). Graft-induced restoration of function in hereditary cerebellar ataxia. *Neuroreport, 6*(14), 1827-1832.

Tsuda, H., Jafar-Nejad, H., Patel, A. J., Sun, Y., Chen, H. K., Rose, M. F., et al. (2005). The AXH domain of Ataxin-1 mediates neurodegeneration through its interaction with Gfi-1/Senseless proteins. *Cell, 122*(4), 633-644.

Tsuji, O., Miura, K., Okada, Y., Fujiyoshi, K., Mukaino, M., Nagoshi, N., et al. (2010). Therapeutic potential of appropriately evaluated safe-induced pluripotent stem cells for spinal cord injury. *Proc. Natl. Acad. Sci. USA, 107*(28), 12704-12709.

Ueda, H., Goto, J., Hashida, H., Lin, X., Oyanagi, K., Kawano, H., et al. (2002). Enhanced SUMOylation in polyglutamine diseases. *Biochem. Biophys. Res. Commun., 293*(1), 307-313.

Vig, P. J., Hearst, S., Shao, Q., Lopez, M. E., Murphy, H. A., 2nd, and Safaya, E. (2011). Glial S100B Protein Modulates Mutant Ataxin-1 Aggregation and Toxicity: TRTK12 Peptide, a Potential Candidate for SCA1 Therapy. *Cerebellum.*

Watase, K., Gatchel, J. R., Sun, Y., Emamian, E., Atkinson, R., Richman, R., et al. (2007). Lithium therapy improves neurological function and hippocampal dendritic arborization in a spinocerebellar ataxia type 1 mouse model. *PLoS Med, 4*(5), e182.

Wernig, M., Zhao, J. P., Pruszak, J., Hedlund, E., Fu, D., Soldner, F., et al. (2008). Neurons derived from reprogrammed fibroblasts functionally integrate into the fetal brain and improve symptoms of rats with Parkinson's disease. *Proc. Natl. Acad. Sci. USA, 105*(15), 5856-5861.

Xia, H., Mao, Q., Eliason, S. L., Harper, S. Q., Martins, I. H., Orr, H. T., et al. (2004). RNAi suppresses polyglutamine-induced neurodegeneration in a model of spinocerebellar ataxia. *Nat. Med., 10*(8), 816-820.

Yoshida, H., Yoshizawa, T., Shibasaki, F., Shoji, S., and Kanazawa, I. (2002). Chemical chaperones reduce aggregate formation and cell death caused by the truncated Machado-Joseph disease gene product with an expanded polyglutamine stretch. *Neurobiol. Dis., 10*(2), 88-99.

Yu, J., Hu, K., Smuga-Otto, K., Tian, S., Stewart, R., Slukvin, II, et al. (2009). Human induced pluripotent stem cells free of vector and transgene sequences. *Science, 324*(5928), 797-801.

Zhang, W., Lee, W. H., and Triarhou, L. C. (1996). Grafted cerebellar cells in a mouse model of hereditary ataxia express IGF-I system genes and partially restore behavioral function. *Nat. Med., 2*(1), 65-71.

Zhou, H., Wu, S., Joo, J. Y., Zhu, S., Han, D. W., Lin, T., et al. (2009). Generation of induced pluripotent stem cells using recombinant proteins. *Cell Stem. Cell, 4*(5), 381-384.

Zoghbi, H. Y. (1995). Spinocerebellar ataxia type 1. *Clin. Neurosci., 3*(1), 5-11.

Zoghbi, H. Y., and Orr, H. T. (1995). Spinocerebellar ataxia type 1. *Semin. Cell Biol., 6*(1), 29-35.

Zoghbi, H. Y., and Orr, H. T. (2000). Glutamine repeats and neurodegeneration. *Annu. Rev. Neurosci., 23*, 217-247.

Zoghbi, H. Y., and Orr, H. T. (2009). Pathogenic mechanisms of a polyglutamine-mediated neurodegenerative disease, spinocerebellar ataxia type 1. *J. Biol. Chem., 284*(12), 7425-7429.

INDEX

B

basal ganglia, x, 36, 139, 140, 143, 144, 145
base, 79, 141, 142, 147
beneficial effect, viii, 29, 38, 86, 89, 174
benign, 65, 82
bias, 127
biomarkers, 143
biomolecules, 78
biopsy, 30, 87
biosynthesis, 86, 89
bipolar disorder, 180, 185
births, 30
blood, 32, 83, 86
body size, 170
bone, 181
boutons, 52, 61, 69
brain, xi, 35, 36, 43, 52, 53, 54, 55, 61, 72, 74, 82, 84, 86, 96, 132, 137, 141, 142, 144, 145, 147, 167, 168, 170, 172, 175, 176, 179, 180, 181, 182, 184, 188
branching, 53
breast cancer, 21, 33, 42
breathing, 47, 56, 63
breeding, 169
bronchiectasis, 33
budding, 14, 23
building blocks, 152
bystander effect, 15

C

caffeine, 56, 63, 65
calcium, vii, 57, 64, 68, 69, 75, 117, 135, 136, 150
cancer, vii, 1, 2, 13, 14, 16, 17, 18, 22, 23, 25, 26, 31, 33, 37, 39, 41, 42, 43, 121, 130, 182
candidates, 89, 174
carbamazepine, 63
carbohydrate, 105
carcinogen, 15
carcinogenesis, 18, 25
cardiomyopathy, 81, 87, 97, 99, 110, 114, 120
catalytic activity, 158
cation, 71, 88
cerebellum, vii, viii, x, xi, 29, 30, 35, 36, 39, 52, 53, 64, 66, 71, 82, 83, 90, 96, 109, 110, 111, 113, 139, 141, 142, 143, 144, 145, 147, 149, 167, 168, 170, 173, 174, 180, 182, 184, 185, 187
cerebral cortex, x, 43, 111, 139, 144
cerebral palsy, 32
cerebrospinal fluid, 104
cervical cancer, 22

chain transfer, 78
challenges, 48
channel blocker, 66
chaperones, 179, 186, 188
chemical, 24, 33, 161, 179, 185, 187
chemotherapeutic agent, 16, 33
chemotherapy, 19, 20
chicken, 106, 161
childhood, 47, 56, 63, 65, 83, 85, 90, 91, 96, 97, 113, 115
children, 32, 37, 41, 56, 84, 89, 94, 105, 114
chimera, 49
chorea, 65, 114, 115
choreoathetosis, 47, 56, 65, 72, 73, 74
chromosomal instability, 12, 39
chromosome, x, 10, 11, 14, 20, 30, 36, 47, 57, 64, 65, 67, 70, 71, 73, 74, 110, 112, 113, 114, 115, 116, 118, 119, 120, 121, 122, 125, 132, 135, 139, 140, 160
clarity, 49
class switching, 34
classes, 34
classification, x, 80, 81, 116, 149, 151, 161, 162, 163
cleavage, 9, 132
cloning, 15, 48, 120
coding, ix, 69, 90, 91, 123, 124, 125, 126, 139, 150
codon, 37, 64
coenzyme, viii, 77, 78, 80, 82, 86, 88, 89, 93, 94, 95, 97, 111, 113, 118, 119, 120
collaboration, 186
collateral, 52
colon, 20, 25, 26
communication, 15, 81
communities, 106
community, 108
comorbidity, 146
comparative analysis, 133
complement, 159
complexity, 15, 150
complications, 38, 85, 130
composition, 54
compounds, 16, 44, 82, 171, 187
comprehension, 128
computed tomography, 148
computer, 62
conductance, 51
conduction, 68, 69, 80, 83, 110, 112
configuration, 51, 54
confinement, viii, 29
conjunctiva, 32
connectivity, 55
consciousness, viii, 103, 104, 105
consensus, 153

F

G

H

M

N

O

P

W

walking, 56, 170
water, 78, 88
wavelet, 161, 165
weakness, 57, 65, 70, 83, 110
web, 171
wheezing, 56, 63
white matter, x, 101, 139, 141, 147, 181
windows, 155
workers, 56, 60, 82, 83, 85, 86, 88, 89, 91, 107
worldwide, 124, 137
worms, 106
wound healing, 171

X

xeroderma pigmentosum, 10

Y

yeast, 14, 91, 93, 100, 111, 117, 122, 179

Z

zinc, 61, 69, 71, 73, 74, 91, 175
zippers, 186